OPIUM

Noelle would have noticed him even if he hadn't driven his Packard through the bar of the Hotel Constellation. He was outrageously handsome, even when he was drunk. He had blue-black hair swept straight back from the forehead, although a dark comma of hair fell rakishly over one eye. He wore a white linen suit, an affectation which in Laos was usually seen only in visiting potentates and ambassadors. It looked as natural on the Corsican as his own olive dark skin.

Yes, Noelle decided, I would have noticed you even without this dramatic entrance.

The careering Packard quickly scattered the occupants of the bar, mostly bored foreign correspondents and diplomats, splintered the rattan tables and chairs, and demolished half of the bamboo bar. Dusty bottles of vermouth, byrrh and black rum toppled off the shelves and shattered on the floor.

There was a deathly silence.

Then Baptiste Crocé leaned out from behind the wheel and beckoned the startled Lao barman. 'I'll have a large cognac,' he said in French.

Also by the same author
and available from Coronet:

Venom
Deathwatch
Harem
Fury
Triad
Dangerous

About the Author

Colin Falconer was born in London in 1953. He is a journalist and has written for many national magazines and newspapers. He has travelled widely in Europe and South-East Asia and now lives in Western Australia. He is the author of seven acclaimed thrillers, all available in Coronet paperback.

Opium

Colin Falconer

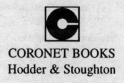

CORONET BOOKS
Hodder & Stoughton

First published in paperback in Great Britain in 1994
by Hodder and Stoughton
A division of Hodder Headline PLC

A Coronet paperback

British Library C.I.P.

Falconer, Colin
Opium
I. Title
823.914 [F]

ISBN 0 340 60992 3

Typeset by Phoenix Typesetting,
Ilkley, West Yorkshire

Printed and bound in Great Britain by
Clays Ltd, St Ives plc

Hodder and Stoughton
A division of Hodder Headline PLC
338 Euston Road
London NW1 3BH

This novel is respectfully dedicated to Alfred McCoy, who was first to argue for the truth.

AUTHOR'S NOTE

This is a work of fiction, and none of the characters or events are intended to reflect the lives of real people. However, the background of the story is now a matter of public record. Anyone interested in knowing more about the politics of the drug trade should refer to Alfred McCoy's books on the subject; United States involvement in Laos has been well documented by Christopher Robbins.

I acknowledge only one discrepancy as a fictional convenience; Vietnam reversed its policy on opium in 1958, not 1959.

ACKNOWLEDGEMENTS

I would like to thank Tim Curnow and Anthea Morton-Saner for their unswerving support for this project. Thanks also to my editor, George Lucas, for his boundless enthusiasm and advice.

Many people gave freely of their time during my research of this book, and I owe them a great debt of gratitude. I am indebted to David Wilson and Jane Gillman in Sydney for their interest in the book and for helping· me track down some of those who assisted me.

In Perth I am grateful to Henry "Slim" Giblett for his reminiscences of police work in Hong Kong during the sixties; to Joe White for advice on certain technical aspects of flying; and to Doug Kirsop who helped me with the more colourful aspects of spoken French.

In Vientiane I am very grateful to Michel Somsanouk, for allowing me access to his newspaper library and for his recollections of the city in the sixties and seventies. In Hong Kong I owe thanks to Senior Superintendent Robert Nicoll, Detective Superintendent Clive Tricker, Chief Detective Inspector Peter Ip Pau-fuk, and Senior Inspector Kevin Chen who all freely gave of their time.

I am greatly indebted to Chief Detective Inspector Trevor Collins, for his hospitality, and for his advice on the background and organisation of the triads in Hong Kong.

Thanks once again to Anne Mullarkey and her staff at Busselton Library for tracking down everything I needed.

Finally, I owe a special debt of thanks to Chief Inspector John Chetwynd-Chatwin, for his generosity and boundless assistance.

All these people I thank; however this book does not necessarily reflect their recollections or opinions. Where my portrayals are accurate, the credit is theirs; any errors, omissions or conclusions are mine and mine alone.

Hong Kong, March, 1994.

PART ONE

Air Opium

'We gave up the drug war in favour of a war against communism.
In fact, we made a conscious choice.'
– former senior DEA agent Michael Levine

1

Vientiane, April 1959

Noelle would have noticed him even if he hadn't driven his Packard through the bar of the Hotel Constellation. He was outrageously handsome, even when he was drunk. He had blue-black hair, with a pronounced widow's peak, swept straight back from the forehead, although a dark comma of hair fell rakishly over one eye. His skin was olive dark and there was a reed-thin black moustache on his top lip. He wore a white linen suit, an affectation which in Laos was usually seen only on visiting potentates and ambassadors. It looked as natural on the Corsican as his own skin. Underneath the suit was a black silk shirt.

Yes, Noelle decided, I would have noticed you even without this dramatic entrance.

The bar of The Constellation was open to the street, so there were no walls to absorb the impact; but the careering Packard quickly scattered the occupants, mostly bored foreign correspondents and diplomats, splintered the rattan tables and chairs, and demolished half of the bamboo bar. Dusty bottles of vermouth, byrrh and black rum toppled off the shelves and shattered on the floor.

There was a deathly silence.

Then Baptiste Crocé leaned out from behind the wheel and beckoned the startled Lao barman. 'I'll have a large cognac,' he said in French.

There was a smatter of cheers and applause from the western journalists, who were also drunk. Any madness was a welcome

11

diversion. Crocé turned to them and, standing on the bench seat of the Packard, gave them a low bow.

'*Imbécile*,' muttered Noelle's escort. 'He's drunk. A disgrace.'

Marcel Rivelini had been her father's choice as her companion that evening; he was certainly not her own. A business associate of Rocco's from Bangkok, he was wealthy, sophisticated and insufferable. He was also almost as old as her father. I would not have minded that so much if he had a sense of humour, she decided. Because a man has money and experience does not necessarily make him an interesting companion. Even in Vientiane.

It was then that the Corsican saw her. He raised his cognac in salute and climbed out of the Packard. He made his way, a little unsteadily, across the bar towards her. She felt Rivelini tense.

This should be interesting.

'May I have the pleasure of this dance?'

Noelle smiled. 'But, monsieur, there is no music.'

'That is beside the point, mademoiselle. All I want is the exquisite pleasure of having such a lovely young woman in my arms.'

Rivelini stood up and punched him on the jaw. The Corsican fell backwards, breaking another rattan table. There was a hiss of disappointment from the gathered journalists.

Noelle stood up.

'I'm sorry if he offended you,' Rivelini said to her.

Then, without really understanding why she did it, she threw her Pernod at him. He gasped in surprise, and stared at the spreading stain on his shirt. The journalists cheered again.

'You little bitch,' Rivelini muttered.

Noelle pushed him in the chest, harder than she intended. He fell backwards, his legs tangled in his chair, and landed in a sprawl among the tables. He screamed, clutching at his knee which had twisted as he fell.

Noelle went to the Corsican.

'Are you all right?' she whispered.

He was bleeding from the lip. He felt around the inside of his mouth with his tongue. 'Are any teeth missing?' he said.

'You're lucky he didn't kill you. He's a gangster from Bangkok. Are you crazy?'

12

'Look, my suit's ruined. Bastard!'

'Here, I'll help you up. You're drunk.'

'Just a little.' As she held out her hand he pulled her towards him. 'But not so drunk that I don't know I've just met the most beautiful woman in Asia.'

'Get back in the car.'

Rivelini struggled to his feet. His knee would not take his weight and he had to lean on a table for support. 'Where are you going?'

'Thank you for an entertaining evening, Marcel,' she said, and helped the Corsican into the Packard. Then, to a final chorus of cheers from the journalists, she got behind the wheel and reversed out of the bar.

Noelle drove the big-finned car slowly through the darkened streets. Dogs and pigs sometimes slept in the middle of the roads. The night was warm, and smelled of ripe fruit and kerosene.

The Corsican rested his head on the back of his seat and took out a packet of Gitanes. He lit one and let it hang insolently from his lower lip. He groaned.

'Are you all right?' Noelle asked him.

'A little headache, that is all.' He looked at her and grinned, his teeth powder-white in the darkness. 'Do you like how I seduce women? I have them fight for me then offer to take me home.'

'This is not seduction,' Noelle said. 'Where to?'

'The Bungalow.'

She knew it. It was a hotel less than a hundred yards away, it's real name was the Settha Palace. 'You could have walked. Why didn't you tell me?'

'I'm drunk but I'm not crazy.' As she turned the car around in the street, he took a silk handkerchief from his jacket pocket and dabbed gingerly at his lip. 'Will you sleep with me tonight?'

She felt herself flush to the roots of her hair. 'If you were not already beaten up, I would break your nose!' she hissed. She took one hand off the wheel and cuffed him across the face. She was already regretting her impetuosity at The

Constellation. What boredom could make a girl do! 'What do you think I am? Some kind of whore?'

. 'No, I don't think that. Not at all. I think you are the most beautiful woman I have ever seen.' She could see his face in the glow of the dashboard light. He was grinning at her.

What's your name?' she said.

'I am Baptiste. Baptiste Crocé.'

'Well, Monsieur Crocé, you are going to wake up in the morning and you are going to regret very much tonight.'

'I don't think so.'

'They will probably lock you up for making so much damage. What were you thinking of? *C'est fou!* Do you always drive that way?'

'Only when I'm very drunk.'

He reached out and stroked her arm with the back of his hand.

She jerked her arm away. 'Don't do that!'

'I can't help it. Your skin is like velvet. If you won't sleep with me, will you marry me?'

They had reached The Settha Palace. It was no palace but actually an old colonial guest house that had fallen into decay. Noelle drove to the front steps. Several of the guests, mostly junior foreign diplomats, came out on to the porte cochère to stare. This is how starved we are of entertainment in Vientiane, she thought. A man with a bleeding lip and a woman driving a battered American car will be the main talking point at tomorrow's breakfast.

'Tell me, Monsieur Crocé, what are you? Some sort of diplomat?'

'Do I act like a diplomat?'

.'Frankly, no.'

'I'm a pilot.'

'A pilot?'

'I was the Air Force's greatest hero during the war with the Viet Minh. Now I have my own airline – Wattay Air. Perhaps you have heard of it?'

'No, I haven't. And I'm amazed you can persuade anyone to get into an aeroplane with you. How do you land? Do you just crash through the terminal doors?'

14

'It depends if I'm drunk or not.'

Noelle allowed herself a smile. 'Goodnight,' she said. She got out of the car and walked towards the clutter of *siclos* that were parked on the other side of the courtyard. The driver was asleep on the cracked leather seat of his machine. She kicked the tyre to wake him. He sat up with a start. Still rubbing his face, he climbed on to the seat of the bicycle.

Crocé stumbled out of his car and ran over. 'Wait! You can't go. I don't even know your name!'

'Bardot. Brigitte Bardot. And next time you wish to make love to me, monsieur, make sure you are sober. All right?'

Crocé watched the *siclo* disappear into the darkness. He grinned. Well, he thought, I won that round.

2

Rocco Bonaventure sat on the balcony of his villa to enjoy his breakfast of eggs and rice. He was in his fifties, with a mane of silver grey hair and a close cropped beard. His hair was pushed back from a high, tanned forehead and trailed over his collar at the back of his head. In repose he looked almost benign. But the clue to his real nature was his hands. They were a wrestler's hands, huge and large-knuckled, and covered with a thick mat of hair that pushed under the cuffs of his white shirt. There were chunky gold rings on each finger.

He affected an air of stillness as he watched the Lao women hurrying along the green arcade of the road, their babies in shawls on their backs, rattan baskets of vegetables balanced on their heads. A flock of heron flew out of the mist, and settled in the rice paddi that bordered the road.

He thought about Noelle.

Rivelini had reported her behaviour of the previous evening. It was outrageous. His hands shook as he picked up his coffee cup. Daughters were a curse. Good for nothing except causing trouble. And Noelle caused more trouble than most. The nuns at Les Oiseaux Convent in Saigon had charmingly described her as 'wilful'.

An understatement, Bonaventure decided.

He sipped his coffee, and grimaced. Impossible country. You couldn't get fresh milk for the *café au lait*, and you couldn't keep your daughter away from adventurers and idiots.

How could she embarrass him this way? Marcel Rivelini was the nephew of a man he was pleased to call his friend. She had humiliated him in front of a room full of foreign journalists, and had even damaged him to the extent that he was unable to rise from his bed. His knee had swollen up like a melon.

Noelle!

As if he didn't have enough troubles to contend with.

The previous year the United States had withdrawn economic aid, forced the leftist government to resign, and put their own man in power, as they had done with Diem in Saigon four years before. This time Bonaventure had a little more sympathy with the American cause. He didn't suppose the communists would look all that kindly on his business. Somebody had to stop them and it might as well be Eisenhower. But in January, Prime Minister Phoui Sananikone had asked the National Assembly for emergency powers to deal with the rebels, and there were reports of more fighting along the border at Sam Neua. For Rocco Bonaventure it was a worrying, if not unexpected, development.

His own Air Laos had been established as a legitimate operation, carrying freight and passengers – mostly spies and missionaries admittedly – around a landlocked and mountainous country. Northern Laos had few roads, and those that existed were no more than tracks hacked through jungles infested with tigers and poisonous snakes. There were less than a thousand telephones in the whole country and air transport played a major role in its development.

But it was not the legitimate but modest proceeds from aviation that kept Rocco Bonaventure in Laos. Honest profits did not pay for the fleet of twin-engined Beechcraft or the villa in Saigon and the bullion on deposit in the Banque de l'Indochine. It did not account for the weekly flights Air Laos made to Bangkok during the spring poppy harvests.

Rocco Bonaventure's real business was opium.

Noelle's appearance shook him out of his brooding. It seemed she had deigned to honour him with her presence for breakfast. She looked radiant, damn her. In the manner of a highborn Lao woman, she wore fine gold chains at her wrist and neck, a traditional silk *pao sin* and a broad silver belt around her long waist. Noelle was one of the few western women Bonaventure had ever seen who could adopt eastern customs to accentuate her own natural beauty. And she is beautiful, he thought. Too damn' beautiful. There was also a colour in her cheeks this morning that he had not noticed before.

I'll have to marry her off soon.

'Papa, tu es troublé?' You look worried.

'Of course I'm worried,' he growled. 'I have just been hearing from Marcel about what happened last night.'

She smiled sweetly at him and joined him at the table. 'Where *is* Marcel?'

'He decided to take breakfast in his room.'

'It's rather childish when men sulk, don't you think?'

Impossible girl! He wished she was still of an age when he could spank her bottom. But then, he had never done that. As a child she had manipulated his anger just as adroitly as she did as a woman.

She took a slice of papaya with her fork.

He glared at her. 'Well?' he said, finally.

Her eyes widened. 'Yes, Papa?'

'What have you got to say for yourself?'

'About last night? Oh, that was nothing. You shouldn't worry.'

'Nothing? That was nothing? You expect me not to worry when my own daughter behaves like a tramp?'

He recognised the hurt on her face and immediately regretted his temper. 'I'm not a tramp, Papa,' she said, softly, and with great dignity.

'I know that, I'm sorry,' said Bonaventure, amazed to hear the apology coming from his lips and not hers. How had she done that? 'But what am I to do when my own daughter behaves this way? What do you think Marcel thinks of us?'

'Marcel is a bore.'

'He says you hit him, and then drove away with some cowboy.'

Noelle giggled, covering her mouth with the back of her hand like a schoolgirl. Infuriating! 'I didn't hit him. I pushed him perhaps.'

'And this other gentleman...'

18

'He is no gentleman, Papa. But it's all right. I was very careful.'

Bonaventure had lost his appetite for his breakfast. He lit a cigarette and regarded his daughter. Probably her mother – may God keep her always in His mercy – and the peasant blood in her were responsible for this wilful streak. And he supposed he must accept some of the blame also. He had indulged her. Noelle had grown up the very image of his Anne-Marie, and perhaps that was why he had been too soft with her.

'This gentleman who is not really a gentleman – do you know who he is?' He tried to sound stern.

'His name is Crocé. He's a pilot. That's all I know.'

'Crocé!'

'You know him?'

'I know every pilot in Indochina, it's my business to know them.' He exhaled a blue-grey stream of cigarette smoke. Crocé! 'What on earth possessed you to behave in such a fashion?'

'He intrigued me.'

'Intrigued you!'

She poured some coffee from the silver pot and drank it black. She dabbed at her lips with a linen napkin. Her eyes were wide and innocent. 'What do you know about him?'

'He is a former Air Force pilot, stayed behind after Dien Bien Phu. He worked for a small freight carrier in Bangkok for a few months, but they sacked him because he was unreliable. Unreliable! That means he drinks. When he came to Laos he wanted to work for me. I told him I didn't have any planes to risk with cowboys. Somehow he made some money and bought a Cessna with another young man called Jean-Marie Pepin. He has a reputation as a womaniser and a gambler.'

Noelle smiled. 'He sounds almost too good to be true.'

'Don't mock me, Noelle.'

She pouted and touched his cheek with her hand. 'Papa, you have to trust me. It was just a little fun. I am bored. I have nothing to do here. What you want me to do? Sit around and pound rice like the peasant women?'

'Perhaps you need a husband.'

19

She smoothed an errant curl from her cheek. 'Perhaps. But not Marcel Rivelini. I would rather join a Convent.'

'Something else I have considered.'

She laughed at that.

Oh, you can laugh, Bonaventure thought. But sometimes I think it's the only solution. How else am I going to control you, my adorable little minx?

A few hours later Jean-Marie landed his Cessna at Wattay Airport and taxied to the cluster of sheds at the far end of the field. One of the Air Laos pilots, Louis Jourdain, was tinkering with the engine of his Beechcraft. He waved Jean-Marie over.

'I suppose you heard about your *ami?*' Jourdain shouted.

'I stayed overnight at Phong Saly.'

Jourdain wiped his hands on a rag. 'So you don't know?'

Jean-Marie suppressed a groan. 'What has he done now?'

'Only driven your car right into the bar of The Constellation. Drunk, of course.'

'Merde alors!'

'That's not the best of it. Guess who was there?'

'De Gaulle?'

'Noelle Bonaventure. Get this – she drove him home.'

Jean-Marie ran his fingers through his blond curls. *Imbécile!* Idiot! He must have been out of his mind to go into partnership with a man like Crocé. A good pilot but a crazy human being.

'What happened?'

Jourdain shrugged. 'Do you think he fucked her?'

'Not even Baptiste is that crazy.'

'Yes, he is.'

'Thanks for the warning, Louis.'

Jean-Marie walked back to the road. There was a taxi parked under a simpoh tree. The taxi was actually a World War Two jeep. The passenger side door was broken and held in place with a lady's pink garter. An ominous portent in the circumstances, Jean-Marie thought. He woke the Lao driver, who was asleep on the front seat, and told him to take him to The Settha Palace.

It was a gentle ride into town, the only obstacles a few water buffalo that had wandered on to the road from the *paddis*, and a handful of high-wheeled oxcarts on their way back from the morning market. The road entered Vientiane along an arcade of flowering trees.

Nestled on the flat rice plain of the Mekong, the capital of Laos was no more than a sleepy rural town. Most of the houses were made of sandalwood, thatch and plaited bamboo, built on stilts of teak, surrounded by stands of mango trees or coconut palms or oar-bladed banana trees. Chickens and black razorback pigs lived under the houses. Great wooden temples with their upswept eaves were everywhere. Automobiles were still something to be stared at.

The commercial heart was no more than three parallel streets of weathered one-storey wooden shops, offering a bizarre selection of merchandise. Indian merchants sold saris and gentlemen's suits, while the Chinese shops displayed Roy Rogers T-shirts, dried herbs and tinned pâté de foie gras.

'*La Baraque Indienne*,' the driver said in French. 'The Bungalow.'

The Settha Palace – or The Bungalow – had the slightly dilapidated air of an old aunt, gone to seed, surrounded by photographs of a riotous past. If everyone moved out tomorrow the gardens would surely reclaim the villa in weeks, Jean-Marie decided. Moss had been allowed to grow without hindrance on the long, gabled roof, and the flamboyants in the courtyard grew unchecked, the questing fingers of their branches stretching across the façade.

He went inside. It was just after lunch and the room boys were curled up like a litter of kittens on a double bed in the hall, under some torn mosquito netting. Four other members of the hotel staff were sitting at the bar. A black telephone was ringing at the other end of the counter. They watched it with detached fascination, like an exhibit in a zoo. None of them moved.

A British journalist was asleep in a rattan chair, looking pale and dehydrated in his tropical whites, a copy of *Lao Presse* open in his lap. His head was thrown back and his mouth gaped open while a fly circled the cavern of his open mouth.

He found Crocé in the back garden sitting under a spreading flamboyant, apparently asleep, in a little courtyard someone

21

had created with thousands of upended beer bottles. He was wearing a white shirt and white linen trousers, both carefully pressed. The only clues to his previous night's activities were a pair of dark glasses and the shadow of stubble on his cheeks. Jean-Marie resented Crocé's ability to look like a Hollywood film star even when he was hungover.

'You idiot,' he said.

Crocé opened one eye. 'Jean-Marie, it's you. What time is it?'

'Time you got some brains. How's your head?'

'It aches a little. And look at this.' He pointed to his lip, which was swollen and cracked. 'Some *espèce de con* hit me.' He took off the sun-glasses and squinted up at his friend. 'You heard about it, I suppose?'

'I was only on the ground two minutes and I got the whole story. Where's my car?'

'Your car's all right. Nothing's broken.'

'What about the bar? How are you going to pay for the damage?'

Crocé replaced the dark glasses. 'Don't worry so much. I'll work something out.'

'*Tu es con.* Do you know who that girl was?'

'Noelle Bonaventure.'

Jean-Marie threw himself onto a chair beside him. 'Noelle Bonaventure, yes! *Merde!* Her father's *un vrai monsieur*, one of the biggest gangsters in Indochina. You'll get your throat cut playing with those people!'

'I'm not playing, Jean-Mar'.'

'Then what are you doing?'

'You know what I heard the other day? The Vietnamese are planning to re-open the opium trade. That's going to mean a lot of money for someone. Perhaps it's time we formed a strategic alliance.'

Jean-Marie stared at him, bewildered for a moment, before he realised what Crocé was thinking. 'You're out of your mind! Go near his daughter and he'll cut your throat.'

He shrugged his shoulders. 'Perhaps. Can you move a little to the right? I'm working on my tan, and you're blocking out the sun.'

3

Noelle stood at the windows, listening to the rhythm of the night, the chirrup of cicadas building to a crescendo then dropping away, building again. The monsoon was still two months away, but already the humidity was oppressive, and a sultry patina of sweat clung to her skin.

'La Vie en Rose', sounding scratchy and sad on the gramophone: Edith Piaf. Noelle hugged herself and thought about the Corsican in the white linen suit. 'Baptiste,' she murmured. Such easy charm. So alive, and so dangerous. He wanted to sleep with her and he just came right out and said it! A part of her was outraged, another part of her...

But that was impossible. Her father would never allow her to see him again.

She stole a glimpse of herself in the mirror. The dark blue of her blouse accentuated the soft violet of her eyes. Her hair was loose, and fell in glossy curls around her face. She tossed it over her shoulders. She was aware of her own beauty, and it tormented her. What was the point of beauty if there was no one to share it with? Papa was right, she thought, I do need a husband.

But one of my own choosing.

Rivelini had returned, sulky and limping, to Bangkok; and that morning her father had flown to Saigon, leaving her alone in the villa. Another long tropical night of boredom and *longueur*. The restlessness she felt was like a physical ache. She wanted to go out. She wanted to flirt. Perhaps if she was back in France...

France was a dream, a jumble of childhood memories and fantasies. They had left just after the war, when she was nine years old. All she remembered of Marseille now was the smell of fish at the docks, the grey rows of stone buildings, the biting cold.

Her whole adolescence had been Asia, the cycle of monsoons, the alien rituals of *les jaunes*, the loneliness of luxurious, echoing villas. She had gone to a Convent school in Saigon, and there had at least been a few French girls of her own age there. In Vientiane the only French females she knew were either married to diplomats or were still at school. And there were no places a young European woman could go alone without exciting comment.

The men she met and that her father approved of did not excite her; those who did – like Crocé – he frowned upon. I wonder if that is more than just coincidence? she thought. Sometimes she wondered at the quixotic and contrary nature of her own character. I love Papa, she thought. So why do I sometimes go to such extraordinary lengths to spite him?

Perhaps we are too similar. We never like anyone telling us what to do or how to live our lives. Perhaps that is it.

Suddenly she heard the clamour of a car horn from the driveway at the front of the house. Who could it be at this time of the night?

She ran on to the balcony of the upstairs dining room, and looked down into the courtyard. Baptiste Crocé was standing on the bonnet of the Packard, holding a dozen red roses.

'For you!' he shouted.

'What are you doing here?'

He ignored the question and tossed the flowers up to her. 'They're plastic. I got them from the hotel. But they're the only roses in all of Laos.'

'What do you want? My father will kill you!'

'He's in Saigon. How will he ever know?' He wore his trademark white suit and his hair was slick and gleaming. 'I have come to take you to dinner.'

'You cannot. Don't be absurd!'

'You have another engagement?'

'That is not the point!'

'I am sober. Look!' He jumped off the bonnet and walked beside the car as if on a tightrope. 'You said I should be sober the next time I made love to you. You don't know what an endurance it is for me not to drink in a lousy place like this! But now I have found you, I would do anything!'

'You must go away!'

Crocé pointed to the ground-floor windows. 'The servants are all staring. If you do not come down, I will stay here until your father returns. You want him to shoot me down like a dog on your own doorstep?'

Noelle hesitated. Oh, to hell with Rocco! 'If I come, you must promise to bring me home by ten o'clock.'

Crocé grinned and bowed. 'My word as an officer and a gentleman!'

Maxim's, unlike its more glamorous namesake in Paris, had latticed bamboo walls and a leaking tin roof. It was one of the new honky tonks that had recently sprung up all over Vientiane. The clientele was mainly French: sunburned men with rolled up sleeves and lank hair, former soldiers or airmen who had not found their way back from the war and were now involved in some way in smuggling gold or piasters or opium. The taxi girls squirmed against them on the dance floor or twittered around them at the tables, trying to entice them to their cribs in the back room.

But now that Noelle had entered, their efforts were largely ignored. She felt every eye on her as they walked through the bar, the men's eyes hungry, the taxi girls' glassy with spite.

Noelle knew it was not the kind of place a girl like herself should go. 'I cannot be seen in here,' she said.

'You don't like it?' he asked her.

'Are any of those girls virgins?'

'Not now, perhaps. But once!'

'I doubt even once!'

Crocé shrugged his shoulders. 'I'm sorry. I've never been here before, of course. I just heard the music was good.'

'You're a liar.'

'Just one drink. We'll sit at the back.'

She hesitated. 'One drink only.'

Crocé found a table in a dark corner and they sat down. He ordered two Pernods with water.

'All these men are watching me,' she hissed.

25

'They are admiring you.'

'I don't think admiration is the word.'

'They all want to sleep with you. That is a form of admiration. But you can relax. You are with me.' And he took out his Gitanes and grinned at her as he lit one.

Noelle picked up her Pernod and studied him over the rim of her glass. 'You should not smoke so much. It is bad for your health.'

'Whoever told you that?'

'I read it somewhere.'

'Nonsense. Anyway, I enjoy it. It is just a little habit I picked up in the war.' He began to tell her about himself. It was much the same story as her father had told her, she noted, but for a few little embellishments; by Croce's accounts he had been decorated in Indochina more times than any French pilot since World War One. He conveniently omitted to mention his brief career in Bangkok.

'And now you have turned to a life of crime?'

He feigned outrage. 'I am an airline executive.'

'You have a fifty per cent share in one Cessna. Which you use to smuggle piasters out of Vietnam.'

'Who doesn't? Maybe a little opium too. But opium is more dangerous. The Vietnamese don't like it. Their President Diem is a Puritan. Either he'll have to change his mind or Viet Nam will change their President. Asia is no place for people with morals.'

'Indeed, monsieur? Then perhaps I'd better be going home.'

'I mean men. Women ... it is different.'

'How is it different, Baptiste?'

'You have to pretend harder.'

'Sometimes I think I should just slap your face and have nothing more to do with you.'

He held up his hands in mock horror. 'No, please. I have seen you fight before. I give in now.'

'You're playing with fire, Baptiste. Don't treat me like a taxi girl. There'll be people lining up to kill you soon enough. And I'll be at the front of the queue.'

'Anyway, how is it you know so much about me?' he asked her.

She raised an eyebrow.

Then he realised. 'Your father, of course.'

'How did you raise the money to buy the plane?'

'Me, I won a little money at cards.'

'And Jean-Marie?'

'He was even luckier. He has a rich father in Lyon. Do you believe in luck, Noelle?'

She shook her head.

'You should. Being lucky is everything. Do you want to know about your luck?' He took her hand and examined her palm. His touch was cool and gentle. 'You see, your luck's written right here in these lines. Look at this. This is your love line, Noelle. Just one deep line. Only one. That's me.'

She snatched her hand away. 'I'm not going to sleep with you, Baptiste. Not tonight. Perhaps not ever.'

He leaned forward so that his face was inches from her, the dark eyes glittering like coal. 'Don't say that. I would kill myself. Come on.'

There was a brass band from Saigon playing Afro-Cuban dance classics. He led her to the dance floor. It was a samba, a brassy trumpet leading the melody, very slowly and very badly. Crocé moved against her. She was uncomfortably aware of the smell of his sandalwood aftershave, the heat of his body, the grins of the men around the tables, the bitter glances of the girls. She pulled away. 'Take me home.'

'What's wrong?'

'I told you, I'm not one of your taxi girls. You said just one drink. Now take me home.'

'But I also promised to buy you dinner.'

'I'm not hungry.'

She went back to their table, found her purse and hurried outside to the car. The *siclo* drivers laughed and chattered beside their cabs. She beckoned one of them.

Crocé followed her outside. 'I don't understand. What's wrong?'

How can I explain it? she thought. You're not a woman, and you cannot understand. I am torn between loneliness and guilt but I am not so desperate that I will become just another of your conquests. I never will be.

27

'I have to go home,' she said.

'You are crazy. First you hit your boyfriend because he hits me –'

'I didn't hit him, I pushed him.'

' – then when I come to take you dancing, you act like you're a nun or I don't know what.' He stubbed out his cigarette with his shoe. 'When will you get it in your head, huh? I fell in love with you the first moment I saw you. I may have been crazy that night, but I wasn't so drunk I didn't know I'd met the most beautiful girl I have ever seen in my whole damn life.' He moved closer and took her face in his hands. He kissed her hard on the mouth. As the kiss went on, his manner became gentler. She felt his tongue exploring her mouth.

Finally she pulled away, breathless. 'No! Just take me home.'

'You are the best fighter of anyone I know,' he whispered. 'I want you by me always, to protect me from danger.'

She looked at him. He was laughing at her now. Impossible, just impossible.

'You're playing with me, aren't you?'

'But isn't it a great game?' He dismissed the *siclo* driver with a nod, led her to the Packard and opened the door for her. 'Please.'

'What do you want with me, Baptiste?'

'I told you. I want to marry you.'

'You hardly know me.'

'I know everything about you. I know you were a little girl who thought she was a princess. I know that little girl thought her papa was the strongest, bravest, cleverest man in the whole world, and now you are disappointed. I know you are bored and lonely and you are looking for a way out.'

She blushed in the darkness. 'You talk nothing but shit,' she muttered.

He pretended to be shocked. 'Where did you learn such language?'

'The nuns at school. Now shut up and drive.'

When they reached the villa he hurried around the car to hold open the door. He took her hand to help her out. 'An officer and a gentleman.'

'Goodnight, Baptiste.'

28

She went up the steps to the screen door. On an impulse, she turned around, ran back, and threw her arms around his neck. She kissed him hard on the lips, forcing him backwards over the hood of the Packard.

She pulled away from him just as suddenly. 'Not tonight,' she said, and then hurried inside, slamming the door behind her, leaving him breathless and amazed.

4

Saigon

Saigon reminded Rocco Bonaventure of a French provincial town that had somehow been scooped up by a giant hand and set down in the middle of an Asian swamp.

The streets were broad, lined with tamarind and lime trees, and the villas behind the painted stucco walls had huge white porte cochères and red-tiled roofs. But the traffic very much belonged to Asia. There were bicycles and putt-putt motorcycles, with whole families balanced precariously around Papa on the handlebars and behind him on the seat; ancient open touring cars that the Saigonnais used as jitneys; and dilapidated Renault and Peugeot taxis that looked as if they were held together with bits of wire.

And often were.

Bonaventure watched from the terrace of the Continental Hotel, inside one of the great arches that screened the tables. He always came here when he was in Saigon. The terrace was supposed to be relatively safe from the grenades that were still occasionally tossed into the cafés by the Viet Minh.

Across the table from him, Colonel Tran van Li gulped an ice cube from his cognac and soda and crunched it between his back teeth. He was a cheerful, round-faced man with a goatee beard, and the lazy demeanour of a government translator. 'So, how was the opium harvest?' he asked.

Bonaventure's expression betrayed nothing. 'Adequate.'

Li grinned. 'Perhaps it will be the last one for a while.'

'You mean the Pathet Lao? Don't worry about them. Savages with bows and arrows.'

'My information is that they have attacked Lao outposts around Sam Neua and Phong Saly. And that the Chinese are conducting manoeuvres along the border.'

'The Americans will never allow the communists to take over in Laos.'

Li said nothing but his eyes speculated. The Americans' passionate war against the communists had saved Vietnam from Ho Chi Minh after partition. Perhaps Eisenhower would make a stand in Laos as well. It was an outcome he desired as fervently as the Frenchman. Laos was still Saigon's main source of illegal opium, thanks to Rocco Bonaventure and Air Laos. Of course, Bonaventure could not have operated so profitably without Li's protection, but then the colonel considered he was being generously rewarded for his services.

Tran van Li was in an ideal position to help Bonaventure. Since 1955 he had been one of President Diem's closest advisers, as well as director of the Military Security Service, an organisation responsible for investigating corruption inside the military. In practise, it put him in charge of the graft; and Li was a man who led by example. For the past three years he had been a silent partner in Bonaventure's Air Laos.

'There may be a new wind blowing through the Doc Lap palace,' he said casually. 'The Viet Minh have not been as easily contained as the Americans thought. There are those who are becoming a little nostalgic for the days of the Binh Xuyen.'

Bonaventure smiled. He remembered the Binh Xuyen from his own days in Saigon; originally just a gang of river pirates, they had later become Vietnam's largest and most efficient private army. They had guaranteed the security of the city, in exchange for the nation's opium concession. When the French left in 1955, after Dien Bien Phu, the Americans had moved in and put the puritanical President Diem in the Doc Lap palace. His CIA advisers had persuaded him to crush the Binh Xuyen; the opium trade had offended the sensibilities of the cold war warriors.

Ridiculous! Had they really believed they could govern Saigon without opium?

Denied secure access to Saigon, Bonaventure had been forced to use drop zones in the Northern Highlands and the Gulf of Siam to smuggle in his opium cargoes. The ban had been in place now for over three years, and trade had been seriously hampered. At last some good news. Bonaventure was not altogether surprised that Diem and the Americans had abandoned the high moral ground, only at how quickly the Viet Minh had forced the change.

'So the Americans have lost their virginity in Asia?' he said.

Li nodded. 'Indeed. It is the morning after and they are very sore. Diem also. He has spent his whole life in palaces and he does not understand the realities of Saigon any more than they do. To have security here, one must have spies and information. But to have spies one needs money. And in Viet Nam, money is opium.'

They heard the siren from the Post Office. It was noon, and soon all of Saigon would shut down until mid-afternoon. As they watched, the streets flooded with people; pretty Vietnamese secretaries and shop assistants cycling gracefully home down the leafy tunnel of the Tu Do in their *ao dai* – flowing white silk trousers and long flowered robes, slit to the waist – their palm leaf hats tied with bright coloured ribbons; siclo drivers pedalling towards the river with Vietnamese businessmen in western suits balanced under the canopies in front of them; hawkers on their way back from the market, flat bamboo springing on their shoulders, piled with cabbages and bananas.

Two men in crew-cuts and orange and green Hawaiian shirts came out of the hotel lobby and were immediately surrounded by children peddling cigarettes and garlands of flowers.

'Americans,' Bonaventure said with a slow smile. 'I sometimes don't know whether to love them or hate them.'

'They have asked me to put all the old machinery back in place,' Li said. 'From now on you can bring in as much opium as you want. It will all be carefully controlled, and you split the proceeds with us. You will still have to use your landing strips up at Pleiku, but now there will be ARVN trucks waiting for you on the ground, and we will bring the opium into Saigon under military escort.'

Bonaventure nodded with satisfaction. If the Pathet Lao could be kept out of the northern mountains for a few more seasons, there was a fortune to be made. 'What about competition?'

'We intend to create a government monopoly. That does not allow for competition. You will be our exclusive supplier.'

Bonaventure raised his cognac in toast. 'To a mutually profitable partnership,' he said.

Li returned the toast with his own glass. 'Indeed.'

5

Vientiane

Bonaventure employed five servants: a cook, a houseboy, two *boyesses*, and a gardener. By nightfall only the cook and the houseboy remained in the house, and after dinner Noelle told them they would not be required for the rest of the evening.

Just before nine o'clock she stood on the balcony overlooking the back of the house and listened. The sing-song chatter of voices from the servants' quarters faded away. By quarter past, all the lights were out and she was satisfied they were all asleep. She went back inside.

Before she went down the stairs, she briefly re-examined her reflection in the gilt mirror in her bedroom. Her hair was braided in what the French called a *baguette*, but one errant curl had worked loose, and teased her cheek. She brushed it back impatiently. She had deliberately refrained from using make-up. There was just a little gloss on her nails, a concession to her education by the French nuns at the Les Oiseaux. Not too provocative, she decided.

But alluring enough.

The night was humid and still, and the white calico dress clung damply to her body. In all the wrong places, she thought, and her cheeks felt suddenly hot. There was nothing she could do about it now. There was a hollow tingling in her belly and her pulse was racing.

Tonight. Perhaps tonight.

She picked up the glass bottle of Joïe perfume and dabbed at her wrists, her elbows, her throat. They said it was the heat and the pulse that activated the scent. One of the girls at the

34

Convent used to put a little on the skin inside her thighs. Tramp!

She took a deep breath.

Tonight.

She tried to stay calm and went slowly down the stairs. She closed the screen door as gently as she could, saw the silhouette of a car parked on the other side of the road, and started to run.

'Baptiste?'

He leaped out and held the door for her. 'I thought you had forgotten.'

'I had to wait until the servants were asleep. Where are we going?'

As she climbed in he bent down and whispered. 'Into the night.'

She whispered a quick prayer to the Virgin to forgive her. It would probably be the last time they spoke. She guessed that after tonight they would have nothing left in common.

Saigon

Cholon was Saigon's ugly twin. The city stank of mud and petrol and sewage.

Rocco Bonaventure wrinkled his nose and held his breath. He would never understand why a man like Chen Giai Han did not remove himself to a better quarter of the city.

Cholon slept by day and worked by night. As the sun dropped low over the rooftops, the city began to come alive. Hawkers set up at the roadside, fanning the little charcoal fires under their portable kitchens; fortune tellers with grey goatee beards squatted against the walls and laid out the ancient playing cards that were the tools of their trade; dentists and barbers were busy under the kerosene lanterns that were slung from the boughs of the tamarind trees that lined the streets.

Vertical signs with Chinese characters hung from the shop-houses, announcing that this was the Chinatown of Saigon. The chiu chao speakers, from the Swatow province of China, ruled here. Chiu chao: they dominated commerce like the Jews, ran the underworld like the Sicilian Mafia. And the man Rocco Bonaventure had come to see, Chen Giai Han – better known as Sammy Chen – was overlord of all chiu chao in Cholon.

They passed the Qan Am pagoda, and Bonaventure ordered the siclo driver to stop outside the Trung Mai Hotel, a sad and decaying four-storey tenement with an evil-smelling *bac si* on one side and a restaurant on the other. The restaurant, Bonaventure knew from previous visits, was very popular. The house speciality was boiled dog.

The foyer of the Trung Mai was gloomily dark. The lights had not yet been turned on. The wooden floor was partly covered by a tattered Chinese rug; the exposed boards around it had been polished to a dull sheen by bare feet. Male guests in black pyjamas lounged in the variety of furniture in the lobby. Two taxi girls, slouching by the desk, studied him with the practised weariness of a *tai tai* examining fish at a market stall.

'*Excusez-moi. Il faut que je vois Monsieur Chen,*' Bonaventure said to the desk clerk.

The man nodded and hawked and spat over his shoulder. For a moment Bonaventure thought he had spat on the floor, but then he heard the ring as the clerk's detritus landed accurately in a brass spittoon somewhere under the desk.

The man went through a curtain that led to a small anteroom behind him. Bonaventure heard a brief exchange in the harsh chiu chao dialect, and then a Chinese woman in flowered silk pyjamas came out and peered at him through thick black-rimmed spectacles.

'*Comment vous appelez-vous?*'

'*Je m'appelle Bonaventure, Rocco Bonaventure. Il faut que je vois Monsieur Chen. C'est très important.*'

The woman considered a moment, then indicated that he should follow her. A doorway under the stairs led to the rear of the hotel; coloured plastic strips hung from the frame to deter the flies. Bonaventure followed her through.

The back room was airless and hot. He was invited to sit on one of the hard-backed uncomfortable chairs he was accustomed to finding in every Chinese anteroom, and then the woman shuffled off again, shouting at some unseen interlocutor in her own dialect.

There was a single low-wattage bulb hanging on a flex from the ceiling. Bonaventure realised the room was not an office, as he had at first supposed, but living quarters, possibly for Chen's extended family. An old grandmother in black pyjamas sat on a bamboo cot while a child crawled on the floor at her feet. Two middle-aged men in white vests and brown trousers played mah-jong at a card table, while another, older man lay on a cot in the far corner of the room, smoking opium.

Bonaventure watched him heat a ball of the black, jelly-like drug over the flame of a lamp, then knead the hot opium into the convex bowl of his pipe. Bonaventure could smell the smoke, sweet and rich. There was no other smell like opium, he thought, you could never mistake it for anything else. Personally it made him want to retch.

The old man reversed the bowl of the pipe over the lamp flame and the little bead of opium bubbled as he inhaled. His eyes were glassy and unfocused.

'Monsieur Bonaventure!' The squat, bespectacled man in the doorway pronounced it 'Bon Van Chao'. Sammy Chen wore a crumpled western-style suit over a white open-necked shirt stained with the day's sweat. He had worn brown sandals on his feet. 'You do me great honour to visit.'

Bonaventure got to his feet. 'The honour is all mine, Sammy.'

They shook – Sammy's hand was clammy and plump, Bonaventure noticed – and then the Chinese pulled up a chair next to Bonaventure's and sat down. He clapped his hands and the old woman on the bed stood up and hurried off.

Sammy immediately launched into long enquiries after Bonaventure's health and the well-being of his family. While they talked the old woman reappeared holding a tray with a teapot and two handleless porcelain cups. The tea was pale and bitter and scalding hot.

After observing the usual conventions, Sammy Chen ventured to business. 'So why you come to Cholon, okay?'

'I came here to discuss a little business with you, Sammy.'

Bonaventure was certain Sammy Chen already knew the change of tide in the Doc Lap palace.

'I had a discussion today with Colonel Li,' Bonaventure went on. 'It seems someone has persuaded President Diem that perhaps he has been a little too harsh in his policies.'

Sammy rubbed his thumb and index finger together. 'Need opium money.'

Bonaventure nodded. 'Perhaps the Viet Minh have simply illustrated to him the realities of the political situation in Saigon.'

'Double lucky for us. Opium is good business. If you can supply, I can sell *beaucoup* here in Saigon. Perhaps I can sell Hong Kong also.'

This was what Bonaventure had hoped to hear. He already sent much of his opium to Bangkok where Rivelini smuggled it to his uncle's heroin laboratories in Marseille. But the market there was saturated, the *Union Corse* getting most of their raw supplies from Anatolia. But if Sammy could offer an expanding market, Bonaventure could buy up all the opium the hill tribes could produce, and more. The potential profits were limitless.

'Look at him,' Sammy said, indicating the old man on the bed. He had drifted off into an opiate reverie, his eyes half open, his body utterly still. 'Does no harm. Is okay when you are old man.'

The baby crawled across the floor and hoisted himself to his feet, clinging to Chen's trousers. His hands left dirty fingermarks but Chen did not scold him. The Chinese rarely scolded their children. 'Number two son,' Sammy said, and picked the child up and sat him on his knee. 'Very good to have many children. Children are the future. Take care of us in wrinkle time, clean our bones when we are dead. Their prayers make sure we are honoured in heaven.'

Bonaventure thought about Noelle and his face set like stone.

'Man should have sons,' Chen said.

Bonaventure did not venture a comment.

Chen bounced the child on his knee and he gurgled happily. 'Daughter is good. Son is better.'

Bonaventure thought about Noelle. You're probably right, he decided.

Sammy put the child back on the floor and the conversation returned to business. But as they discussed prices and quantities Bonaventure found it increasingly difficult to concentrate.

He kept thinking about what Sammy had said about sons and daughters, and wondered what Noelle was doing right now.

Vientiane

The ruins of the ancient *wat* appeared in the splash of the headlights. The demons and heroes of the *Ramayana* were resurrected for just a moment in the phosphorescence, clambering along the eaves, clawing at the invading creepers of the jungle. When Crocé switched off the beam they returned to the jungle shadows. He lit a paraffin lantern and they climbed out. He came around the car and Noelle felt his hand on her shoulder. It was somehow comforting. 'You know this place?' he whispered.

'I came here once with my father, years ago. He told me it was abandoned last century.'

'Do you know why?'

'No one remembers. Bad *phi* perhaps.'

The Lao were great believers in *phi*, the unseen spirits who governed the material world. They believed *phi* lived in everything – in mountains, in rivers, in animals, in people, even in the sky. Rainbows were the sky spirits bending to drink, thunder and lightning the voice of their anger. The local version of Buddhism had absorbed the *phi* cult to make a unique amalgam of beliefs. A great deal of a Lao's time was spent consoling and cajoling these spirits with sacrifices of rice and elaborate rituals. A provoked *phi* could sprain ankles or break limbs, even bring sickness and tragedy.

Their footsteps echoed on the stone flags of the courtyard as Crocé led her further into the ruins. The swinging yellow light of the lantern briefly illuminated the dragons that snaked along the curlicues of the roof, the stone lions that stood guard at the arches, the serpents on the balustrades. Two putty-coloured lizards froze in the light of the lamp before scampering away into the darkness. The play of the shadows made it difficult for the mind to distinguish between what was carved and what was real.

They sat on the cool stone inside the *sala* and Crocé put the lantern at their feet. His face was half in shadow.

'You're quiet tonight,' he said.

'I'm nervous.'

'About what?'

'About my father.'

'Let me handle him.'

'You don't know what he's like.'

He picked up her hand, held it in his lap, stroked the soft skin inside her arm with his other hand. He found the dark blue string tied around her left wrist. 'What's this?'

'Last year I was very sick. The local doctors did not know what was wrong. Tao Koo, our houseboy, fetched his uncle. He's a sort of shaman. He performed this little ritual over the bed. The Laos think all illness is a bad *phi* luring the souls from the body, and if they cannot be persuaded to return you will die. So he calls on the friendly spirits to summon the lost souls and call them back to the body. The string is meant to bind them there so they can not wander any more.'

'You sound like you believe all this?'

'Perhaps I do.'

His fingers traced the contour of her arm to her shoulder. She shivered.

'How can a person have more than one soul?' he asked her.

Keep talking. Try to pretend this isn't happening. I don't want to do this now, I'm too scared. 'The Laos say we have many souls. When we die they fly away to different places to be reincarnated in different bodies.'

'You believe it?'

She shook her head. He was very close now. She felt his breath on her neck. She was shocked to hear herself utter a soft whimper of pleasure as his lips brushed gently against the soft skin of her throat.

'Then what do you believe?' he whispered.

'I believe you just have one soul and when you die it returns to the one you love. When I die perhaps my spirit will come back to you, Baptiste.'

There, it was said now. She had known from the moment she had seen him what would happen between them. Perhaps he was right. It was written in their hands.

The night closed around them, the chirruping of the jungle insects a cacophony of sound. He pushed her gently back on to the stone, and she felt his weight on top of her.

'Do you love me?' she whispered.

'No. No, I do not love you. Love is too simple a word. I am obsessed by you. I can think of nothing else but you. I am going to turn your life into a raging storm.'

She stared at the vaulted shadows of the pavilion, the *nagas* dancing along the eaves, the geckos rustling in the roof, hunting for lust, for murder.

The male smells of sandalwood and tobacco.

The hardness of the muscles of his body.

The *phi* whispering from the darkness, spirits good and bad.

She felt her own spirit being coaxed away. Too late to return now.

6

When he'd first arrived in Asia over ten years before, Rocco Bonaventure had quickly adopted the daily routine of the French colonialists; he rose at eight, enjoyed a leisurely breakfast, and rarely conducted any business before ten o'clock. After lunch he rested during the hottest part of the day, and concluded the day's affairs by six o'clock. The evening was the time to drink apéritifs.

It was now his habit, at *l'heure d'apéritif*, to sit in the upper-storey room he used as a study, and watch the sunset. Tonight Marcel Rivelini kept him company during his vigil. Bonaventure reached for the bottle of Pernod and refilled two glasses, one for himself, and one for Rivelini.

'They say there's been more fighting around Sam Neua and Phong Saly,' Rivelini commented.

Bonaventure nodded.

Rivelini seemed anxious. 'Communists. They get in the way of business.'

'The Americans will not let them take over in Laos, Marcel. They saw what happened in Eastern Europe. They won't let it happen here.'

'I hope you're right, Rocco.'

'Don't worry about it.'

Bonaventure added a little water to his Pernod, and the golden liquid immediately turned the colour of milk. He returned his attention to the window. The monsoon had begun, and the twilight was dirty and grey; even the city's gilded stupas looked drab. The banana palms and bamboo in the garden wilted under the assault of the rain.

Rocco looks so smug, thought Rivelini. So smug here in his

42

retreat, the bookshelves filled with leather bound volumes, plays by Corneille and Racine, his bronze statues of the Buddha and Hanuman on the polished teak desk. So civilised. A pirate of culture and refinement. Such a shame to prick his balloon.

But I shall.

'How is Noelle?'

Something in his tone jarred Bonaventure from his complacency. He frowned. 'She is well, as far as I know. Why, Marcel?'

Rivelini shrugged, affected an air of discreet concern. 'It is just, well ... one hears things. I would hate to see her hurt.'

'How could she be hurt, Marcel?'

'Rocco, I apologise. Perhaps one should not listen to rumours.'

'What rumours? Stop talking in riddles.'

'Look, I suppose you should know. I have heard reports that she has been seen in the company of a certain gentleman. You were in Saigon, I believe. Perhaps it was innocent. But it is not good for her reputation to be so careless.'

'Who?' Bonaventure snapped.

'His name is Crocé. Baptiste Crocé.'

The glass cracked in Bonaventure's fist. Dark red blood welled through the knuckles and dripped on to his white linen trousers, mixing with the milky Pernod.

He fumbled in his pocket for a clean linen handkerchief and wrapped it around his hand to soak up the blood. Then he reached with his good hand into the pocket of his jacket for his Gauloises and lighter. He lit the cigarette one-handed, his fingers shaking.

'Rocco? Are you all right?' Rivelini sounded alarmed.

Bonaventure ignored the question. 'What else did you hear?' he snapped.

'They were only rumours, Rocco.'

'Did the rumours say she has been sleeping with him?'

'People will make up any lie, you know that. But she cannot afford even to be seen with him. This man does not enjoy a spotless reputation in Vientiane.'

'Or anywhere else,' growled Bonaventure.

There was a long silence. Rivelini stared at the scarlet blossoming on the handkerchief. A better reaction than he had imagined. That will teach the bitch to make a fool of me, he thought.

. 'I thought you should know,' he added.

Bonaventure nodded. I bet you couldn't wait to get straight round here and tell me, he thought. A salve for your wounded pride, I suppose. But I don't blame you, in the circumstances.

'Thank you, Marcel. I appreciate your concern. Now I'd like to be alone for a while. I need to think about this.'

Rivelini took his cue to leave. He finished his Pernod and stood up. '*Bientôt*, Rocco.'

Bonaventure nodded, but did not look up. He did not even hear the door close. Already he was thinking about Noelle, and Baptiste Crocé.

She had made a fool of him. He had tried to arrange suitable companions for her, and she had spurned them all. He had warned her about this Crocé, and she had disobeyed him. The moment his back was turned she had chased after him, like a bitch in heat.

And Crocé? Did he really think he could get away with this?

Perhaps they both needed to be taught a lesson. And Rocco Bonaventure was a very good teacher.

7

Every year, during the poppy harvest from February to the first weeks of May, local Chinese traders went into the northern mountains with salt, iron bars, and silver coins to barter for the tiny bundles of raw opium that the hill tribes – mainly the Hmong – grew in the sweet, friable soils.

The Corsicans flew to provincial capitals like Ban Hoei Sai or Sam Neua or Phong Saly to barter with the Yunnanese traders for the opium they had collected. They would then fly it to Phong Savan or Vientiane to be stored until a buyer could be found in Bangkok or Saigon.

The airport at Wattay had no Immigration or Customs controls, and the airfield was no more than a cleared pasture. There was a handful of sheds at the eastern end of the strip, warehouses and hangars for the handful of pirate airlines that flew the treacherous skies over Laos. In the dry season the airfield was a dust bowl; now, in the monsoon, it was a cloying swamp.

The sky was overcast, the air like steam. Baptiste and Jean-Marie were soaked with perspiration and rain. They had three hundred kilos of raw opium to load into the Cessna. Some of it oozed jelly-like from splits in the burlap sacks.

'There's rumours going all around Vientiane, Baptiste.'

'About what?'

'About you and Rocco Bonaventure's daughter.' Jean-Marie grunted as he lifted another sack. 'You have to be out of your mind.'

Baptiste grinned. 'Jealousy.'

'Why won't you listen to me? She's out of bounds, Baptiste! He'll cut off your balls when he finds out!'

Baptiste slid another sack into the hold. 'His daughter's in love with me. What can he do about that?'

Jean-Marie shook his head. He admired his business partner, but sometimes he found he didn't like him very much. His coldness frightened Jean-Marie. There was an edge to Baptiste Crocé, a steel that was camouflaged by the velvet of his charm. If ever he was asked his opinion of the man, he declared that Baptiste Crocé was both calculating and ruthless.

And Jean-Marie was his friend; he wondered what Baptiste's enemies said about him.

'I'm telling you, you're crazy, Baptiste. When he finds out, he'll want to kill you.'

His partner grabbed him by the shoulders. Sweat ran freely off his face, and the dark comma of hair hanging over his eyes made him look raffish and just as crazy as Jean-Marie had suggested.

'You're not listening to me. I'm telling you, she loves me. She wants to marry me. What do you think Bonaventure is going to do, huh? If he hurts me, his daughter will make his life unbearable.'

'This guy is a gangster, Baptiste.'

Crocé was not listening. 'What do you think about a merger, Jean-Mar'? Rocco Bonaventure's Air Laos and our little Wattay Air? Bonaventure is getting to be an old man. He'll want someone to take over his business, a clever son-in-law to keep his daughter in the proper manner, huh?'

'He won't do it, Baptiste.'

Crocé gave him a lop-sided grin and patted him on the shoulder. 'Yes, he will. Now let's load the rest of this mud. And don't worry so much. I know what I'm doing.'

Rocco Bonaventure was breakfasting on *café au lait*, croissants and papaya with lime juice. A copy of the French language edition of *Lao Presse* lay open on the linen tablecloth in front of him. His right hand was heavily bandaged.

He looked up as Noelle joined him on the balcony. She sat down. Bonaventure examined his daughter anew in the light of last night's revelations. She looked pale and fretful.

'What's the matter, *chérie*? Is there something wrong?'

'There is something I have to talk to you about.'

He raised a single eyebrow in enquiry. So. She had decided to confess.

'It concerns a certain ... gentleman.'

'A gentleman? Not Monsieur Crocé then?'

'You knew?'

Bonaventure watched her, a mocking smile on his lips. 'Vientiane is a small town, *chérie*.'

'Why didn't you say anything?'

'I pay no attention to rumours.'

'You attend to nothing else.'

He nodded, conceding the point. 'Perhaps you had better tell me what's been going on.'

She thought about that night in the temple ruins, almost six weeks ago. It had hurt, and the physical sensations had been far more muted than she had expected. But every movement, every whisper, had seared itself on her memory. And Baptiste had been so gentle. Somehow the act had forged a bond between them, a bond she knew could never be broken.

'I think I love him, papa.'

'Love him?' Bonaventure mused. 'Love? How long did you say you have known this man?'

'Does it matter?'

'It depends what you intend to do about this ... *love*.'

'I want to marry him.'

'Well then, perhaps it does matter. Especially if you want the marriage to last longer than a week.'

He seemed far more sanguine than she had expected. After all, her confession was tantamount to admitting she had defied him. Noelle had anticipated one of his rages. She had witnessed them before – terrifying, violent episodes when nothing in the house was safe. Not that he had ever struck her, of course; she had never been frightened of him in that way.

'Papa, I'm serious about this.'

Bonaventure threw down his napkin. 'I cannot pretend I am happy,' he said. 'But if there is one thing I have learned with you, *chérie*, it is that you are a very stubborn woman. I think you are misguided, and blinded by appearances. That is what I think. But if you are determined to go ahead, with

47

or without my approval, then I suppose I had better talk to this ... gentleman. You have my permission to invite him to dinner tomorrow night. Now if you do not mind, I shall retire to my study and sulk.'

After he had gone, Noelle sat for a long time staring at the dregs of her coffee, listening to the rain falling on the tin roof. She had not anticipated that he would capitulate so easily. If that was indeed what he had just done.

Near Ban Me Thuot, Central Highlands, Vietnam

There were no radio beacons in Laos, and the maps had been drawn in the time of the French and were sometimes inaccurate by as much as fifty miles, so a pilot had to learn to navigate his machine by dead reckoning. Even the Catholics among them wore little jade Buddhas around their necks as good luck charms beside their Saint Christophers. They felt they needed all the luck they could get.

Baptiste searched for a break in the gauzy white clouds, then glanced back at the altimeter. Eight thousand ASL. He dared go no lower. The Cessna lurched in the monsoon. The jungles below were invisible. Like flying through a milk bottle, he thought.

He spotted a gap in the clouds and dived towards it. The Highlands appeared just a few hundred feet below, verdant green forest wreathed in mists of wispy cloud, savagely beautiful. The montagnards who lived in those forests still used bows and poisoned arrows, he reminded himself. Not a good place to get lost.

Another flurry of rain spattered across the windshield.

He searched the horizon for the tell-tale smudge of the beacon that would give him his final bearing on Ban Me Thuot. After five minutes he was almost ready to give up and take a compass bearing for home when he saw the skein of dark smoke perhaps five miles away on his starboard side. The south west monsoon had carried him further north than he had anticipated.

He banked gently, came in low. He saw the thatched roofs

of Ban Me Thuot in the distance, and below him the airstrip, a track three hundred yards long, carved from the raw jungle. A truck was parked at the far end of the strip and he saw a man in a white T-shirt waving him in.

He circled once, checked the air-sock at the far end of the runway, and lined up for the descent.

The Cessna bounced once, and then Baptiste felt her settle on to the strip. The wheels skidded in the mud and his fists tightened on the controls as he anticipated the unseen bog that would clutch at the wheels and send the Cessna over on her spine. But his luck held. The Cessna slowed, splashing to a stop fifty yards from the tarpaulin-covered lorry.

The man in the white T-shirt jumped in the truck's cabin and roared through the mud to meet him. Baptiste cut the engine and stepped out. He waved to the driver of the truck, a man he knew only as Hung.

But Hung did not wave back. He did not even smile. He looked scared.

Merde!

Baptiste felt a stab of panic. He ran for the Cessna's cabin, groped for the revolver that was hidden under the pilot's seat. When he turned around a dozen ARVN soldiers had their carbines and submachine guns pointed at him, others jumping from the tailboard of the truck to surround the plane.

Putain!

He dropped the revolver in the mud and raised his hands.

Tran van Li stepped forward, his own revolver still holstered, his hands on his hips. 'Monsieur Crocé?' he said in French.

'How did you know?'

'These gentlemen told us to expect you.' Li indicated Hung and his two companions. They were soaked and miserable.

'But how did you know about the drop?'

'I keep my ears to the ground.' He sauntered over to the cockpit and peered into the hold. 'What sort of cargo are you carrying?'

'Toys for orphans and medical supplies for the poor.'

Li smiled. He liked a man with a sense of humour. 'I imagine there is a certain amount of contraband in there also.

49

Would that be correct, monsieur?'

And then he knew: Bonaventure!

Well, okay. He kept a certain amount of gold under his seat for just such an occasion. 'How much?' he said.

But Tran van Li shook his head. 'Smuggling opium and offering graft to a member of the military are both considered very serious offences in the Republic of Vietnam, Monsieur Crocé. You are under arrest.'

8

Vientiane

Noelle found Jean-Marie at The Bungalow. He was sitting on the porch outside the dining room, staring at the rain dripping from the roofs of the kitchens and servant quarters. The green tangle of the garden looked sodden and forlorn.

He heard her but did not turn his head. 'Noelle Bonaventure,' he said softly in greeting, and swigged at the cognac bottle he had cradled in his arms.

'Is it true?' she said.

Jean-Marie nodded.

'How?'

'He was arrested by the Vietnamese police yesterday afternoon. That's all I know. They impounded the plane.' He gave her an accusing look. 'That plane was everything we had. Everything.'

The broken ceiling fan laboured noisily on a broken blade. A few slow flies followed its journey.

'What's going to happen?'

'He's going to prison. Two years. Five years. Who knows? *Les jaunes* can be little bastards when they want to be.'

Noelle could not imagine spending another two hours without seeing him, never mind two years. Five was unthinkable. 'There has to be some way to get him out. I'll talk to my father.'

Jean-Marie gave a hollow laugh and drained the cognac bottle. He tossed it towards the pile of old whisky bottles that had been stacked next to the chicken coop. He missed and it smashed on a broken toilet bowl that lay against the wizened trunk of a banyan tree.

51

'What's the matter?' asked Noelle.

'You don't get it, do you? Do you think this was an accident? A coincidence?'

'Baptiste always said there were risks.'

'Risks? If there are such risks, how is it your father never loses a plane? Have you never thought about that?'

She didn't answer.

'Haven't you worked it out yet?'

'Worked it out?'

'Your father! Rocco arranged this. I warned Baptiste about you but he wouldn't listen to me. He thought he was so smart. I told him you were bad news!'

Her legs felt weak. She remembered her father's easy capitulation the day before Baptiste was arrested. Could he really have been so devious? 'No,' she whispered.

He put his head in his hands. 'Everything we had was in that plane. I warned him to stay away from you!'

'You're wrong,' she said, and turned and walked away. *No!* Her father was many things. An adventurer, a pirate perhaps. He smuggled gold and piasters and opium, sometimes used his influence with the Laos and the Vietnamese unfairly, but he would never do something like this. He would prove it to her; he would help her get Baptiste Crocé out of jail.

She found him upstairs, in his study. He was sitting at his lacquered writing table, *en smoking*, the crushed velvet of his jacket worn at the sleeves from purple to silver grey. It was late afternoon. The crystal wall sconces threw a dull yellow glow over the teak floorboards and walls. The gold-embossed leather volumes of *Voyages dans l'Indochine* glowed on the bookshelves.

He looks the perfect French *gentilhomme*, she thought, a little roguish perhaps with that long silver grey hair and grizzled beard, but civilised, a man of sensibility. Not a man who would condemn another to incarceration in the black hell of a Vietnamese prison because he did not approve of him.

And yet what did she really know of her father's real nature? She had never defied him before; not on something that really mattered to him. She had never known him not to have his own way.

He looked up as she entered and laid his fountain pen to one side. His expression changed from pleasure to concern. Her eyes were sore from weeping and she knew her face must look a mess. He jumped to his feet and came around the desk. '*Chérie*, what is the matter? You have been crying. What is wrong?'

She allowed him to lead her to a chair. 'Baptiste has been arrested.'

'Baptiste?'

'Baptiste Crocé. You know who I'm talking about.'

His voice became frosty. 'Forgive me, but he and I are not on such intimate terms. We do not generally refer to each other by our Christian names.'

'What else could it have been to hurt me like this?'

Bonaventure ignored the question. 'What happened?'

'He was arrested at an airfield somewhere in the Central Highlands, on the other side of the border. The Vietnamese were waiting for him.'

'I suppose his cargo was not legitimate?'

'Do you ever carry legitimate cargoes?'

He shrugged his shoulders. 'Sometimes.' He rested his weight on the edge of the desk. Then he leaned forward and raised her chin with the forefinger of his right hand. 'So this is the reason for these red eyes?'

'I told you, I love him.'

He grunted, and offered no further comment. She twisted her head away.

Bonaventure got up and went to the window. It had stopped raining. The sun was flat on the plain, the Mekong a ribbon of liquid platinum. Almost time for his apéritif. 'They will imprison him, of course. That is usual. It is bad luck.'

She took a deep breath. 'Did you have anything to do with this?'

He was still for a long time, but she could see the tension in his shoulders. Finally he seemed to relax. 'Is this what you think of me?'

'Did you?'

'No.' He turned around. 'I am outraged that you could accuse

53

me of such a thing. But, as you demand an answer, no. No.'

'Don't lie to me, Papa.'

'And don't you dare interrogate me! I have given you my answer! I would not lie to my own daughter!'

Noelle wanted to believe him. Perhaps Jean-Marie was wrong. But she loved Baptiste and would not let him languish inside a Saigon prison. 'Then help me get him out.'

'Get him out?'

She watched for some clue to what her father was really thinking, but his face remained inscrutable.

'It will not be easy,' he said at last.

'Papa, you know everyone who matters in Laos and in Viet Nam. You must be able to do something.'

He rested his great hands on her shoulders. 'Is he really so important to you?' he whispered.

She placed her hands on top of his. 'Please, Papa. Do this for me.'

A long silence, a sigh of regret and weary acceptance. 'I do not like this man, Noelle. I have told you before, I think you have chosen poorly. He is going to break your heart.' When she did not reply, he added. 'But it is your life. Next week I go to Saigon. I will see what I can do.'

'Thank you, Papa,' whispered Noelle. She kissed him tenderly on the cheek.

'See, it is settled. Now come and have an apéritif with your papa.'

'I'm not in the mood. I just want to be alone.'

'You will be down for dinner?'

'I don't think so.' She went out, closing the door gently behind her.

Bonaventure stared after her. Baptiste Crocé, you must have the wiles of the devil to bewitch my daughter this way! But it hasn't done you any good, has it? I wonder what a few years in a Vietnamese prison will do for your looks and your charm?

Saigon

A week later Rocco Bonaventure was once again enjoying a vermouth cassis on the terrace of the Continental Hotel with Lieutenant Colonel Tran van Li of the Military Security Service. A woven bamboo canopy protected them from the torrential monsoon. The drains were overflowing in the Tu Do and the tyres of the Renault and Peugeot taxis ploughed furrows through the water.

'What happened to that pilot I told you about, Li?' asked Bonaventure. 'What was his name ... Crocé?'

'His case has not yet come before the courts. But opium smuggling is a very serious offence in Vietnam.'

'How long will he get?'

Li raised the cognac to his lips and considered. 'Two years. Maybe even five.'

'Try and make it five,' said Bonaventure, and then the conversation turned to other matters.

9

Hong Kong, October 1960

The blue and white globe of Pan Am Airlines glittered in the late-afternoon sun as the Boeing 707 swooped down towards Kai Tak. The rumble of the Rolls-Royce engines shook the grimy cocklofts and airless workshops in Mongkok just two hundred feet below, where immigrant Chinese hunched over their benches assembling cheap transistors and artificial flowers. Cocooned inside the thin metal skin of the modern jet airliner, the pampered air travellers could not smell their sweat or imagine their misery.

Just one of the passengers in the airliner's first-class compartment understood a little about it. Sammy Chen had been born in Dao Yung in the Swatow province of China. His father had made a living as a street hawker, his mother as a charwoman. Alone among the men and women on the flight that afternoon, he had experienced the crushing humiliation of poverty. Dao Yung was over forty years ago but he could still sometimes smell the open sewers and taste the sticky rice that had nothing to flavour it except a few roots and some pieces of cabbage.

It was the triad who saved him from that life. His half-brother ran errands for the Fei Lung, and when he was fourteen he had encouraged Sammy to join him. They were both hired as look-see boys at an opium den.

When Sammy's family emigrated to Vietnam in 1938, Sammy had quickly identified himself to the local hong of the Fei Lung, and his quick brain had helped him rise quickly through the ranks. For the last five years he had run the Cholon chapter

56

of the Fei Lung, and now his personal wealth was close to half a million dollars.

Not that any of Sammy Chen's fellow travellers would have identified him as a man of great means. The black western-style suit he wore was shiny from wear, and the white open-necked shirt was not of exceptional quality. You could find one for a handful of coins in any street market in any city in Asia.

Sammy Chen considered it unwise to flaunt his wealth.

He looked out of the window, saw the tiny landing strips of Kai Tak, like two chopsticks in the folds of the Kowloon Hills. He caught a glimpse of the press of sampans and junks in the harbour, and allowed himself a moment of private satisfaction. Down there was the key to his fortune. The trail that started in the mountains of Northern Laos ended here among the maze of islands off Hong Kong, where chiu chao fishermen smuggled Sammy's opium to his triad connections in Aberdeen and Mongkok. From there it was transported to the opium divans or cooked into a low-grade heroin in the factories of Kowloon.

It was a simple import and export business, and for years the trade had been a thriving but unspectacular part of the family interests. But two separate developments had changed that. First, Sammy's brother had become Incense Master and deputy chief of the Fei Lung in Hong Kong. And then President Diem had abandoned his stance on opium, making transportation easier and more profitable. The trade was suddenly ripe for development.

Sammy Chen's only concern was the increasing instability in Laos, source of his opium supplies. If the communists should take over, his business might be threatened. But if the Americans kept them out, even for just a few more years, Sammy Chen and the Fei Lung would make a fortune.

All they needed was a little joss.

The Boeing dropped alarmingly over the city, then the engines roared once more as the pilot groped for the concrete apron. The road crossed near the end of the runway and Sammy Chen saw coolies, backs bent under their loads, risk their lives to duck under the red and white striped barriers and race the aircraft across the tarmac as it taxi-ed to the terminal.

They could not wait for it to pass, even for a few seconds. There was a living to be made. Every minute was precious. Nothing else mattered.

It was a philosophy he understood well.

But although Sammy Chen did not know it, his destiny was not in the hands of a few Pathet Lao rebels in the hills of northern Laos. His nemesis was actually struggling for his life in the cold waters of Mirs Bay, just a few miles to the north.

At the narrowest point of the bay, the People's Republic of China is just fourteen hundred metres from the New Territories of Hong Kong, north of Starling Inlet, and Ho Kuan-ling was confident of his ability to swim far greater distances than that. But when he had originally planned his escape, he had not counted on the strength of the current that day. Freedom was not as close as he had imagined.

He had set off just before sunset; but the current carried him away from the far shore, and as night fell he was still struggling in the water, short of his goal. He drifted south of Robinson Island into Crooked Harbour, almost four and a half kilometres from where he had set off. He was a strong swimmer, but cold and fatigue began to sap his reserves. He had never considered failure, it had never occurred to him that he might die...

Now, for the first time, he began to feel real fear.

Several times he passed tantalisingly close to land. But each time he thought he was within a few hundred yards of the beach, the currents swept him on and the green headlands disappeared into the gathering gloom of evening.

By now there was no direction to his strokes. It was all he could do to keep his head above the water. His leg and arm muscles were starting to cramp. He searched the night in desperation but there were very few lights, and those he could see were so far away they might just as well have been the stars in the velvet dark above him.

But he would not submit.

He tried floating on his back, conserving his strength for one last effort. He began to pray to Kuan Yi, Goddess of Mercy, Goddess of the Sea. Save me, he promised. Save me and I will burn a thousand incense in your honour. I will build a whole temple...

Just save me ...

Then he heard it: the low rumble of boat engines, carrying to him on the stillness of the night. The sound grew louder, rising and falling like the rhythm of cicadas in a forest. Where was it coming from? So hard to identify the direction at night. He flapped at the water, trying to bring his body above the white-caps, searching the darkness.

He did not see the fin in the water, heard only a splash close by as the great fish made its first pass. He felt a moment's panic. What was it?

Had he just imagined it?

He could see the red and green navigation lights on the cross trees of a motor launch, perhaps no more than two hundred yards away.

I'm not going to die, he thought. Tonight I am lucky.

He sensed something flash by him in the water, very close.

He slapped desperately at the water and perhaps it was his frantic thrashing that finally gave the fish the confidence to attack.

There was no pain, just a sickening blow to his left leg and then he was being dragged below the surface.

It was a small one, no more than five feet, a hammerhead. A larger one would have taken his whole leg. Instead it shook him like a dog with a bone.

He had no idea what was happening to him. Choking, he scrabbled desperately at the thing that held his leg, trying to tear himself free. The fish tore a chunk of meat from his thigh and veered away with its prize. He bobbed back to the surface like a cork.

It was his shrill scream of panic and horror that attracted the attention of the duty watch on *Police 48*.

Sergeant David Tarrant was one of three white officers aboard the police launch 48 that evening. Their work involved the random interception of junks and sampans, to search for contraband. The chances of coming across a lone swimmer at night were remote, but the launch passed within less than twenty yards of Ho and his screams carried clearly to Tarrant on the bridge. He ordered the patrol boat about immediately and within minutes the searchlight had picked him out in the water.

Three Chinese crewmen used a gaff to pull the exhausted man aboard. Ho Kuan-ling was shaking from hypothermia and shock and there was a dark and jagged tear in his trousers at the level of his left thigh muscle. Watery blood poured on to the deck. The ship's medical orderly covered him with a blanket and put dressings on his leg to staunch the flow.

'Another poor bastard trying to get away from Mao's utopia,' Tarrant muttered.

Tarrant's commanding officer had emerged from below decks. 'Will he live?' he said.

'Looks like the sharks have been having a go at the poor bleeder. I doubt it.'

Police 48 turned about and headed for Northern Division base at Tai Po Kau. Tarrant radioed ahead for a helicopter to take Ho to Kowloon. Perhaps, if they were quick, he might make it.

10

Vientiane, December 1960

It was Noelle's father who inadvertently presented her with the means of obtaining Crocé's release.

It was the day of her twenty-first birthday, and the scene was Bonaventure's traditional nativity celebrations. She had been born on Christmas Day, 1939 – hence the name Noelle – and every year Bonaventure invited *le tout Vientiane* to his home, an occasion that had become one of the city's grandest social gatherings. As Noelle looked around the lawns, she recognised some of the most important politicians: King Savang Vatthana, his huge frame draped with the uniform of Commander in Chief of the Army, looking more like an admiral from a comic opera; General Ouane Rattakone, resplendent in his white uniform, emblazoned with so many decorations Noelle feared that he might topple over on to his face; the Prime Minister, Phoui Sananikone; and General Phoumi Nosovan, an American in a seersucker suit clinging to his heels like a bird-dog. Rumour was that Nosovan was the CIA's man in Laos.

Ever since the Pathet Lao had won the 1958 elections, the Americans, with their crew-cuts and Bonds Brothers suits, had been very much in evidence in Vientiane. You could see their money and influence everywhere. They had introduced the first telephone book, and replaced the colourful and beautifully lithographed French banknotes with their own drably functional little bills.

Noelle despised them.

Her father's attitude to the Americans surprised her. Privately, he too was scornful of their arrogance and their naïvety in Asian affairs; but publicly he courted them, nodding his head sagely at their opinions, lauding their anti-communist crusades.

Just business, he told her whenever they were alone.

A red silk pavilion had been erected on the lawn, with food laid out for the guests in hand-wrought silver bowls. There was chicken cooked in coconut milk with fennel, cinnamon and mint, and diced raw fish marinated in lemon juice and herbs; for the Lao guests there were delicacies such as pig's feet, bat's wings, buffalo steaks, and *lao*, a strong white spirit distilled from rice.

Many of the French guests had taken shelter from the heat inside the pavilion; diplomats and their wives from the French Embassy mingling with members of the Corsican *milieu* from Bangkok and Saigon who had flown in especially for the occasion. Marcel Rivelini was deep in conversation with a woman Noelle recognised as a relative of Rattakone's. When he saw Noelle he excused himself and came over.

He kissed her hand in greeting. *'Bon Noël, belle Noelle.'*

She had heard that joke more times than she could count. 'Thank you, Marcel.'

'Your father spares no expense.'

Noelle forced a polite smile. She still suspected it was Rivelini who had told her papa about Baptiste Crocé.

'I hope you liked your present?' he said.

Noelle remembered. Some trinket of jade. 'I cried over it,' she said, and looked around the pavilion, searching for an escape.

'Perhaps I might see you during this visit. If you are not too busy.'

He's not easily put off, thought Noelle. 'Perhaps.'

She was about to move away.

'How is your friend? The one with the car. Is he still a guest of the Vietnamese?'

'I think you know the answer to that, Marcel.'

'It was very bad luck. But then, no man is above the law.'

'Whose law, Marcel?'

Rivelini smiled at that, and confirmed her suspicions. You could not go against the *milieu*. That had been Baptiste's real crime.

'You know your trouble, Marcel?'

Rivelini gave her a mocking smile. 'Tell me.'
'You were born.'

Rocco Bonaventure watched the celebrations from his study window. A week ago, such a gathering would have been unthinkable. Back in August, a captain in the paratroopers, a man named Kong Le, had staged a coup, citing corruption as his reason. Phoumi had fled to Savannakhet with his American advisers. His army was still deployed against the Pathet Lao in the north, and he had not been able to move against Kong Le until late-November. It was only a week ago that government troops had finally retaken Vientiane, after three days of street fighting.

It's not over yet, Bonaventure decided. While Phoumi's officers celebrated their great military prowess in the brothels, Kong Le was making an orderly retreat north, with all the trucks and artillery he had captured in the coup, as well as the supplies the Russians had flown in to him over the last four months. The Americans still expected him to take Route 13 towards the ancient royal capital of Luang Prabang. But what if he took Route 7 and headed north to the Plain of Jars? If he captured the air strip at Phong Savan, opium supplies would be cut off, just when there was a real opportunity to expand the business through Saigon.

Communists! May they all rot in hell.

Noelle's entrance distracted him from his brooding. She looked glorious, a breathtaking melding of East and West; she wore a silk blouse of rich blue, a broad silver belt, and dark *sin* bordered with three or four inches of gold or silver trim, picked out with scarlet and blue. There was an ivory Buddha at her neck, and her hair hung in a long braid down her back. She had that poise and hint of arrogance that all beautiful women possess. Sometimes when he looked at her, all he saw was her mother. And what a bitch she could be when she set her mind to it!

But he understood why Rivelini wanted her so badly; he and every other eligible Frenchman in Vientiane, bachelor or not. Another problem to be solved.

'You wanted to see me, Papa?'

63

'Come in,' he said, and gave her his most indulgent smile. 'Are you enjoying your party?'

'But of course,' she said, in such a way that he understood she was hating every minute of it. Sometimes she was so damned difficult to please.

She had changed somehow. Ever since she had met that man Crocé. She was always pleasant, but also somehow vague, as if her mind was somewhere else. She showed no interest in any of the distractions he arranged for her. All right, he understood how she felt about Rivelini. Perhaps he was too old for her. But he had introduced her to a number of suitable young diplomats from the embassy, as well as some well-connected young Corsicans from the *milieu* in Saigon; and while she had not actually been rude, she had treated them with a casual indifference that must have lacerated their budding egos.

Surely she was not still carrying a torch for Monsieur Crocé?

But he did not regret anything. Why should he? Everything he had done, he had done for her own good. She was young and impetuous. Someone had to save her from herself.

'I want to give you something.' he said.

'Not advice, I hope,' she murmured.

'Good God, no.'

A hint of a smile.

He unlocked the drawer of the lacquered bureau and took out a long, black box. He came around the desk, kissed her lightly on the cheek and handed it to her.

'Happy birthday, Noelle.'

She took the box and opened it. A necklace nestled on a bed of soft purple velvet. It was eighteen-carat gold, set with diamonds. The centrepiece was a huge Burmese ruby, pigeon-blood red, cabochon-cut. It was breathtaking.

She took it out of the box and held it in her fingers. Heavy and very, very expensive. 'Oh, Papa, it's beautiful.'

'I'm glad you like it,' he whispered. He held it to her neck, and fastened the clasp. Then he turned her to face the gilt mirror on the wall.

'It must be worth a fortune.'

'A small one, I suppose. But you are worth it. I wanted to give you something special.'

64

'I don't know what to say,' Noelle murmured.

'You don't have to say anything. You know I love you, don't you? Sometimes I know you think I am just a blustering old bully, but I only ever want the best for you.'

She put her hand against his cheek. 'You know I love you too. Despite everything.'

He had seen the caveat on its way. Despite everything? Did she still blame him then, for this business with Crocé? 'We had better go back out and rejoin our guests,' he said.

But the day was ruined for him. *Despite everything*. Damn this Crocé. Perhaps he should have had Li put him against a wall and shoot him.

11

Jean-Marie Pepin thought he knew why Noelle had asked to meet him at The Settha Palace on New Year's Eve, but still held on to a slim hope that the conversation might not revolve solely around Baptiste Crocé. But he was prepared to be disappointed.

Rocco Bonaventure's daughter was achingly beautiful. In the five minutes since they had sat down to dinner he had made love to her in his mind a score of times, though they had discussed nothing more erotic than politics and the weather. He reminded himself of his own advice to Crocé: This girl is bad news.

No wonder Baptiste had told him to go to hell. He would have done the same.

Jean-Marie tried to concentrate on the menu.

Settha Palace:
New Year's Eve, 1960

*

Cold consommé with port

*

Rabbit roasted with prunes
Asparagus vinaigrette
Goose with truffles
Endive salad

*

Camembert
Custard in liqueur
Coffee

The dining room had the weary atmosphere of a civil service canteen when all the supervisors were away on holiday. There was a scattering of foreign journalists who were already in the sleepy stages of drink, a few diplomats with their bored wives and unhappy children. The waiters moved around the room with the dreamy expressions of postal clerks.

One of them approached the table. He took their menus with a deferential smile. 'So sorry,' he said in French. 'Cannot get.'

'Cannot get?' Jean-Marie echoed. 'What? None of it?'

The waiter shook his head and kept a determined smile.

'Not even the soup?'

'What *do* you have?' Noelle asked.

'Chicken,' the waiter said.

'Then that's what we'll have,' Noelle said to the man with a gracious smile.

There was always the wine. Jean-Marie raised his glass. 'Happy New Year,' he said.

Noelle touched his glass with hers in toast.

'How are things with you, Jean-Marie?'

He shrugged his shoulders. 'I get by.' He was working for Christian Mittard, one of her father's competitors. It was not as rewarding as owning his own plane, but he could still make up to fifteen hundred dollars a month, perhaps more when the government and the Pathet Lao were shooting at each other. How much longer he would have a job he would have to wait and see.

'I know you still blame me for what happened.'

Jean-Marie shook his head. Her lips were wet from the wine. How long could a man really stay angry with you? he asked himself. 'Baptiste knew the risks. We all know the risks.'

'But it was because of me that you lost your aeroplane.'

'That's life.' Jean-Marie began to feel a little ill, as he always did in the company of a woman he wanted so utterly and suspected was beyond him. 'But while we're on the subject, does your father know you're here with me tonight?'

She shook her head. 'He had to go to Phong Savan. He said it was urgent.'

Jean-Marie understood. Kong Le's Army had entered the Plain of Jars. All the Corsican airlines were trying to evacuate their planes and their stocks of opium from Phong Savan while there was still time.

'Why did you want to see me? It's about Baptiste, isn't it?' She nodded.

Oh, well, he thought. No point in fooling myself. 'Have you heard from him?'

'He writes me letters,' said Noelle. 'He's going through hell.'

Without women, without cognac, without a guaranteed supply of cigarettes ... yes, I suppose he is, thought Jean-Marie. 'I have a friend in Saigon. He smuggles in cigarettes and money occasionally. He'll be all right. You intend to wait for him?'

Noelle shook her head and for just a moment Jean-Marie felt a surge of hope. 'I want to get him out,' she said.

Jean-Marie shook his head. 'Impossible.'

'I don't think so, Jean-Marie. Not if you'll help me.'

Careful. You need this lady's help like Laos needs more communists. 'Help you? How?'

'Will you fly me to Saigon? I'll pay you, of course.'

Jean-Marie frowned. 'Why don't you go on one of your father's planes? He has his own airline, remember? It won't cost you anything.'

'I don't want him to know.'

Jean-Marie hesitated. Mittard would not object to a paying passenger, if the price was right. He did not have to know her identity. And he wanted to help Baptiste.

But a man does not easily cross Rocco Bonaventure, he reminded himself. 'I'll have to think about this.'

'Sure. I'll give you till the chicken arrives. That would be appropriate.'

Jean-Marie felt himself flush. The little bitch! 'How are you going to get him out?' he hissed.

'Perhaps it's better you don't know. Just get me to Saigon, Jean-Marie. Then I'll make up for everything I've done.'

He gave his assent, an almost imperceptible nod of the head. The chicken arrived soon after but he found he had lost all appetite, and the wine tasted sour and acid in his mouth. A formidable young woman, Noelle. Perhaps Baptiste Crocé had met his match after all.

He drank to the New Year without his customary enthusiasm and was at home in bed by eleven. He had an early flight in the morning.

12

Saigon

Noelle had not been back to Saigon since the French defeat in
1955. She remembered it as a city of bicycles. It had changed
utterly in the five years that the Americans had been there.
Now it was a city of Vespas and Lambrettas; of crew-cut,
red-faced men in bright Hawaiian shirts; of huge, finned
Chevrolets with red, white and blue stickers on the chrome
bumpers showing an American and Vietnamese handshake.
What had not changed was the barbed wire around the US
Embassy, the sandbagged machine guns outside the Doc Lap
palace and the tanks in the streets.

They met in the Vieux Moulin. There was a bridge beside
the restaurant and after sunset diners ate there knowing that
the far, dark bank was a rustling nest of Viet Minh guerillas.
There was iron mesh on all the windows to keep out grenades
and the windows were unglazed so diners would not be
lacerated by flying glass in the event of an attack. To eat
at the Vieux Moulin was to sample the rich, sensual flavours
of Burgundian cooking and fear.

The restaurant was redolent with the aromas of roasting
capons and melting butter. Colonel Tran van Li was already
waiting, at a table overlooking the coffee-coloured river. He
ordered a pastis for her, a cognac and soda for himself. He chose
her lunch from the menu for her – Chapon Duc Charles.

And then he settled back to decide how best to deal with
her.

So this was Rocco Bonaventure's daughter.

Li was impressed. She was everything he had anticipated:

statuesque, elegantly dressed, exquisite as fine porcelain. There was no plumpness about her, the thing he detested about most Western women. She had all the svelte qualities of an Asian, but with the wonderful roundness of her eyes and paleness of skin that made her a delectable prize.

This should be a very interesting afternoon.

'Your father did not tell me you were coming to Saigon,' Li said. 'I would have prepared a more formal welcome.'

'My father does not know I'm here. Nor do I wish him to know.'

Li digested this information. He took a packet of Lucky Strike cigarettes off the table. 'Do you smoke?'

Noelle shook her head.

'This is a great surprise. But I am most honoured that you should have thought to contact me. I am a great friend of your father's, as you probably know.'

'Of course.'

She was watching him steadily. He had the uncomfortable feeling that he, too, was being assessed. 'What can I do for you, Mademoiselle Bonaventure?'

'I want your help, Mister Li.'

'As a friend and business associate of your father's, I will do all within my power, of course.'

'This has nothing to do with your relationship with my father.'

Li allowed himself a moment's reflection. He wondered what it was the girl had to trade, if she had not come at her father's request. He leaned forward and allowed his eyes to drop insolently to her body. He exhaled a long stream of cigarette smoke and smiled. 'Perhaps you had better tell me what you want.'

'It's about a man called Baptiste Crocé.'

'I've never heard of him.'

'He's a pilot. Last year, before the monsoon, he was arrested by your men at Ban Me Thuot and his plane was impounded.'

'He had broken the laws of the Republic of Viet Nam?'

'He had a certain amount of opium on board his plane.'

Li shook his head. 'Very bad. A great evil in our country, Mademoiselle Bonaventure. A great evil.'

'He was sentenced to five years' imprisonment.'

Li made no comment.

'I want to know what I can do to get him released.'

The Colonel drew on his cigarette. He raised an eyebrow. 'And you say this request is not from your father?'

'It's from me.'

Li shook his head. 'Impossible.'

Noelle reached into her purse and withdrew the black box her father had given her. She opened it. Li stared at the ruby, glinting in the nest of velvet like an ember in a slow fire. He picked up the necklace with the fingers of his right hand, felt its weight.

'Nothing is impossible, Colonel Li.'

'You're serious?'

'I would not want to waste your time. I realise you are a busy man.'

Li's manner changed. He realised he had underestimated this girl. She had a great deal more to bargain with than he had imagined. 'This is a very unusual situation,' he said.

'Unusual?'

'I believe your father does not like this man very much.'

'Then you recall him a little better now?'

'Perhaps.' He replaced the necklace in the velvet-lined box. It snapped shut between her fingers.

'What did my father tell you to do, Colonel?'

'Your father is a citizen of another country. He has no influence on the internal affairs of the Republic of Viet Nam.'

'Of course he has.'

The drinks arrived. Li raised his glass in toast but Noelle ignored him. 'I am not at liberty to discuss my conversations with your father. Even with you.'

'All right then, I'll ask a much simpler question. What do you want in return for the release of Baptiste Croce?'

Again Li picked up the black case and opened it. He could not even begin to guess how much the necklace was worth, but it would be a considerable amount. Was it enough to risk losing the friendship of Rocco Bonaventure?

'If you should find a way to release Baptiste, I would be happy to present you with this gift as a token of my appreciation. For your wife perhaps.'

72

Li slammed the lid shut and pushed the case away from him. 'It's not enough.'

Noelle bit her lip. 'Then how much do you want?'

'It might perhaps serve as a down payment, a token of your appreciation. But I am already a rich man. What would I want with more jewellery?'

'What are you saying?'

Li shrugged and again allowed his eyes to travel over her body. 'There are still some things that interest me.'

Noelle felt suddenly cold in the stifling heat of the afternoon. 'Such as?'

He leaned towards her and she could smell on his breath the taint of tobacco and cognac and betel nut. 'How badly do you want to see this man again, Mademoiselle Bonaventure?'

Noelle felt as if a snake had slithered across her skin. She took a deep breath. She thought about Baptiste, rotting away in a tropical prison. 'Tell me what you want,' she said.

The light was diffused through the bamboo blinds, slivers of hot yellow sunlight angled through the dusty wooden slats. The gentle rumble of the overhead fan, the clicking of mah-jong tiles from the next room, the cry of the hawkers from the street outside. The strong taint of incense and anise and ginger.

Noelle hugged her arms to her breasts as if she was cold. She had come this far for a man she hardly knew. What if her father was right? What if Baptiste Crocé was a waster and a drinker and a womaniser?

Worse – what if she were to live the rest of her life without passion? Surely this fear was better than the stultifying boredom I have lived with for the past five years in Vientiane?

To hell with it.

And she would go to hell too, if need be. But she knew what she wanted.

Tran van Li picked up the hard-backed chair next to the ancient armoire and straddled it, resting his arms on the back. He would have liked to have taken her to a better hotel than the Trung Mai. But what could he do? He could not take her home – if she ever found out, his wife would attack him

73

with scissors – and if he had gone to The Continental he would have risked being recognised.

'Take off your clothes,' he said.

He gripped the chair to still the trembling in his limbs. Noelle pulled the dress over her head. Her body was oily slick with sweat, gleaming like burnished bronze. She took off her underwear and stood in front of him, naked. Just a few bands of gold at her wrist and throat, and the Cartier wrist-watch.

His mouth was dry, he couldn't swallow. 'Lie on the bed,' he rasped.

What was it the French believed in? *Liberté, egalité, fraternité.* Liberty, equality, brotherhood. Well, what could be more equal than a well-educated Vietnamese like himself sleeping with a beautiful French girl? That was liberty. That was brotherhood.

He got up and came to sit on the edge of the bed. 'Put your hands above your head,' he said.

Noelle hesitated then obeyed. Li ran his hand over her body, from her shoulder to her thigh. The flesh was firm, he could feel the spring of the muscles, the damp-warm of her perspiration. It was hard to breathe.

He would be gentle, of course. Perhaps she thought he was a generation from the *paddis*. Because he was a policeman, she probably thought he had no sensitivity, no skill. She could not know his father had been a highly respected businessman in Dalat, his mother educated in France. How the world turns.

He took off his clothes and lay down beside Noelle on the bed. Some of his family despised him, but if they could see him now they would realise that public office had far more compensations than they had ever realised.

13

A crowd had gathered around the charred corpse that lay in the middle of the street. The smell of burned flesh hung in the air, a sweet and nauseating stench that wrinkled Baptiste Crocé's nostrils. A journalist was taking pictures. Saffron-robed monks stood to one side, their expressions indecipherable.

'What's going on?' he said.

'A monk barbecue,' Li commented. They drove past.

'Why?'

'The Buddhists are making trouble for President Diem. They are protesting against government policies by setting light to themselves.' Li giggled. 'It is very obliging of them. Why should we get rid of them if they do it for us?'

'They actually set themselves alight?' murmured Baptiste. He could not imagine the kind of courage a man must possess to do such a thing.

'Difficult job being a monk. Burn out very young.' Li giggled again.

They were in the back of a green MSS jeep. It had all happened so quickly. This morning Baptiste had woken as usual in prison, then without warning two guards had dragged him out of the exercise yard and through the gates. For a few terrified minutes he thought they were going to shoot him. Instead they had thrown him in the jeep with the Vietnamese Colonel whom he recognised from the day of his arrest at Ban Me Thuot.

Tran van Li turned his head and hawked into the street. He took a deep lungful of air. 'Very sorry, but I don't know which smells worse. You or that monk.'

'I must excuse myself, Colonel. Normally I bathe in asses' milk, but your boys interrupted my toilet this morning.'

Li prodded him with his swagger stick. 'Sit a little further over that way.'

'May I ask where we're going?'

Li ignored him. 'I hope you have learned your lesson, Monsieur Crocé?'

'I learned next time not to get caught.'

For the first time it occurred to Baptiste that he was going to be released. But why?

They had left Saigon and crossed into Cholon. The streets became narrower, and life moved from the offices and the shophouses out into the streets. The air was ripe with the taint of the sacks of dried fish by the wharves, the streets clamoured with the squawking of ducks in the open air markets and the din of motorcycles and *siclo* bells.

'Where are you taking me?'

Li again pretended not to hear. He pointed to the red, white and blue bumper sticker on the big-finned Cadillac in front of them. 'So many Americans coming here now, Monsieur Crocé. I think I like it better in the old days, when the French are still here. I like their women. You like women, Monsieur Crocé?'

'What do you think I've been thinking about for the last eighteen months?'

Li laughed, a brittle sound like a bark. 'Of course. It must be very hard for a man like you. All you can think about is women.' A Vietnamese woman cycled past them, in a beautiful *ao dai*, a long mauve smock, split to the thigh, over ankle-length diaphanous silk trousers. 'So beautiful, yes? Beauty is a question of balance, isn't it Monsieur Crocé? I can talk to you about this, I know. You are a connoisseur, like me.'

Baptiste watched him, wondering where this might lead.

'Yes, a question of balance. Nothing too big, nothing too small. The eyes, the lips, the nose, the breasts. They say breasts should not be too big, same as rice bowl. Bigger and it is all wasted; smaller and not enough to hold, to weigh in the hand.' A beat, and then: 'Like Noelle. Everything is perfect. In balance.'

Noelle.

'*Petit salaud*,' muttered Baptiste.

Li grinned at him.

76

Noelle had come through for him. She had bought his freedom. And now he knew the trade.

They stopped outside a Chinese hotel. The shabby lobby was open to the street. A man in brown peasant pyjamas came out and hawked into the gutter.

Li reached into the breast pocket of his uniform and handed Baptiste his passport. 'Well, goodbye, Monsieur Crocé.'

'I can go?'

'Of course.' As Baptiste got out, Li leaned forward and whispered, 'She is waiting for you, inside. Room 23. If she is wet, Monsieur Crocé, it is not because she is happy to see you. It is because I have only just got out of her bed!'

Li tapped the driver's seat with his swagger stick and the jeep lurched away into the noonday traffic.

The door was not locked.

As he went in, he saw his own reflection in the cracked mirror of an ancient dressing table. His face was shaded by a dark stubble, and he looked gaunt and desperate. A criminal, a gypsy.

The shades were down and the room was in semi-darkness. There was little furniture; just an armoire and a native wooden platform bed covered with a thick cotton pad.

Then he saw her silhouette by the window, watching him.

'Noelle.'

She came towards him and gently put her arms around him. 'Baptiste.' She looked up at him, and he saw the hurt and injury in her face. 'You're so thin.'

'I'm all right.'

'I thought I'd never see you again.' She reached up and brushed the hair out of his eyes. '*Mon pauvre.*'

He looked down at his clothes. They were encrusted with dirt. 'I need a bath.'

She nodded and led him through to a cool, white-tiled washroom. Pale chinchook lizards chirruped high on the walls. There was a water jar in one corner, almost as high as his waist, with a long-handled dipper resting on its edge.

She unbuttoned his shirt and peeled it off him, then unfastened the cracked leather belt and let the rest of his clothes

77

drop on to the wet, stained tiles. She scooped up some of the cold water with the dipper and poured it over his head. Crocé leaned against the tiles and gasped with pleasure.

Noelle worked soap into a rich lather in her hands and started to soap down his body. She was wearing just a sheer cotton shift. Her hands were warm, and the tiles on his back were cold.

'He has missed me,' she whispered.

'Please,' he murmured. She lathered the soap around his groin, pulling rhythmically down the shaft of his penis. He gasped aloud, every nerve jangling and raw.

He pulled her towards him, tore away the cotton shift, gripped the cheeks of her bottom and lifted her easily. He was panting, like a runner. 'Noelle...'

'Go on,' she whispered.

Hard to breathe, just this uncontrollable, desperate need. His weight pressed her against the wall, and he forced his way inside her. Almost as quickly it was over.

It had been so long that in the final moment there was no sensation, just a sudden, terrible release. Then he felt her trembling, her arms curled around his neck. She was crying.

'It's all right,' he whispered.

'Baptiste, I would do anything for you.'

Well, you have proved that already, he thought. For the first time in his life Baptiste Crocé wondered if it was possible for him to love someone besides himself.

They lay on the bed, their limbs intertwined. Her head was on his chest, her fingers entwined in the short, dark hair, listening to the pounding rhythms of his heart. Should I feel ashamed or smug? she wondered. She had run away from her father, bought her lover out of prison, had two men in one day. She felt reckless and terrified, a whore and a saint.

'Did they hurt you?' she whispered.

He reached for the Gitanes beside the bed and lit one. 'I couldn't smoke a cigarette whenever I wanted to. Wasn't that torture enough?'

'You're thinner.'

'All they ever fed us was rice, and now and then they slopped some sort of meat on top. Funnily enough it was always the day after one of the inmates died.'

She thought he was serious but when she looked up he was grinning at her. She slapped him. 'Don't joke about it.'

'Why not? Everything's funny once it's over.'

She wondered if he knew about her bargain with Colonel Li. That was over, and it still wasn't funny. 'Don't you want to know how I got you out?'

'Li said you bribed him.'

She tried to read the expression on his face. 'Yes, a bribe,' she said.

'It's almost as if you missed me.'

'I dreamed about you every night for the last seventeen months.'

'I never thought about you once,' he said. She hit him and he laughed. She raised her hand to slap him again and he caught her wrist. He rolled on top of her. She struggled for a moment, but then her struggles became sinuous and her laughter earthier, her breathing ragged.

It had been too long and there was so much time to make up. At that moment Noelle did not think there would be enough time in the rest of her life to drink her fill of him.

14

Late evening, the hour of the apéritif. Kerosene lamps glowed from the hawker's stalls in the side streets. On the Tu Do, the East and the West met without touching; a noodle seller fanned a charcoal stove at the roadside, surrounded by his Vietnamese customers, while behind him, sprawled on bentwood chairs in front of the cafés, Corsicans of the *milieu* drank pastis and played dice, and laughing American engineers drank cognac and sodas.

The bells in the basilica summoned the faithful to Mass.

Noelle and Crocé found a table at the Café Verlain and ordered Pernod. He lit a Gitane.

'You smoke too much, Baptiste.'

'I can't help it. I'm addicted. Like I'm addicted to you.' He grinned and kissed her softly on the neck. Two Americans in loud shirts looked over and their faces were hard with envy.

'Don't make love to me no more, Baptiste,' she whispered. 'I can't keep up with you.'

He slouched in his chair, saw the Americans watching. He winked at them, and they turned away, scowling.

So handsome, Noelle thought. Devastating. A smile that could melt butter, eyes like a gypsy, a face like the devil. She could hear her father's voice: *I hope you know what you're doing, Noelle.*

She could not believe that they had only been together again for eight hours. It could have been a lifetime. They had made love all afternoon; then, while he slept, she had left the hotel to buy him new clothes from the Indian tailor on the street corner – a white linen suit, a navy blue silk shirt, and a broad black leather belt.

A few hours before he had looked as hollow as a shadow, but already the arrogance and shout at the devil set of the shoulders had returned.

A white-jacketed waiter brought the Pernod. Crocé tipped him outrageously. Why not? Noelle thought. It's not his money. It's my father's.

'What are you going to do, Baptiste?'

'I am going to make this day last for ever. I never want the spell to end.'

'But it will. Tomorrow is tomorrow.'

He shrugged his shoulders.

'You don't have to stay with me. I didn't pay for your freedom to make you feel as if I had trapped you.'

'Don't talk crazy. I want to spend the rest of my life making love to you.' He grinned again and ran the tip of a finger lightly along her bare shoulder. She shuddered. There was gooseflesh all along her arms.

'Stop it.'

'Never.'

'I'm serious, Baptiste. I don't have much money left. We can't stay here for ever. I have to know what you want to do.'

He looked sulky. She had reminded him about reality. 'I want my own airline again.'

'Airline? One Cessna and a bag of spanners?'

He frowned at her. 'It's a living.'

'You can't be a pilot for ever.'

'Why not?'

'And spend the rest of your life chasing clouds?'

It was the first time she had ever seen him uncomfortable. 'I'll do what I damned well like,' he muttered.

'No, Baptiste. You just spent the last eighteen months in prison. While you were there, Papa did what *he* damned well liked!'

He concentrated on his Pernod and cigarette. 'So what are you suggesting?'

'I don't know. But we can't run away for ever.' The moon rose over the tamarinds, floating against wisps of white cloud. 'He needs a man like you, Baptiste, he just doesn't know it

81

yet. When you have my papa behind you, then you can really do what you damned please.'

'He'll never be behind me. Right now I hate him so much it makes my teeth ache.'

'But if we run, he'll find us.'

Baptiste stubbed out his cigarette viciously. 'I don't want to talk about this,' he said. 'Tonight we celebrate. Tonight there is just me and you. Tomorrow I will fight the world.'

She took his hand. 'All right. But please don't underestimate my father. Tomorrow may be closer than we think.'

It was a dimly lit room, no more than three paces wide and five paces deep. There was just one window, with a shabby curtain drawn across. The only light the eerie glow of the opium lamps.

The air was pungent with opium smoke.

There was a row of bunks, like a school dormitory. Two middle-aged Chinese were squatting on one of the wooden platforms doing business, sipping tea, their pipes laid to one side. On another, a gaunt Chinese, bare to the waist, lay with his head on the wooden head-rest, his sunken eyes glazed with the effects of the drug. A naked Chinese girl lay beside him, her arms around him. He ignored her, speared a small ball of opium and held it over the flame of a spirit lamp. When it was on fire he jammed it into the bowl of his pipe and held it over the lamp. As the opium cooked, he inhaled the sweet smoke.

It had been Baptiste's idea to come here. Noelle had never been in an opium den, and she was curious. As always, it had been Baptiste who had brought the fantasy to life for her.

'Come on,' he said.

Noelle held back. 'I'm not sure.'

'You have to try some, even if it's only once in your life. With opium you stand at the gates of heaven and peer through. The chiu chao have a saying: "If god made anything better than opium, he kept it to himself." '

She allowed him to lead her to one of the platforms.

The Chinese proprietor prepared the pipes for them. He brought a small packet containing the treacle-like opium, scraped off a small portion and put it over the end of a needle, then held the needle over the flame of a spirit lamp. Noelle lay down, Baptiste on the wooden platform beside her. He smiled reassurance.

She examined the opium pipe; it was a bamboo rod, just over a foot long, with a bowl set a few inches from the end. The bowl was round like a ball, with a small hole in the top. Opium! After all she had done, defying her father, trading her body, giving herself to Baptiste, opium was the last taboo to be thrown aside. This was an Eastern sin. She was spinning off the edge of the world now.

The two businessmen had returned to their pipes, their business done; the other Chinese had dropped his pipe and was lost to his morphiate dreams. The girl was going through the pockets of his trousers.

There was silence except for the gurgling of the opium pipes.

The pellet was bubbling on the end of the needle. With practised skill, the Chinese proprietor rolled the pellet into the aperture of the pipe bowl.

'Suck it deep into your lungs,' whispered Baptiste. 'Hold your breath as long as you can.' The first time she tried, she choked on the smoke. He was grinning. 'Don't breathe in quite so hard until you are used to it.'

Noelle tried again. The black bead of opium bubbled gently. The blue-grey smoke drifted towards the ceiling.

Noelle did not remember how they got back to the hotel. After a half dozen puffs of the pipe, the pellet was gone. She remembered she had been disappointed; it had had no effect on her. She had three or four pipes, and was aware of nothing more dramatic than a growing sense of calm, a warm glow that sloughed away her terrors. The whole world became a wonderful place and her worries evaporated. She wished her father had been there, she would have told him how much she loved him. She knew now that everything was going to be all right. She even felt a growing affection for two Chinese businessmen in their undershirts. They were her friends, companions on a wonderful night-time journey.

When they got back to the hotel she let Baptiste undress

her. When he lay on top of her his skin felt like damp velvet. Every sensation was exaggerated, every little pleasure almost unbearable. They were spinning through space, a vortex of light and exquisite sensation, swollen blue veins pounding like drumbeats, sweat smooth as warm oil, her nipples engorged, hair triggers to a vortex of light and colour, the small hairs on her arms sparkling like static, skin as tender as a bruise. She fell into a red gelatin world of erotic fantasy, and when he ejaculated inside her it was like hot waves of molten lava in her belly, and when the eruption subsided she was carried over the edge of the world into a black vortex, without dreams.

15

When Noelle woke her head felt wonderfully light. She was surprised to find there was no hangover. The sounds that filtered through the shuttered windows – the cries of the hawkers, the clamour of car horns and bicycle bells, the thump of electrical generators – were of crystal clarity. Baptiste was asleep. She kissed his shoulder and slid naked out of the bed.

The room was airless and hot. She went to the washroom and poured the cold water over her head with the long-handled dipper. She felt the stickiness between her legs and the memories of the previous night that rushed over her were poignant with sweetness and guilt.

She brushed out her wet hair and dressed in a thin blue gingham frock before going downstairs to fetch their breakfast. Some chicken congee from the toothless old hawker outside, or perhaps some fresh fruit, melon and papaya and some sweet, plump bananas...

The street was a riot of noise, the sing-song shouts of the chiu chao and the bleat of a horn as an olive drab ARVN truck tried to barge its way past a snarl of siclos. A barber was at work in the centre of the boulevard. The broken mirror he had nailed to the trunk of a plane tree caught the morning sun and hurt her eyes. An old Tonkinese in a mollusc hat pushed past her, two baskets of ducklings slung on a pole over her shoulder.

Noelle did not pay any attention to the black Mercedes parked at the kerb a few yards away. Suddenly two Europeans in dark suits were beside her, their hands gripping her elbows so tightly she cried out in surprise and pain. They propelled her towards the limousine and bundled her inside.

Rocco Bonaventure was reading a French language edition

of *L'Indochine*. He looked up and smiled at his daughter, as he did every morning at breakfast time. 'Good morning, Noelle. I have been looking everywhere for you.'

The thin wooden door crashed open, snapping one of the hinges. One of the men grabbed Baptiste and threw him naked on to the floor. Baptiste woke from his drugged sleep to see a huge Corsican standing over him. His shoes were of expensive black leather. One of them swung into his stomach.

He doubled over, gasping for breath. The other Corsican grabbed a handful of his hair, lifted his head from the floor, and smashed his fist into his face.

After that, he was only semi-conscious and remembered little about the beating. One of the men pinned his arms behind his back and braced him against the wall. The other one took his time, picking the targets for his blows with elaborate care. Baptiste could not remember if he had cried out during the process. He hoped not, but he could not remember.

It seemed to go on for ever, but he supposed it must only have been a minute or two or he would have been dead. Finally they let him drop to the floor.

He did not know how long he was unconscious. Perhaps seconds, perhaps hours. He came to in a pool of dark blood.

He dragged himself to his knees and retched painfully. He looked around. The door was still yawning open, on its broken hinge. No one had even bothered to come and stare.

He crawled to the washroom, and examined his reflection in the broken mirror. No one that he recognised; eyes almost closed, nose a pulpy mess. No gaps in his mouth, although several of his teeth were loose.

He forced himself to urinate. No blood, thank God.

He splashed water on to his face. His ribs made it an agony to breathe. He slid down the wall to the floor, brought his knees up to his chest to try and ease the pain.

Everything hurt. He was going to be sick again.

He knew what had happened, of course. He had not expected Bonaventure to find them so quickly. But if he thought that one beating ended it, he had misjudged his man very badly.

16

Vientiane

The loudspeakers were grinding out music for the *boun*, the religious festival that every *wat* held at least once a year. The *wats* were not just temples, they were also schools and community and cultural centres, and the festivals, which ran day and night, were a means of raising funds. There were so many temples in Vientiane that it seemed to Noelle there was a boun in progress every day during the dry season. If you lived next door it was impossible to sleep for the crashing of cymbals and the wailing of flutes.

She moved among the crowds, edgy, alert. It was her *boyesse* who had brought her the message. A man had approached her in the market, said the maid, and asked her to give Noelle a note. She had read it quickly, before burning it over a candle. It had said, simply: *Wat Si Saket.* 1800.

She recognised Baptiste's handwriting.

Her father would not suspect. Not here.

Groups of villagers danced around the *sim* to the clamour of flutes and drums and cymbals, carrying the decorated money trees they had brought from their villages as an offering to the temple. They clapped and sang in time with the music while the bonzes watched, chattering and laughing like women at a water hole.

The Laos were in their festival clothes, the men in their white jackets and *sampots*, baggy knee-length trousers of iridescent silk; the women in traditional *sins*, with wide bands of intricately woven silver and gold trim around the hems.

She anxiously searched the faces for him.

Where was he?

He appeared suddenly at her side, moving from the shadows to take her arm. 'This way,' he whispered.

He pulled her into the cloister. Thousands of Buddhas in stone, silver and bronze filled the niches and shelves along the walls, offerings of bright yellow and crimson paper flowers garlanded at their feet.

'Baptiste,' she murmured.

She turned to look into his face.

It was a mess. One eye swollen shut, his lips cracked, still weeping watery blood. She threw her arms around him and he gasped and pushed her away. 'I'm sorry. My ribs are a little sore.' A swollen, crooked grin.

Noelle could not find the words. Her father had done this.

He seemed to read her mind. 'I'm all right,' he said.

She was too shocked to speak for a long time. She touched his face gently with her fingertips.

'It looks worse than it is,' he said.

She moved closer, more gently. She held him for a long time. 'What are we going to do?' she whispered.

'Come away with me.'

'He'll find us. No matter where we go.'

'Then what's the point?' he hissed. 'I only came here for you! He'll kill me if he finds me in Vientiane! What do you want me to do?'

She shrugged, helplessly.

'Just go then!' he said.

Noelle hesitated. He looked too broken to do what was on her mind. But what other choice was there if she was not to lose him?

'There is another way,' she said.

He fumbled in his shirt pocket for his cigarettes and lit one one-handed, still clutching at his ribs with his left hand. He drew in the smoke but said nothing.

'My father still has six hundred kilos of opium stored in the Snow Leopard Inn in Phong Savan, but because of Kong Le he can't get it. The Pathet Lao and Kong Le's paratroopers have encircled the town. One of Papa's pilots was killed this afternoon. Now the other two are refusing to go back.'

'Kong Le's paratroopers have taken the airfield?'

'Not yet. But to make the approach you have to fly over Kong Le's soldiers and they have anti-aircraft guns. But if someone were brave enough to do it, what kind of reward do you think he might get from my father?'

'*Dis donc!*'

She watched him. 'Six hundred kilos is a lot of opium. My father wants it very badly.'

She saw the play of emotions across his face. *He thinks I have set him up.* 'What kind of idiot do you think I am?'

'I'll come with you, Baptiste! If anything happens to you, I don't want to live anyway.'

She watched his expression soften. 'Your father knows about this? He would let me fly one of his Beechcraft?'

'He would rather put a snake down his trousers than let you near one of his 'planes! Besides, he thinks it is too dangerous also. He has lost one Beechcraft, and does not want to lose another.'

He drew on his cigarette and was about to walk away. Then he came back. 'It's suicide.'

'I have faith in you, Baptiste.'

'Have you ever been in an aeroplane that is being shot at? It is not a very pleasant experience. We could both be killed. Have you thought about that?'

'I feel lucky.'

He shook his head. '*Non, absolument, non! C'est fou!*'

Again, he turned to leave.

'You want to drift around Asia the rest of your life, Baptiste? Do you have any capital?'

'I have my life.'

'And what have you done with that so far?'

For a moment she thought he was going to hit her. Then the fury in his black eyes faded. 'You have no idea what you're asking.'

'I want you, Baptiste. I am prepared to take a risk. Are you?' When he did not answer, she went on: 'This could seal your future. Both our futures.'

'How will I get to Phong Savan. On a bicycle?'

'What about Jean-Marie?'

He shook his head.

'Then you'll have to fly Air Laos.'

'You just said your father would not let me near his aeroplanes.'

'They are not guarded at night.'

'You mean we should steal one?'

'Borrow it.'

Baptiste threw back his head and laughed. The Laos worshipping at the feet of a Buddha turned their heads to stare at the crazy Corsican. 'You would really risk so much? Just to have me?'

'I have done more things in the last week than I ever thought I could. I would not have done anything if I had not met you. You said that night in the temple you would turn my life into a raging storm. I want to keep you to that promise.'

He shook his head.

He was tempted. Why not? If you did not gamble a little in life all you got back at the end was the stake you started with. *Eh, bien*. Danger and women; they were the only things that made life worth living anyway.

'It's suicide,' he said. 'You'll get us both killed. I won't do it. Goodbye, Noelle.'

She was too stunned to follow him, and within moments he was lost in the crowd. She had never thought he might refuse her. A Buddha watched her, inscrutable, through the blue-grey coils of joss smoke. He offered no solace.

17

The sun had not yet risen and the airfield was blanketed in mist, the rice and tapioca fields still shrouded in the monochrome colours of the dawn. Gilbert Pépé arrived at Wattay aerodrome in an ancient jitney. He clambered out with his canvas flight bag over one shoulder, a survey map of Cambodia held in the other. A squadron of ducks took flight suddenly out of the haze and fluttered into the air, startling him.

He was scheduled to fly to Pnom Penh to pick up some American geologists. Legal work for a change. Better than flying to Phong Savan. He had made three trips in the last two days and each time had been convinced he was not coming back. It had taken Paul Sarti's death to persuade Bonaventure to call a halt to the madness.

As he walked towards the sheds he stopped suddenly and gaped as a Beechcraft appeared out of the haze. It roared along the airstrip and took off, banking almost directly over his head. The plane had the familiar tiger decal of Air Laos painted on the fuselage. He read the identification sign on the tailplane.

'That's my fucking plane,' he muttered.

Then it was gone, lost in the low blanket of cloud. The drone of the engines was muted and soon swallowed up by the heavy mist.

Pépé jumped back in the jitney and told the driver to return as fast as he could to Vientiane. Monsieur Bonaventure was not going to like this.

Noelle heard the buzz of the engines as the Beechcraft passed very low over the house. She jumped out of bed and threw open the shutters. The navigation lights winked in the chill dawn, a silhouette that hung for a moment in the mist over the coconut palms before disappearing into the mist.

Baptiste!

Her hands balled into fists – frustration, relief, pride, anger, fear all welling up at once. He had gone without her! He could be killed!

But he had changed his mind. He loved her enough to do this.

But he could be killed ... she might never see him again.

Why had he gone without her?

She stared at the grey dawn in an agony of frustration and helplessness. The chill moisture settled on her skin and her nightdress, making her shiver. She waited until she could no longer hear the drone of the Beechcraft's engines.

She knew she might just have sent the only man she had ever wanted to his death.

Baptiste flew north-east over the Mekong plain. Through the smudges of cloud and mist he made out a jigsaw of green rice *paddis* below, small black earth dams dividing one field from another. Occasionally he would glimpse purple, jagged towers of limestone striking out through the clouds to the north.

It was growing lighter, and a golden glow suffused the cabin as a milky sun rose through the mist.

He kept climbing. The journey would take a little less than an hour, but there was no easy flying. He was navigating time and distance. He would have to climb to ten thousand feet to clear the mountains, on a bearing that would take him over the ancient capital of Xieng Khouang. When he reached the city he would start his approach to Phong Savan, on the edge of the Plain of Jars. With luck his route would not take him over Kong Le's anti-aircraft batteries; with luck the airstrip would still be in Royalist hands.

With luck he would live to see the sun set at the end of this day.

18

The mountains were covered in thick, verdant jungle. Come down in that and you would simply disappear, thought Baptiste. No one would ever find you. Just once he saw a village high on a mountain slope, a cluster of thatched huts raised on stilts as protection from the monsoon rains.

Sweat glistened on his forehead, residue of the constant gnawing pain. It was this pain that inspired him. It reminded him of Rocco Bonaventure and how he wanted to spit in his face when he delivered his opium.

Baptiste checked his watch. By dead reckoning he should be almost over Xieng Khouang. The mountains below were again obscured by cloud. He eased back on the throttle and the Beechcraft fell another five hundred feet, dropping through the cloud ceiling. He saw the city still far away to the north-east. He altered course and followed the brown pencil line of Highway 4 through the drab green of the jungle towards the Plain of Jars.

The plain was a vast plateau in the shape of a heart. It had taken its name from the giant earthenware jars that had been found buried there, the legacy of earlier Chinese inhabitants.

There was a lot of traffic on the road below, long convoys of trucks carrying Loyalist soldiers heading south, fleeing from Kong Le. He did not attempt a closer look. Those bastards were likely to fire at him with their rifles, just for the hell of it.

Over Lat Houang he banked to the north and started his descent towards Phong Savan. He had no idea if the Army was still in control there. Perhaps Kong Le had taken the garrison with its American advisers already. They could be waiting at the end of the airstrip to blow him out of the sky.

He looked down, saw the thatched roofs of Phong Savan, glimpsed the red Lao flag hanging limp over the garrison. A good sign, but he decided to circle the airfield first. No movement but he spotted an American DC-3 parked at the end of the dirt strip, near a cluster of Quonset huts. If the Americans were still here, it should be okay...

A sudden pap-pap-pap, a noise like an electric sewing machine. He looked down and saw a stitching of bullet holes in the floor of the Beechcraft. He reacted instinctively, threw the rudder of the plane hard to port. He clutched at his ribs as the plane lurched sickeningly in the sky.

Tracers flashed past the cockpit windshield in a green arc. 12.7-millimetre, he thought. *'Ah, putain!'*

Altitude, altitude. They had taught him in pilot training it was the only thing that could save him from ground fire. No matter how cleverly you weaved and turned the aircraft they would track you eventually.

Altitude.

He boosted the engines to full power, pulled back on the stick and climbed hard to port.

'Merde!' he gasped, felt a sharp pain in his left leg. He looked down. There was dark blood all over the floor.

Altitude.

The pitch of the motors rose to an agonised whine, and he fought the nose to keep from going into a stall.

Baptiste looked over his shoulder. The green tracers were arcing through the sky, falling short, bending away as they spent their force.

'Bastards!' Check the gauges. Oil pressure was good, the rudder and stick still responding easily, fuel gauges steady.

Everything else was agony. His ribs, his leg. Where was the blood coming from? There was nothing he could do about it now, he had to fight the controls.

He levelled out, instinctively brought the Beechcraft around, and banked steeply over the airfield, lining up the dirt runway. There was still time to abort, and return to Vientiane. And then? Bonaventure would be waiting at the aerodrome with his assassins. No, there was no point in going back without the opium.

The anti-aircraft fire had come from the north-east. This time his approach would be from the opposite direction, landing into the wind. He could still get her down. But he would not be able to fly her much longer if the leg wound was bad.

What was it Noelle had said to him: Do you want to chase clouds for ever?

He lowered the flaps and began the descent.

Baptiste held his breath against a wave of nausea. He felt light-headed. Whenever he moved his left foot he heard the blood squelching in his boot and felt a shrill stab of pain.

He looked at the altimeter. One thousand feet AGL.

He eased back on the throttle, concentrated on keeping the wings straight and level. He waited for the ground batteries to find him again, but this time there was nothing.

A few feet from the ground he cut power and lifted the nose. The Beechcraft's wheels touched almost at once, and the plane bounced down the strip towards the jungle. He was down.

Fuck you, Rocco. I did it.

The Beechcraft rolled towards the wall of green jungle at the end of the strip. He relaxed, shivered with sudden cold. There was sweat all over him, like cold grease.

He almost fainted, willed himself to stay conscious. He taxied the Beechcraft around. He looked out of the cockpit, there were three wooden stakes driven into the ground at the edge of the strip. They each had a human head impaled on them.

'Welcome to Phong Savan,' Baptiste murmured aloud. 'We hope you enjoy your stay.'

Gerry Gates was one of two Americans who watched in amazement as the aircraft touched down on the dirt. Who the hell was this idiot? Kong Le's troops were on the outskirts of the town. They were planning their own departure within hours.

The Beechcraft taxied over to the ramshackle collection of huts at the edge of the strip and the pilot shut off the engines. But no one stepped out of the cockpit. When Gates and his partner reached the aircraft, the pilot was unconscious, slumped over the controls.

19

Gérard Petrovski had the seamed face of a street fighter, long, lank grey hair and a beard like the sable of a silver fox. He had been in Asia almost all his life and the heat and the sweat had aged him. His skin was the colour of Mekong whisky, and the flesh hung in pouches under his eyes and his chin. He wore a dirty red bandana and combat fatigues.

He bent down to peer closer at Crocé's face, and shook his head. The pilot looked as if he had come straight from a bar-room brawl. *Merde alors!*

'I don't know this one,' he said to Gates.

'It's one of Bonaventure's planes.'

'Sure. But I don't know him.'

They had propped Baptiste on the floor, his head lolling on a rice sack. They had treated his leg wound as best they could, a combine dressing packed over the wound, held in place with a thick swathe of crêpe bandage. The leg was propped on an old orange crate.

'Shot out some calf muscle,' Gates said. 'Lost a lot of blood. No damage to the artery or he'd be dead.'

'How long's he been unconscious?'

'Not long. Could be shock, could be he just fainted. Not much we can do for him here anyway.'

Baptiste began to recover. He started to gag. Gates reacted first, stepped forward, and kicked him over on to his side. Baptiste retched painfully, then clutched his ribs. He uttered a string of obscenities and Petrovski and Gates laughed.

Baptiste rolled painfully on to his back. His mouth tasted foul, his head pulsing with pain. Everything hurt. He looked around. He was in some sort of warehouse – the place smelled of grease and opium and urine. A Cessna, plundered for spare parts, skeletal and rusted, took up most of the space. Wooden crates were stacked along the walls.

Two men stood over him. One was an American, with short, brown hair and a thin moustache, wearing a startling orange and green Hawaiian shirt and black cotton trousers. The other was a bearded nightmare with bad teeth.

Another man stood in the corner. American too, guessed Baptiste. He looked bored. He was smoking a cigarette and leaning on one of the hangar doors.

Baptiste tried to focus on the grey-haired man in the bandana. 'Petrovski?' He slurred the name, his tongue feeling twice its normal size. He tried again. 'Petrovski?'

'Perhaps,' the nightmare said, after a moment, in French.

Baptiste was having trouble breathing. He brought up his left arm to splint his ribs and rolled onto his left side. 'Baptiste Crocé.' He held out his hand.

The man ignored it. 'Is that supposed to mean something to me?'

There was the sound of small arms fire from the town, followed by the crash of mortars. Petrovski and Gates looked at each other, their faces taut with strain.

'Monsieur Bonaventure wants his opium,' he said.

'So he sent you here to get it?' said Petrovski. 'He must be paying you plenty. You know what happened to your comrade yesterday?'

'He liked it here and decided to stay?'

'He circled the airfield before he landed, just like you did this morning. Only he didn't react as fast as you and the Pathet Lao blew him out of the sky.'

'Communists?'

'They're helping Kong Le for now,' Gates said. 'Classic pincer movement. It's only the Meos that are holding them off. The Lao soldiers just cut and run. They don't like real wars.'

Baptiste forced himself painfully up on his elbows. He didn't give a damn about who owned Phong Savan. 'Where's the opium?'

'Where's Rocco's regular pilots?' Petrovski asked him. 'Where's Gilbert and Marius?'

'They wouldn't come back.'

'You were the only one crazy enough to do it, *hein?*'

'Where's the opium?' repeated Baptiste.

'Forget it, *ami*. You can't walk, never mind fly an airplane. We'll put you on the Dakota, you'll fly out with us.'

You want to chase clouds the rest of your life?

Baptiste tried to get on to his knees, but the hangar seemed to spin around him. He clutched at Petrovski's leg for support, waited till the dizziness had passed. Petrovski did not try and help him.

He put his weight on his uninjured leg. Sweat ran down his face in beads. He found his balance and released his hold on Petrovski. 'I want Rocco's opium.'

A mortar round landed in the middle of the airfield and a spray of dirt bounced on the wings of the Dakota parked outside on the grass next to the Beechcraft.

'I haven't got time to argue with this stubborn bastard all day,' Gates said. 'We're leaving in an hour. If you want to come with us, get your ass on the Dakota.'

The two Americans walked out.

'Rocco wants his opium,' repeated Baptiste. He took the revolver from the pocket of his flight jacket and aimed it at Petrovski. 'He's paid for it, he wants it. You don't want to disappoint him, do you?'

Petrovski looked at Gates and shrugged his shoulders. 'There's no talking sense to some people, is there?' he said.

Petrovski drove back to the Snow Leopard Inn in an olive drab jeep that was coated with ochre dust. After he was gone Baptiste dragged himself back to the Beechcraft. There were holes peppered through the fuselage and the starboard wing, but the hydraulics appeared to be intact and neither engine had sustained damage. He hauled himself up into the cabin, and sat at the controls to wait for Petrovski.

Another mortar round landed on the strip, throwing up a drifting spray of dirt. Black plumes of smoke rose behind the coconut palms at the northern edge of the airfield, the sound of small arms fire getting louder.

His leg was bleeding again.

Fuck you, Rocco. I'll get your opium.
And then it will be your turn to bleed.

Bonaventure had his driver park the Mercedes in the shade of a pipal tree at Wattay airport. It was hot inside the car, and Bonaventure sat with his legs stretched out of the open door. Noelle sat beside him, fanning herself gently with the morning's copy of *Lao Presse*.

Neither of them spoke for a very long time. Out on the airfield a flock of vultures were picking over the carcas of a buffalo.

It was Bonaventure who broke the silence first. 'I cannot believe you did this,' he hissed.

'Don't preach to me, Papa. Not after what you and your gangsters did to him.'

'He deserved it. So did you. You behaved like a whore. I should have had him dumped in the Saigon river.'

'If you did, I would have killed myself.' She fanned herself even more furiously. 'Or perhaps I would have killed you.'

Bonaventure did not doubt it for a moment. It was the peasant blood again. In the name of the Holy Virgin, why was he ever cursed with such a daughter?

'He's getting your opium for you. I thought you would be satisfied.'

'He isn't back yet,' Bonaventure said. And perhaps he wouldn't be. That would solve all his problems.

Baptiste taxied the Beechcraft to the end of the runway. Another mortar round landed less than fifty yards away and he felt the Beechcraft tremble from the aftershock. That was the fourth round to hit the airfield, but the strip itself was still serviceable. But not for much longer.

Behind him the Dakota rumbled away from the Quonset huts with the last Americans in Phong Savan on board. Petrovski was with them.

Baptiste swung around on to the strip, the three captured Pathet Lao heads grinning at him, already rotting black in the sun. He pushed the engines to full throttle and bounced along the runway. He eased back on the controls and felt the familiar rush of adrenalin as the wings lifted him clear off the ground.

He had done it...

He did not hear the rattle of the machine gun fire over the roar of the engines. The perspex canopy split with holes, and the Beechcraft seemed to lurch in the air. For a moment he was blind, and when he put a hand to his face it was wet with blood.

20

It was almost sunset when Rocco Bonaventure heard the distant whine of an aircraft coming from the north. He had all but given up hope. He murmured a quick prayer of thanks; he could not afford to lose another aircraft.

The Beechcraft was a grey speck in a violet sky. As it swooped towards the coconut palms at the edge of the strip, he got out of the Mercedes and ran across the airfield.

Noelle waited by the car. There was something wrong. She knew by the beat of the engines even before she saw the trail of oil spewing from the port engine. She crossed herself.

'For the love of God,' Bonaventure shouted. Then Noelle saw it too. There were jagged holes in the fuselage and the tailplane. Only God and Baptiste Crocé's luck was holding the frame together.

'Please God,' Noelle whispered.

Baptiste had cut the port engine, the remaining propeller laboured to keep the plane airborne. The port wing dipped suddenly.

He was not going to make it.

'My plane,' Noelle heard her father shout in an agony of loss.

Somehow Baptiste corrected the descent. The wings wobbled and shook but a few feet from the ground he levelled her out and set her down on the dirt in a perfect three point landing. The Beechcraft bounced to a halt at the end of the runway.

Noelle whispered her thanks to the Virgin. She suddenly realised she had been clutching the crucifix at her throat so tightly it had left a livid imprint in the flesh of her palm.

Baptiste shut down the engines. Eerie silence.

Bonaventure ran back to the Mercedes. 'Get over there,' he said to Tao Koo.

Baptiste had bled all over the cabin.

Noelle cradled him in her arms. He was unconscious. There was blood everywhere, most from a deep laceration on his scalp. A crust of it had hardened on his face, soaked his shirt and trousers, and the force of the jetstream through the shattered perspex had sprayed more around the cockpit. There was more blood seeping from a soaking bandage on his lower left leg.

But it was his left eye that worried her. The eyelid was split open, and she could see the eyeball underneath, the pupil dilated and misshapen.

Bonaventure was more concerned with the contents of the hold. 'He got the opium,' he said. There was a note of grudging admiration in his voice.

Noelle ignored him. 'Look what I've done,' she moaned. She could not believe she had led him to this. She was as crazy and as cold as her father.

'Is he alive?' Bonaventure asked her, curious rather than concerned.

She could only stare back at him.

'Let's get him in the car,' he said. 'We'll find him a doctor.'

Bonaventure found Baptiste dozing – perhaps – in the garden of The Bungalow, one heavily bandaged leg resting on a rattan chair. There was a thick pad over his left eye. The rest of his face was still misshapen from the beating he had taken in Cholon and there was a thick swathe of bandaging under his shirt splinting his ribs. He held a cigarette in one hand and a glass of vermouth cassis in the other. He looked pale and tired and insufferably smug, thought Bonaventure.

'Crocé.'

He opened his good eye. 'Monsieur Bonaventure. What a pleasure.'

Bonaventure grunted. 'For you perhaps.'

He pulled up a rattan chair and sat down heavily. He took out a silver cigarette case and selected a Black Russian cigarette. His doctor had told him they were not good for him, but he allowed himself one on certain occasions, such as when he had unpleasant duties to perform.

'How is the leg?'

'The bullet broke a small bone, but the doctor says it will heal. It is the eye that is the problem.'

'Oh?'

'He says the fragment of perspex he removed has damaged the cornea and I will probably lose sight in that eye. I shall be one-eyed from now on.'

Like my daughter, Bonaventure thought bitterly. 'Will you be able to fly again?'

'Not without an aeroplane.'

He took the point. 'I don't know whether to shake your hand or cut your throat.'

'A difficult choice for you, I imagine.'

'My daughter seems to be very fond of you, Monsieur Crocé.'

'She is a poor judge of character.'

'Precisely.' Bonaventure drew on the cigarette and studied the other man. I wonder what he wants? he thought. I can guess. But perhaps I shall be able to accommodate him. He has shown himself to be far more resourceful than I imagined. 'You are either very brave or very foolish. I cannot make up my mind which.'

'Perhaps both. Anyway, it was Noelle's idea.'

'She says she is going to marry you. Is that her idea also?'

'No. It was mine.'

'What are you in love with, Monsieur Crocé? My daughter – or my business?'

'I don't know.'

Bonaventure was startled by the candour of the reply. He hadn't expected that.

'My daughter is a highly intelligent girl, Monsieur Crocé. But this time, I think she has been something of a fool. But...' He spread his hands in a gesture of helplessness. 'It makes no difference what I think. She has made up her mind. I have decided to make the best of the situation.'

'Oh?'

He looks so sure of himself, Bonaventure thought. What does my Noelle see in this arrogant bastard? 'I could perhaps use a pilot with skills such as yours. Especially as it appears I will have to accept you into the family.' He reached into his jacket pocket and handed Baptiste a heavy gold coin. It was embossed with a Napoleonic eagle and a Corsican crest.

'It is your passport to the *Union Corse*. It may be perverse of me, but I believe you have earned it. Come to dinner tonight. Nine o'clock.' He got up to leave. 'By the way, I assume you plan to have children?'

'Of course.'

'A word of advice. Don't have daughters.'

21

Hong Kong

Ho Kuan-ling soon realised that freedom would not be as easy as he had imagined. When he had first been brought to the hospital he had been confused by the language: in his own province of Swatow everyone spoke a chiu chao dialect of Mandarin, but here in the hospital the nurses and his fellow patients spoke Cantonese or English. He lay awake every night in the crowded ward of the Queen Elizabeth Hospital, listening to the babble of voices around him and stared at the tent of sheets over the lower half of his body and whispered his supplications to Kuan Yi in the darkness.

Finally, one of the Chinese doctors told him, in halting Mandarin, that the shark had taken a piece of muscle the size of a baby's fist from his thigh. He would keep the leg, but he would be left with a permanent limp. He would be a virtual cripple for the rest of his life.

We'll see about that, Ho had thought.

While the leg healed, he stared at the slow ceiling fans and battled the pain and isolation and planned for his return to a world that remained beyond his view beyond the hospital walls.

But the extent of his alienation did not really impress itself on him until the day he limped from the hospital on Nathan Road and surveyed his new world.

Kowloon was a marriage of colour and noise, of slender, expensive women in tight red and gold cheongsams, bowed amahs in black Chinese pongee tops and trousers, businessmen in western suits. He sniffed at the smells of garlic, barbecued pork, raw fish, kerosene, sweat and sewage. The streets were crammed with scaffolding and people and traffic, and the blur of commerce and construction and hurry. On Hong Kong Island, the pinnacles of the Hong Kong and Shanghai Banking Corporation and the Bank of China stood guard over the harbour like sentinels.

He wandered along Nathan Road, gaping like a country boy. Kowloon's main thoroughfare was a teeming, noisy sprawl of tenements and skyscrapers, the focus of China's collision with the West. The ancient brick, stucco and wood shophouses and apartments with their awnings of oiled rice paper and their balconies crammed with potted plants and caged birds and people, were quickly disappearing. They were being razed one by one, the ugly brown gaps quickly filled with tall concrete towers that seemed to sway dizzyingly over his head.

People rushed past him and around him; they jostled him, and did not spare him a second glance. He was like a cork bobbing on the ocean.

A sixteen-year-old boy could get swept away and be lost for ever in this place, he decided, swallowed up in some tenement or factory. But Ho Kuan-ling knew he would be saved because he had direction and purpose. In Swatow, when he had first begun to plan his night swim over the border, his mother had told him where he should go; she had told him about her brother-in-law, Ho Chan-fu, who lived in a place called the Walled City.

'But if Hong Kong is such a big place, how will I find one man?' he had asked her.

'You'll find him,' was all she had said.

The Chinese called it Hak Nam: Darkness.

The Walled City of Kowloon was an ugly, tenement fortress off Tung Tau Tsuen Road, on the north side of Kai Tak airport. Ho followed a street of glass-fronted shops, the surgeries of unqualified dentists announced by the gold and silver teeth in bottles in the windows, by the pickled abscesses, by the ornamental goldfish that were supposed to be beneficial to their patient's nerves.

This was the southern rampart of Hak Nam, the city within a city, and beyond the reach of the British administration. By the original treaty governing the New Territories, the old Walled

City – which comprised a mandarin's *yamen* and village – was supposed to stay under Chinese Imperial control, but when the British traders had complained, the concession had been unilaterally withdrawn. In the impasse that followed, the mandarin who lived inside the city had governed, but on his death the six acres inside the walls had fallen to anarchy.

For over a century it remained disputed territory with both the British and Chinese claiming sovereignty. The walls had long since disappeared, the stone used by the Japanese during World War Two as core material for the runway at Kai Tak. A tenement slum had grown on the site like a malignant tumour, home to thirty thousand people who, by an aberration of politics, remained beyond the reach of both British and Chinese law.

Ho wandered the street for almost an hour before he found a way inside. It was no more than a slime-covered alley, the stench of rotting food, offal and ordure leaking from the darkness like a bank of fog. The light penetrated only in dismal yellow bolts.

A *tin man toi*, a weatherman, sat on an old wooden crate in a soiled T-shirt, picking distractedly at filthy toe nails. He looked up as Ho approached. 'What do you want?'

'I want to see Ho Chan-fu.'

The boy snorted with derision and returned his attention to his toenails.

Ho was not afraid. Instead, he felt a dawning of contempt. Was this really one of his uncle's sentries? If he wanted he could have snapped the idiot's neck with one kick. He had been taught never to turn away from a potential enemy. 'Ho Chan-fu is my uncle.'

He could feel the man sizing him up. This scrawny little kid with a limp? 'Get out of here.'

He stood his ground. 'Ho Chan-fu is my uncle,' he said. 'I bring him greetings from his family in Swatow.'

The guard got up slowly. He hesitated, then grabbed Ho's arm and pushed him into the alley. 'All right, you'd better come with me. But if you're not who you say you are we'll cut out your liver and throw it down the sewers.'

No light could penetrate far into the alleys of Hak Nam. It was the middle of the day but outside it might as well have been night. And it was filthy, filthier even than the squalid streets of the village where he had been born, *lap-sap* – rubbish – lying everywhere. As they made their way through the gloomy maze, Ho kept his eyes down to avoid stepping in human waste or discarded food. Twice someone threw refuse from a window in a tenement high above them and it landed just a few yards from where they were walking.

There were no streets. Unencumbered by government planning regulations, Hak Nam had become a solid mass of buildings. They had to walk crouched over, for the alley they followed was no more than a concrete tunnel, inches of grime and filth on the stucco walls, the low ceiling a jumble of knotted electricity cables, tapped illegally from the main supplies in the street outside. Water dripped continually from overhead pipes, hissing and sparking on the wires.

Tunnels and alleyways and gloomy wooden staircases led off in every direction, littered with broken slabs of concrete and mounds of mouldering garbage. They passed a wooden sign that said, in Chinese characters 'Rat's Piss Street'. An apt name, Ho decided, for there was certainly no shortage of rats, the biggest he had ever seen, their eyes bright and orange in the shadows. The *tin man toi* clapped his hands at them but they turned their heads in disdain and continued to feast on the devil's banquet arrayed for them in the gutters.

The look-see boys dozed on their haunches in the urine-soaked dirt outside the gambling dens and the opium divans. Ho recognised these places from the look and the smell. He too had been a look-see boy in Swatow.

And there were the prostitutes. They sat on orange crates, their faces powdered to the colour of corpses, the backs of their hands scarred with needle marks. They went deeper into the slippery, stinking maze. They moved to one side to allow a child to pass on a tricycle. Barefoot children played in the dirt, babies strapped to their backs.

Finally they started to climb endless flights of concrete steps, the walls stained with dripping water and the stairwell littered with decaying rubbish, until they reached the twelfth floor, and the Eyrie of the Dragon Fist.

22

The Eyrie of the Dragon Fist was a one-room tenement on the very top floor of the building. The look-see boy knocked on a door with peeling red paint. It opened a fraction and eyes peered out at them. Ho was pulled inside and the door slammed shut.

Men were arguing. Ho realised there was an impromptu court in session. Dragon Fist sat at a table, drinking tea from a small porcelain cup, surrounded on either side by his fighters. A boy was shouting and pleading with him. To Ho's relief, everyone spoke in the same chiu chao-accented Mandarin.

The young man was begging. He kept repeating, over and over: 'I didn't take the opium, *tai lo*. I swear it. I didn't take the opium.'

His uncle was dressed in black jacket and black sunglasses and tight jeans, too tight for him. He was fast approaching middle age. Ho decided he didn't look so fearsome. He looked like a clown.

But just then Dragon Fist gave an imperceptible nod of his head and two of his fighters picked the boy up by the arms, dragged him across the room and pushed him out of the open window. They grabbed his ankles at the last moment.

The boy was screaming.

'Ask him again if he took the opium,' said Dragon Fist.

'I didn't take it! I swear!' He was squealing like a pig on a stake.

'Black Mai – ask him who has my opium,' Dragon Fist said, in a tone that suggested he was quickly becoming bored with the proceedings.

'He says he doesn't know, *tai lo*,' one of the interrogators answered, the one called Black Mai.

Dragon Fist sipped his tea. 'Wash him anyway,' he said.

The two men let go and came back to the table, laughing.

Ho Kuan-ling's uncle turned away and looked hard at the newcomer. 'Who's this?'

The *tin man toi* propelled Ho further into the room. 'He says he is your nephew, *tai lo*. From Swatow,' the teenager said, in a loud voice. He was enjoying his moment in the spotlight.

Dragon Fist sipped his tea, appearing to be only vaguely interested. 'My nephew?'

'My mother told me to come to you, Uncle,' said Ho, choosing his words with care. 'She said you were the brother of my father, Ho Chen-Li.'

'Where do you live?'

'Tsinwen, in Kwangtung province in Swatow.'

Dragon Fist lit a cigarette and studied him carefully. 'And how is my brother?'

Ho Kuan-ling felt a surge of relief. He had been wondering if perhaps he had made some dreadful mistake. But the question confirmed to him that this Dragon Fist was his uncle after all. 'But he is dead, Uncle. The communists killed him.'

'How?'

'Surely you heard? They executed him for being a triad. A People's Guard officer took off his head with a sword.'

Dragon Fist nodded slowly. Ho Kuan-ling realised he had known the answer, the question was merely a test. 'What happened to your leg?'

'Two months ago I tried to swim across from Shenzhen side. A shark attacked me.'

'Bad luck for you. Or perhaps it was good luck since you are here. What's your name, Nephew?'

'Kuan-ling. But I call myself Douglas.'

'Douglas. Why Douglas?'

'After Douglas MacArthur. He commanded a great army. I want to control a great army one day.'

Everyone seemed to think this was a good joke.

When they had all finished laughing, Dragon Fist said: 'What do you want from me, Douglas?'

111

'I have nowhere to go, and no work, Uncle.'

'Do you have any money?'

'No, Uncle.'

Dragon Fist reached into his pocket and brought out a thick wad of Hong Kong dollars. He peeled off two one-hundred-dollar notes and tossed them carelessly across the room. Douglas scrambled to pick them off the floor.

'What can you do, Douglas?'

'I can fight, Uncle.'

More laughter. Black Mai found this so amusing he had to sit down on a chair.

'A skinny pole like you?'

'My father taught me to fight from when I was young. He was still instructing me when the communists came for him.'

The only one who wasn't smiling now was his uncle.

'Then perhaps I can use you,' he said. 'Your father was a good fighter. A good fighter with no brains. If he had been clever, he would have got out of China with me, twelve years ago.' He pointed to one of the men in the room, a man of about fifty with blackened teeth, thinning hair and a big, moon face. 'Go with Tse-ping. He needs a look-see boy for his divan. His last little bird flew out of the window.' The men laughed again. 'Perhaps you can be of some use, Douglas. Or shall we call you Sharkfin?'

Douglas Ho bowed his head. 'I think Sharkfin is a very good name, Uncle,' he said, because even then he realised the value of a good legend.

23

Douglas Ho's first job was as a look-see boy for Tse-ping, who was a *pang-jue* – master of a drug den. The job taught him many of the basic lessons of survival in the Walled City.

The first lesson he learned was never to touch opium or heroin. Many of the triad members he met were themselves addicted to the crude number three heroin. In this form it looked like brown sugar; they would tip it on to a piece of tinfoil, light a screw of toilet paper and heat the tinfoil underneath. The heroin would melt to a dark brown treacle. Then, using a matchbox or a piece of rolled up paper as a funnel, they would inhale the fumes.

They called it 'chasing the dragon'.

They were useful as soldiers – until the drugs made them so dependent they could not think about anything else – but once a man started chasing the dragon he would never rise any higher in the triad. He was no longer chasing the dragon, Douglas decided; the dragon was chasing him.

He quickly learned to despise the addicts who came to the divan, to buy their release from Hak Nam. The divan was a long tin shed, with low, rough tables where addicts could sprawl in blank dreaming, skins waxy like a corpse, thin as stick insects. For fifty cents an addict could buy himself a screw of toilet paper, a piece of tinfoil, and a cardboard funnel. After that, it depended on what each purse could afford.

They knew what the drug was doing to them, but they seemed unable to help themselves. They were like oxen, led by the nose, driven by their own craven desires. Douglas was contemptuous of their weakness.

From the addicts he learned that people were just like everything else, just commodities, to be bought and sold. Beasts of burden.

These beasts provided the cheap labour that fuelled triad businesses; women bowed over ancient manual sewing machines, working in windowless rooms by the light of a single thirty-watt bulb, making the cheap shirts for Temple Street; emaciated men in filthy vests moulding hot metal over pit fires in the bowels of a steaming tenement, cranking out bicycle spares for mass export; toothless old harridans in black pyjamas, crouched in fetid little rooms moulding enormous plastic penises that would be sold to western tourists in Wanchai.

In return for their labour they were packed into flats a few feet square, drew their water from a pump in a filthy courtyard, used the same two street-level cess pools shared by thirty thousand people and the sewer spiders.

And the triad paid them less than a dollar a day.

How was it possible to feel anything but contempt?

Douglas learned too that people were not just valuable for their labour. If a young girl was considered sufficiently attractive, Dragon Fist would arrange to have her gang-raped by his soldiers – he called it 'stamping the merchandise'. The girl was so shamed by the experience that she rarely protested when Dragon Fist paid her family to take this liability off their hands. Depending on the girl, he would then either use her in one of his own brothels or sell her to a 'fishball stall', specialising in pre-pubescent girls.

But the greatest lesson Douglas Ho learned was that the triads were his way out of hell.

There was no shortage of recruits. Boys as young as nine years old were sent to work making plastic flowers and toys in the gloomy factories of the Walled City, and the triads were their passport out. In return for their obedience, they received the triad's protection, and could earn a living as look-see boys in the gambling dens and opium divans – like Douglas – or selling tickets to the pornographic film shows.

Now he shared a room with four others, all teenagers like himself, in a filthy tenement in the heart of Hak Nam.

It was better than the plastics factory, and for Douglas it was a lot better than Swatow and communism.

But at night when he lay on his hard cot, listening to the never-ending clank of machinery from below, the cries of the addicts and the sing-song chatter of chiu chao, he knew the world owed him far more. Douglas Ho did not plan to remain a look-see boy for long. He would use the talents his father had given him and one day he would leave Hak Nam and the smell of raw sewage far behind.

24

Hak Nam was in the control of two triads, the 14K and the Fei Lung. Like nations, they disputed their borders regularly, and there were occasional outbreaks of fighting as wars were fought over possession of a stairwell or a garbage-strewn alley no more than a few inches wide.

Tse-ping's opium divan was on Chicken Fat Street, on the border of 14K territory. A concrete passageway that led off the alley belonged to the 14K, together with a lean-to shed that showed pornographic films – 'yellow movies' – and a restaurant where stray dogs were flayed to death to provide tender dog steaks, considered a delicacy by Douglas' fellow Chinese, and illegal by British authorities.

Appropriately a wooden sign proclaimed it as Half Dog Street.

Douglas had been apprenticed to Tse-ping for more than a month and already he was bored and restless. Police rarely ventured into the Walled City, except in large raiding parties, so there was no real need for a look-see boy. The only real danger came from the 14K, and Tse-ping told him there had been no trouble in the Walled City for months.

Instead of sitting on his haunches and picking at his toe nails – which appeared to be a prerequisite of the job – Douglas occupied his time by learning to use his injured leg again. He was not a cripple, as the doctors had threatened, but his left leg was now useless as a weapon. Every day he practised against the wall of the alley, spinning and kicking, building up the remaining muscle, until he could at least pivot on it as well as he could on his right leg.

The prostitutes, watching him from their perches on the orange crates further down the alley, pointed and laughed.

'Hey, Limpy!' they shouted. 'Want to wrestle us?'

He turned away, scowling with contempt. One day he would show them he was more than just a look-see boy.

Every day his uncle came to the opium den to collect the takings from Tse-ping. Dragon Fist was always accompanied by two of his fighters, the men Douglas had seen the day he first came to the Walled City, the ones who had thrown the thief out of the window.

But Dragon Fist rarely spoke to him, or even looked at him.

'Is he really your uncle?' Tse-ping asked him one day.

'He's my father's brother,' Douglas told him.

'He often asks about you,' Tse-ping said, and seemed as intrigued by Dragon Fist's behaviour as Douglas himself. 'But I notice he never talks to you. I think he is testing you.'

Douglas aimed another kick at the wall. Tse-ping watched, his tight mouth drawn down in a frown. 'I think if you prove to be a weakling, he will disown you.'

'I just need one chance,' Douglas said.

But the prostitutes on their orange boxes giggled and laughed, and Douglas glowered and simmered and waited.

His chance finally came one morning, without warning. Dragon Fist had collected the takings from Tse-ping, and was making his way back up the alley with his two bodyguards, Black Mai and another man Douglas knew only as Benny East Street. Five triads ran screaming out of Half Dog Street, waving meat cleavers. Dragon Fist's bodyguards had barely time to react. The 14K were expert with choppers, and aimed their first blows at the muscles on the shoulders and back, chopping Benny to the ground before he had even turned around.

Black Mai had no time to draw his own weapons. He raised his arms to defend himself, and the choppers slashed down and blood started to pour from his hands and shoulders. He screamed once.

Dragon Fist reacted quickly. He threw his back against the wall of the alley and drew a chain from inside his leather jacket. He dodged a slashing blow from one of the 14K and flicked the chain backhanded, raking it across his adversary's

117

face. The man staggered back blindly, clutching at his eyes, blood welling through his fingers.

Black Mai was now a bloody wreck. The other four triads turned their attention to Dragon Fist.

Douglas launched himself up the alley in the lop-sided, limping run that he had practised every day under the cold eyes of the prostitutes. But this time, instead of the wall, his target was alive and deadly.

25

Pivoting on the left leg.

Strike with the heel of the right.

It rammed into the first triad's kidneys. The boy had not heard Douglas. He screamed in pain and turned to face his attacker. Pivoting again, on his right foot, Douglas pushed the heel of his hand into the other man's face, just below the nose, as his father had taught him to do. It forced the nasal bones up through the skull, lacerating the frontal lobes of the brain and killing him instantly.

But as he fell, already the triad on his left had turned and slashed downward with his cleaver. Douglas leaped back, raising an arm to ward off the blow, felt the electric stab of pain as the cleaver slashed into the flesh of his arm.

Another chop, more pain.

He knew he had to step inside the blows. As the cleaver was raised again, he kicked out and connected with the 14K's knee, knocking him off balance. He stepped inside the arc of the weapon and chopped down on the other triad's nose and his left hand darted out like a snake, the fingers extended, into his throat. The man fell back, chopped again, blindly, catching Douglas a glancing blow to the side of his scalp.

Douglas felt as if he was about to fall, and steadied himself against the wall. If he went down he knew he was dead.

His attack had given Dragon Fist the advantage he needed. He leaped forward, sweeping the chain in a broad arc, pushing the 14K fighters back.

There was a shout from the end of the alley and Tse-ping appeared with more of Dragon Fist's own fighters. The 14K realised the battle had swung against them. They grabbed two of their wounded brothers and fled back into the gloom of Half Dog Street, leaving their compatriot lying at Douglas' feet.

Silence. Douglas could hear his own breathing sawing in his chest. His uncle examined the still and bleeding bodies of Benny and Black Mai. Then he slipped the chain back inside his leather coat and looked up at Douglas.

Douglas could feel himself sliding down the wall.

'You're bleeding, Nephew,' he said, and walked away.

Douglas felt the world swimming in front of him. The prostitutes were staring at him, and they weren't giggling any more.

He blacked out.

When Douglas opened his eyes there were shapes floating in and out of his vision, silhouettes against a white background. His mouth felt gummy, and there was a throbbing pain in his skull.

One of the silhouettes came closer. He made out a face. Sunglasses, black, slick backed hair, a double chin. His uncle.

'One hundred and nineteen stitches,' he whispered. 'Even I never got that many in a fight. Congratulations!'

Douglas tried to focus. He couldn't move one of his arms. One was encased in thick crepe bandage, the other immobilised to the bed, a needle and a long tube in one of the veins.

Dragon Fist leaned forward again. 'If anyone asks you, you fell through a glass window.'

Douglas nodded his head to show he understood.

'You're a tough little pi-dog, Nephew. By the sacred pussy of Kuan Yin, you've had more meat cut out of you than my grandmother's pig.'

'I can fight,' Douglas whispered.

'Better than Benny and Black Mai, at least. When you can walk again, you can take their place.'

The silhouettes faded into a buzzing, gelatin haze. When he woke again, they had gone. There was only a nurse, who barked at him in shrill Cantonese. He wondered if perhaps he hadn't imagined the whole thing.

But then he remembered what his uncle had whispered to him and he smiled through the red mist of pain. He knew he had taken his first steps out of the mire.

26

There was an ancient Taoist temple in the very heart of the Walled City, and around it one of only two courtyards in the whole of the Hak Nam. The whole area had been netted off to keep garbage from the surrounding tenements from falling on to the temple roof.

They were met at the temple doors by two triad soldiers, carrying metal cleavers. Douglas was one of perhaps fifty or sixty new recruits, and each one was greeted individually. When it was Douglas' turn he gave one of the men the secret triad handclasp, as Dragon Fist had taught him, and waited for the questions he had learned to answer by rote.

'Why do you come here?' the guard asked him.

'We come to enlist and obtain rations,' he answered.

'There are no rations for our army.'

'We bring our own.'

'The red rice of our army contains sand and stones. Can you eat stones?'

'If our brothers can eat them, so can we.'

'When you see the beauty of our sworn sisters and sisters-in-law, will you have adulterous ideas?'

'No, we would not dare to.'

'If offered a reward by the government, even as much as ten thousand ounces of gold, for information about your brothers, would you give it?'

'No, we would not dare to.'

'If you have spoken truly, you are loyal and righteous and may enter the city to swear allegiance and protect the country with your concerted efforts.'

Douglas entered the temple to join the rest of his fellow recruits. The interior was heavy with joss, massive coils of incense spiralling down from the ceiling on long chains. Douglas smelled sweat and fear and blood.

There were tablets on the walls, bold characters in black on red, or black on green. Douglas noted shallow Maoist epigrams such as: 'The heroes are supreme; the brave ones have no equal.' There were others, more enigmatic, black on yellow: 'When will be the end of enmity? Regrets will remain for ever.'

There were other banners around the walls, the flags of the heroes of triad legend, such as the Five Tiger Generals, and the pennants of the Four Great Faithful Ones, the fabled guards on the gates of the ancient Triad city of Muk Yeung Shing, the city of Willows.

The main altar was lit by a brass lamp with seven stems, the Seven Stars lamp that signified the seven planets of the heavens. There were other bowls of fruit and flowers and spices. The centrepiece was the *tau*, a large wooden tub, painted red and filled with rice. Each grain of rice, Dragon Fist had told him, was supposed to represent a society member.

The rest of the paraphernalia, Douglas noted, was a mixture of the overt and the mystic. There was a red wooden club, the symbol for punishment; the Sword of Loyalty and Righteousness; and a grass sandal, supposedly one of a pair of magic sandals from triad history. There was also a mirror, the Mirror of Truth, in which a man's innermost soul was supposed to be reflected. There was a bloodstained white robe and rosary, in memory of the rebel monks from the Shao Lin Monastery in Fukien, who had founded the triad almost three hundred years before.

The final icon was an object intricately folded from a single sheet of paper, known as the Gall of the Tau. Once unfolded it was said to be impossible for the uninitiated to reconstruct, and its secret was held by the Incense Master alone. It was placed in front of the *tau*, in plain view, proof of the Incense Master's arcane knowledge.

The temple's interior was supposed to represent the walls and gates of the ancient triad City of Willows. Douglas and his fellow recruits walked solemnly through the paper arches that had been built inside the temple to signify the gates that once existed inside the secret city. They were then invited to kneel in front of the Incense Master.

The Incense Master sat on the right of the altar. He wore a white robe, with a knotted bandana on his head, prayer beads in his right hand, a grass sandal on his left foot. The Vanguard, on the left of the altar, was dressed in black. He carried a whip, symbol of his authority; on his back was a pack, which was supposed to contain the ashes of the thirteen monks who had founded the Hung Mun, the black society of the triad.

The rest of the Lodge officials sat facing each other in two rows. Douglas saw Dragon Fist, solemn and ridiculous in his black robe, but his uncle showed no sign of recognition.

'An order has been issued from the Five Ancestors Altar,' the Incense Master began. 'Investigation must be made around the lodge, and if police are present to spy on us, they must be relentlessly washed.'

It was ritual only. No police officer would venture into the heart of the Walled City, Douglas knew. The two guards nodded to the Incense Master.

'There are no strangers,' the Incense Master announced. 'We will open the lodge.'

The Vanguard recorded the names and addresses and ages of each recruit in a great book, and their initiation fee was paid. The Incense Master then went to the altar and laid the register book next to the *tau*, and returned with three straw figures, each bearing the name of famous triad traitors pinned to its chest. The effigies were forced into a kneeling position and their heads cut off with the Sword of Loyalty and Righteousness.

Then Douglas, with his fellow initiates – or, the 'new horses', as the Incense Master referred to them – crawled under the crossed cleavers of the guards, on their elbows and knees. This first phase of the ceremony, Dragon Fist had explained, was called Passing the Mountain of Knives.

One at a time they knelt in front of the Incense Master. When it was his turn, Douglas felt him rap his neck with the back of the sword.

'Which is harder, the sword or your neck?'

123

'My neck,' Douglas answered, as Dragon Fist had instructed him.

The ceremony went on for hours.

Douglas Ho was captivated by the ritual. Unlike his fellow initiates, he understood why it was necessary. He realised the power of the arcane, the grip that the cabal could take on a man's spirit. He drank it all in. It enthralled him.

The Incense Master burned a sheet of yellow paper to represent the yellow pall that protected the first triad monks from the flames when their monastery was torched by the Manchus. The ashes were collected in a wooden bowl and mixed with wine, cinnabar and sugar.

The Vanguard brought in a live cockerel and handed it to the Incense Master. Its feet and beak were tied with string. It struggled frantically, twitching in the Incense Master's hands. He expertly chopped off the cockerel's head with one blow of the knife, and drained the blood into a large wooden bowl.

Then he went to each of the recruits in turn. They extended their left hands, palm upwards, facing the Vanguard who held a needle threaded with red cotton. He pricked the middle finger of each man's hand until the blood flowed.

'As the silver needle brings blood from the finger, so do not reveal our secrets to others. If any secrets are disclosed, blood will be shed from the five holes of the body.'

The blood was mixed with the ashes and wine and spices and the black blood of the cockerel. As the Incense Master brought round the bowl, each recruit dipped a finger into the bowl and placed it in his mouth.

The blood oath was taken.

When it was done, the bowl was broken on the altar. 'So shall traitors to the triad similarly be broken.'

The Incense Master placed some joss paper on the floor and set it alight. With the others Douglas was invited to leap the fiery pit. 'It commemorates the burning of our founders' ancient monastery,' Dragon Fist had told him. 'Everything in the ceremony has a meaning. Everything.'

Finally, as they knelt on the cold stone floor, a stick of incense held between their joined hands, the Incense Master read to them the thirty-six oaths of the society. They recited each oath back to him, striking the end of their joss stick on the floor.

'I shall not disclose the secrets of the Hung family, not even to my parents, brothers or wife. I shall never disclose the secrets for money. I will be killed by myriads of swords if I do so...'

When he had finished Douglas Ho was a triad. He was no longer an alien. He had a place to belong. He had a family.

27

Laos, May 1962

Baptiste Crocé saw a break in the clouds and began a slow spiral descent into the valley. The altimeter showed four thousand feet ASL, and through the black monsoon clouds he saw the wild green mountains rising all around him, some as thin as knife blades. Another squall spattered against the windshield and the Beechcraft jumped like a rollercoaster.

The ground disappeared behind a blanket of clinging grey and Baptiste felt the familiar tightening in his gut as he searched for another break in the cloud to give him his bearing. For almost a minute he was flying blind, corkscrewing down towards the ground. He could feel the mountain slopes closing in on him on every side. Then a patch of green opened for him and he dived under the cloud and saw the dirt strip almost dead ahead.

It was tiny, a brown scar against the emerald of the surrounding forest. He cut back the throttle and lowered the flaps bringing the Beechcraft low into the valley. Now he could see the bend in the strip, fifteen degrees to starboard. The Americans had hacked the landing strips from the mountains like raw scars, and they suited the STOLs – Short Take off and Landing aircraft – that they used.

For more conventional craft, they were a nightmare. This one, Baptiste remembered, also had a 25-degree upslope.

But it was better than nothing. Without the American presence, there would be no opium.

As he flew over the village he saw the children staring up at him, the dogs and chickens scattering under the poled huts.

A child, sitting astride the back of a water buffalo, waved to him. Crocé brought the Beechcraft along the valley, the wheels almost skimming the forest canopy.

His fists were greasy on the controls, sweat stinging his eyes.

He would have to land with the nose of the Beechcraft pointing at the sky.

As he approached the strip he pulled back on the controls, lifted the nose, stamped on the rudder to correct against a sudden wind sheer, and snatched back the power as the wheel groped for the ground.

Only two hundred yards to make the landing. Less with the bend. The upslope would work in his favour, gravity killing the speed.

Keep the nose up . . .

Vache! Not enough!

The Beechcraft hit the ground hard, skidded in the mud. He gasped as the impact jarred his body, almost forcing his hands and feet from the controls. A spray of mud splattered on the windshield, blinding him. But then the Beechcraft was slowing. He swore harshly under his breath, and the tension drained out of him.

He was down.

There was another aircraft parked under the wind-sock, near a squalid collection of tin sheds. It wasn't one of the CAT's Pipers or Helios; a Cessna 195, with the red and blue insignia of Mittard's Lao Charter.

A familiar figure emerged from under the Cessna's wing and waved. Jean-Marie.

Baptiste climbed out of the cabin.

'That was the tidiest crash landing I've every seen,' Jean-Marie shouted. 'Are you practising for a kamikaze squadron?'

'Wind sheer.'

'It was like dropping an omelette on a plate!'

Baptiste scowled. He didn't make mistakes very often and when he did, he didn't like to be reminded of them. 'It's not a toy plane like yours,' he snapped back. 'You try putting this bitch down on the side of a mountain.'

Jean-Marie was delighted at his reaction. He wrapped an arm around his shoulder. 'You're shaking, *mon vieux*. You look like you need a drink.'

The rain rolled across the valley in a grey sheet, and they ran, slipping, through the mud for the shelter of the huts.

'So how's the eye?' Jean-Marie asked him. They sat side by side on the rice sacks that were piled against the wall of the shed. Steam rose from their backs, their cotton drill shirts soaked through. Baptiste took a swallow from the bottle of Mekong whisky, felt it burn his throat and stomach. He adjusted the black patch he now wore over his left eye.

'Not so good. It's harder to judge distance now. That's why I bumped the landing.'

Jean-Marie drank some whisky. 'Maybe you should find something else to do.'

'Like what?'

Jean-Marie scratched at the sweat itch under his shirt. 'So the eye patch is there to stay?'

'It's good for my reputation.' He took back the whisky bottle and took another pull. The sky was impenetrable and his contact had not arrived. He would not be flying again for a few hours. Maybe not again today.

'How's Noelle?'

'Fine.'

'When's the baby due?'

'After the monsoon.' He pulled a crumpled pack of Gitanes from the breast pocket of his shirt. They were wet. After four or five attempts, he was able to light one. 'You haven't told me what you're doing back in Laos. I thought you were flying for some outfit in Thailand.'

'It didn't work out. Then Mittard came to see me, offered me twice as much as before. He's buying another Cessna.'

Baptiste raised an eyebrow. So far Bonaventure had tolerated the competition, but with Mittard increasing the size of his fleet he might not be so sanguine. 'So you agreed to come back and fly it for him.'

'It's good money.'

'Be careful, Jean-Mar'.'

Jean-Marie screwed the top back on the whisky bottle. 'There's enough mud up here for everyone,' he said, using the local slang for opium.

Baptiste didn't answer. He got up and went outside. In seconds he was soaked through, but he ignored the rain. He walked over to Jean-Marie's Cessna and threw open the cabin door to peer inside. The hold was stacked with canvas sacks of raw opium, perhaps as much as three hundred kilos.

He looked up. Jean-Marie was leaning against the door of the hut, watching him. Neither man said a word. The rain hammered down. Mother of God, thought Baptiste. This could get serious.

28

The end of April had brought Nyam Fon, the season of rains and monsoons. The sun rose unseen in the mornings, the valleys flooded and the fields grew rich with jade green rice. Everything smelled of mould, and at night insects swarmed around the kerosene lanterns and infested every room.

A bat swooped in through the open French windows, hypnotised by the slowly turning ceiling fan. It circled the room, following the whirling blades until it grew tired and flapped and skittered around the floor. It happened often during the monsoon. Noelle had learned to ignore them.

The swallows had built their nests under the eaves, sheltered from the storms. It was raining again now, steadily, without the ferocity of the afternoon. Water dripped steadily from the eaves onto the banana leaves.

It was too hot to be pregnant. She felt the size of a whale. Tiny beads of perspiration glistened on her face, inched along her spine, itched in her hair. She went out on to the verandah, but it was no cooler there. The air was like steam.

After their marriage, Bonaventure had bought Noelle and Baptiste a villa just half a mile away on the western edge of the town, on the banks of the Mekong. It was pale blue stucco with a red tiled roof, and polished teak floors. The courtyard was shaded with pipal and mango trees. And they had servants: a cookboy, two *boyesses*, a gardener.

But for Noelle, life had not changed. In fact, she felt lonelier than she did before.

She heard someone enter the room behind her and turned round. Baptiste. It isn't fair, she thought when she saw him. When he came back from Phong Savan he was almost dead, his face a battered mess, and the doctors thought he was going to lose his leg as well as his eye. Now eight months later he's as handsome as ever, and I'm fat and ugly.

The eye patch was an affectation, of course, pure vanity. Incredible he hadn't thought to blind himself in one eye before, really. It suited him, damn him. His jet hair fell carelessly over his forehead, accentuating the overall effect.

And now he parades in front of me in his royal blue shirt and white suit, looking like a silk pirate, and wants my blessing for his lies. When had he changed? When had she?

'Where are you going, Baptiste?'

'I have to meet Rocco.'

'Rocco,' she repeated, her voice flat.

He looked guilty, like a little boy. 'A man has to have some pleasures.'

'And having dinner with your wife is not one of them?'

'I'll be home later. I need a drink.'

He would not meet her eyes. She knew what it was he wanted, something he no longer seemed to want from her. 'You look at me these days and I see a cloud pass over your face.'

'Noelle, please ...'

'It's your child in here. I can't help it if I'm fat like a whale.'

He pulled out his Gitanes, a nervous habit. He was tapping his foot on the floor, anxious to be away from her. For the love of God, how had it all gone wrong so quickly?

'You don't make love to me no more, Baptiste?'

'The baby ...'

'Just because I have your child in my belly, doesn't mean I'm made of glass! I still love you.' She felt the hot tears in her eyes and she stopped herself. She did not want to look weak in front of him. 'Do I disgust you so much?'

'Of course not.'

'Then I'll ask you just once, Baptiste. Please stay here and have dinner with me tonight.'

'I shall not be long, *chérie*. But I have to see Rocco. We'll have dinner when I get home.'

'When you're so drunk you can't stand up, and you have the stink of some taxi girl on you!'

'I don't know why I ever married you,' he said, and walked to the door.

Noelle was on her feet. 'Because you wanted my father's business!'

She picked up a ceramic elephant her father had bought for her in Saigon. It hit the wall inches from Baptiste's head. Noelle heard the *boyesses*, who had been listening on the other side of the door, shriek and run for the kitchen.

He turned, one hand on the door, his eyes bright points. 'Don't ever do that again,' he growled.

'I won't. Next time it's a knife, and I won't miss!'

She heard the Packard roar out of the courtyard, in the direction of downtown Vientiane. When she was sure he was gone she threw herself into a chair, and wept. What a fool she had been. Baptiste had not changed; he was exactly the same as he had always been. She had simply made the mistake of falling in love with an illusion.

She hated Laos, she hated the baby inside her, she hated her father for being right; and most of all, she hated her husband.

Amicu's was a single garishly lit room, scattered with school desks that served as tables. Journalists in crumpled shirts, American pilots with gold jewellery, and members of the town's Corsican *milieu* in their white tropical suits, lounged in wicker chairs. There was a small bar in the corner where the nightclub's owner, Madame Lola – no one imagined for a moment that this was her real name – propped herself on a stool every night in a sequinned cocktail dress, and got herself lousy drunk. The selection of music was limited, scratchy Edith Piaf and Maurice Chevalier 78s played on an ancient phonogram. After the first bottle of pastis Lola would regale the room with stories of her life, which seemed to consist of bedding a succession of French generals all over Indochina.

But neither Madame Lola nor Edith Piaf was the reason Amicu's attracted such a large crowd of Westerners every evening. There were few other places to go. Only two other establishments in Vientiane stayed open until the early hours of the morning: one was The White Rose, Amicu's only genuine competition; the other was a place called The Vieng Ratray, which was Lao for 'Pleasant Retreat'. It was owned by General Rattakone, filled with dowdy Bangkok hostesses and stank like an Indonesian urinal. It was more commonly known by the nickname the city's foreign community had given it: The Green Latrine.

Amicu's had won a certain reknown for its House Special, which consisted of oral sex in a curtained cubicle in the rear of the club. For two dollars, plus a complimentary drink, a man could surrender to the expert attentions of one of the taxi girls Madame Lola kept on the premises. It was said that each of the girls had been coached in the arcane art by Madame Lola herself, but no one had yet been drunk or desperate enough to test the theory.

Among the American CAT pilots the place was known as the Suck and Soda.

Rocco Bonaventure was playing *vingt et un* with Gilbert Pépé and another of his pilots, Marius Nicoli. When he saw Baptiste he collected his winnings from the centre of the table, picked up his glass of cognac and walked over to join him at the bar.

'Baptiste. How was your trip?'

'Milk run,' he said. A milk run: an hour flying back into the teeth of the monsoon, convinced he was going to die. But there was no point trying to explain dead reckoning and survey maps that were inaccurate up to twelve degrees and faulty drift gauges. Rocco Bonaventure was not a pilot and he could not understand.

Baptiste hoped he might get his cognac and escape to a corner before Madame Lola spotted him, but he was not quick enough. As soon as she saw him, she came over and smothered him in an enormous embrace, leaving a smear of lipstick on his cheek. He was overpowered by the taint of cheap scent and sweat and alcohol. 'I could make you so happy, Baptiste,' she growled.

Baptiste was accustomed to these pawings from Madame Lola. He tried to pull away.

'Free drinks for a month if you come in the back room with me.'

Bonaventure was laughing. Perhaps he put the old cow up to this, thought Baptiste.

'I'm a good fuck,' she whispered, 'you can ask anybody.'

'I'm tired, Lola.'

'Did I ever tell you about the time I fucked three generals at Dien Bien Phu? The first two were killed by shrapnel, but the third one I fucked to death myself!' She cackled and tried to kiss him again.

This time he managed to twist away. He pulled Bonaventure towards a table in the gloomiest corner of the room.

'*Elle est cul de vache!*' Baptiste muttered under his breath.

Bonaventure said nothing. He put a booted foot on one of the school desks and grinned. 'You only play hard to get because your father-in-law is here, Baptiste.'

'I'd rather cut it off.'

Bonaventure raised an eyebrow. I wonder what he knows? thought Baptiste.

'So tell me about the trip?' Bonaventure said. 'You were gone nearly three days. I was starting to worry.'

'About me?'

'About my opium.'

'I was stranded near Sam Thong for two days by the monsoon. Another half an hour and there was no way I could have landed her. I would be a dead man right now.'

Bonaventure shrugged this off as an incidental. 'But you made the drop on the Vietnam side?'

Baptiste nodded. 'Your opium's safe.'

Bonaventure patted his hand, and signalled the little Lao bartender for two more cognacs.

'I met Jean-Marie Pepin,' said Baptiste.

'I thought he had gone back to Bangkok or somewhere.'

'Mittard brought him back. He says he's buying another Cessna.'

Bonaventure looked as if he was about to spit. 'Buying another plane?'

'Jean-Mar' must have had two or three hundred kilos in the back of his Cessna.'

134

'Mittard! His father was a peasant. They say his mother was a mountain goat.' He drained his cognac and slammed the empty glass on the table.

So, it seemed their heavyweight protection would not be enough after all. Baptiste had been landing his shipments in drop zones in the Vietnamese Central Highlands that were heavily guarded by Vietnamese Air Force commandos. Mittard had been frozen out. But he had persevered and was now not only able to compete but to prosper. Just the previous week Baptiste had learned that Mittard had dumped twenty-nine watertight tin crates, wrapped in a buoyant life belt, to a waiting Vietnamese fishing boat in the Gulf of Siam. Inside each of the crates was twenty kilos of raw opium. Such methods were difficult and there were greater margins of risk and cost. But from that one successful drop Mittard had made over fifty thousand dollars.

'They're starting to eat into our profits,' said Baptiste.

Bonaventure nodded. 'What do you think I should do, Baptiste?'

He tried to conceal his surprise. It was the first time Bonaventure had ever included him in his decision making. 'Can the Vietnamese help us?' he said, remembering what Bonaventure had done to him a few years before.

'Mittard's too careful. He never lands inside Vietnam these days.'

'Perhaps the Americans . . .' began Baptiste.

Bonaventure looked up. 'Talk of the devil and one of his closest friends appears,' he muttered.

Baptiste looked around. It was Gerry Gates, the American he had seen with Petrovski on the last day at Phong Savan. Officially he was within Laos under the auspices of something called the Program Evaluation Office but Baptiste assumed he was some sort of spy. The country was full of them these days.

Laos had been on a knife edge these last two years. After the debacle with Kong Le, world attention had focused on the country. Eisenhower had taken the view that if Laos fell to the Pathet Lao, all of Indochina would follow. He called it the Domino Theory.

After Phong Savan the communists had swept southwards

towards Vientiane. Baptiste and Bonaventure, together with the rest of the Corsican community, had been ready to flee across the border to Thailand. It was Kennedy, the newly elected US President, who had saved them, putting the US Marines at Okinawa on alert to intervene; meanwhile, five hundred Marines at Udorn, just across the Thai border, had climbed into helicopters ready to ship out and defend the Lao capital.

The crisis had been averted but ever since the American presence in Laos had increased dramatically. For a long time Baptiste was unsure how to feel about the Americans; he finally decided on a mixture of gratitude and contempt. After all, they had saved the opium business, and not only by staring down the communists.

After Kong Le took Phong Savan in 1961, he had linked up with the Pathet Lao and the Americans could no longer use the Plain of Jars as a staging area. Instead they had carved a number of airfields in the surrounding mountains in order to make rice and ammunition drops to the Hmong. But Air Laos also used these same airstrips to pick up their opium, and keep the trade alive; a trade United States advisers like Gates found it politically expedient to ignore.

'Gerry!' Bonaventure raised a hand and beckoned the American to their table.

Gates ambled over. He was an unremarkable man, Baptiste thought, except for his eyes; it was the thing Baptiste remembered best about him from that day at Phong Savan. His gaze seemed to take in everything in the room, in an instant; the eyes of a man walking point in the jungle.

'Come and sit down,' Bonaventure said in English, playing the expansive host. 'What are you drinking?'

'Cognac and soda, thanks, Rocco.'

'Have you met my son-in-law, Baptiste Crocé?'

'Face is familiar.' They shook hands. Gates' grip was strong and dry. Yes, he remembers me, Baptiste decided.

'Monsieur Gates is with the American Embassy,' Bonaventure was saying. 'Gerry, tell me again, what is it you are doing in Laos?'

'I'm here advising the Meo on agriculture,' Gates said.

136

Bonaventure threw back his head and roared. 'Ah, you people are wonderful! What a sense of humour!'

'I'm glad you think so, Rocco,' Gates said, but his expression did not change.

'We were just discussing the difficulties of the opium business.'

'I have nothing to say on that subject, gentlemen.'

'But it is very important for you,' Bonaventure pressed.

'Not in the least. Because the United States government has chosen to look the other way while you people conduct your affairs, does not mean the United States government approves.'

Baptiste wondered how far Bonaventure would press his point. Theirs was a symbiotic relationship, a marriage of convenience. Baptiste, like the rest of Vientiane, knew that Gates and his fellow advisers in the United States Embassy were not advising the tribes on agriculture but in guerilla warfare, using them as a proxy army to fight the Pathet Lao.

'It's a question of priorities,' Gates added.

'Exactly. You see, I have a small problem. It is about one of my competitors. No, "competitor" is too grand a word. I shall not dignify him this way. He is a tick on the rump of a buffalo.'

'You mean Mittard?'

'You see? My description was adequate.'

Gates shook his head. 'I know what you're going to ask me, Rocco, and the answer is still the same. I can't stop him using those airfields.'

Bonaventure discarded his air of bonhomie, and his grey eyes glittered with anger for the first time. 'I have done everything you ask me. I use my contacts in Saigon and Bangkok to give you reports on the politics there. What else do you want from me?'

Baptiste looked up in surprise. It was the first time he had heard of this part of his father-in-law's business.

'And we appreciate everything you've done, Rocco. You know that. And I don't have to tell you, because I'm sure you realise, that the help you give us is in both our interests. But Mittard's been helping us too. I repeat, I can't stop him using those air strips. Our government built them, sure. But

137

they now belong to the government of Laos. If you got a beef, maybe you better take it up with Rattakone.'

'How much?' Bonaventure said.

Gates shook his head and finished his drink. 'I'd like to help you, Rocco, but I can't. Look, all my government cares about is keeping the reds out of this place. To do that we need the Meo, we need to keep them happy. We've got to get their opium out, and we've got to get guns in. We don't want any part of a vendetta. I'd be happy to take your money, but it's not our call. You go and see the General.'

Baptiste knew Gates was right. All airports in Laos were classified as military terminals and permission to take off and land required a written order from the Royal Laotian Army. Opium runs were considered *requisitions militaires* – military charters – and had to be approved by Laotian High Command. For such permissions Bonaventure had to reach an understanding with the appropriate people in the government.

'Rattakone already has our money,' said Bonaventure.

'I'm sure he'll take a little more. But my guess is if you start a bidding war for exclusive rights, like the arrangement you've got on the other side of the border, it's going to start eating right into your profits.' Gates stood up. 'Thanks for the drink, Rocco.'

He left.

Bonaventure turned back to Baptiste. His face was dark with fury. 'Never trust anyone who can't be bought,' he hissed under his breath.

'Perhaps we should talk to Rattakone.'

'It won't do us any good.'

Baptiste drained his glass. 'I'd better be going home too.'

Bonaventure stood up, put an arm on his son-in-law's shoulder and escorted him outside. Two taxi girls stood in the shadows, smoking cigarettes. They whistled and cat-called, but Baptiste ignored them.

'How are things at home?' Bonaventure asked him.

'Fine.'

'You don't seem sure.'

'I told you, everything's fine.'

'She is a headstrong girl, Baptiste. But she is also my daughter. Take care of her.'

The rain was driving down in grey sheets. Baptiste ran through the ankle-deep water to his car and jumped in. The canvas hood was leaking and there was a pool of water in the driver's seat. Damn this country! The inside of the car smelled of mould. Everything rotted here, everything.

He drove slowly through the rain, and when he was out of sight of Amicu's he doubled back and headed for The Green Latrine. He needed his ego and his body massaged for a little while by expert hands. Flying in the monsoon season made him tense. It was all very well for Noelle to complain, but she didn't understand that it was different for him. To a man, sex was like food and water, and it was hard to raise much appetite when she was the size of a house. Their life would probably return to normal when the baby was born.

But he would have to be careful. He could not afford to lose Noelle. There was an empire resting on it.

29

The rain had stopped, but the night swelled with the boom and tonk of frogs, and the mosquitoes whined outside the netting. Noelle felt too heavy to sleep. She was naked under the single, thin sheet. The child was awake too, and the stirring of life inside her surprised her and made her gasp.

She heard him enter. The door closed gently, but she could smell him in the room, a cocktail of whisky and tobacco and sex. She could make out his silhouette in the moonlight. He fell against a rattan chair and slumped into it.

He undressed quickly and clumsily and staggered into bed.

'You smell of another woman,' she said.

'I did not mean to wake you.' His voice was hoarse from cigarettes and drink.

'How dare you get into my bed when you've just climbed off some taxi girl?'

He lay down. 'No, I just went to Amicu's to see Rocco, I swear it.'

Noelle rolled on to her side. The effort made her wince. She put her feet in the small of his back and pushed. Baptiste, caught by surprise, rolled heavily onto the teak floorboards.

'Sleep in the other room, *cochon!*'

There was a new edge to his voice in the darkness. 'Don't ever do that again,' he growled.

She kicked out once more with her heel. It connected with satisfying force against something soft. Baptiste gave a moan of pain. Encouraged, Noelle rolled out of bed and kicked out in the darkness, again and again.

'Noelle!' He caught her leg and brought her down. She fell heavily to the floor, screaming.

'My God, I'm sorry! The baby! Are you all right?' he said.

'Get out!'

'Did I hurt you?'

She felt his hand on her shoulder and lashed out with her fist, felt it hit something hard, his shoulder or the muscles of his chest. It hurt her hand. 'Get out!'

'I still love you, Noelle,' he whispered. When she did not answer he got up and padded out of the room. The door closed gently behind him.

Noelle lay on the bare boards and listened to the rain. She heard her own breath sawing in her chest. I wish you were dead, she thought. I wish you had died that day over Phong Savan and then at least I would have the bittersweet memory of you. Surely grief is better than betrayal?

The child kicked again, imitating her own fury. She put a hand on her stomach and whispered to still him, as if he could hear her, as if he could understand. And then the rage seeped away, and she was tired, too tired to rise from the floor, and the rain began again. She listened to it drip from the eaves, and wept.

'I tried to warn you about him,' said her father.

Noelle angrily brushed at her eyes. 'You were right. That is little consolation to me now. What am I going to do?'

Bonaventure shrugged his shoulders. 'What do you want to do?'

They were on the verandah of Bonaventure's villa. Mist wreathed the swooping roofs of the surrounding temples. In the distance pirogues slid along the coffee brown river like water beetles. In the garden a flamboyant seed exploded with a crack like gunfire.

Tao Koo brought them a pot of hot tea and poured a little into two handleless porcelain cups.

'I love him, Papa.'

'If you cannot change him – and you won't – and you still love him, then you will have to put up with him. After all, *mon petit chou*, what did you expect?'

He's right. What did I expect? Noelle asked herself. I was utterly disarmed by his charm. Did I really think that after he

141

married me he would become a different creature, stop chasing women, stop drinking? Yes, I did. Which only proves what a fool I was.

But then women love in a different way to men. 'I have his child in my belly, Papa. I could not leave him even if I wanted to.'

'And you don't want to, so why talk about it?' Bonaventure leaned towards her, and the granite of his face softened. 'Look, little princess,' he said, using his childhood name for her, 'I will talk to him for you. But what can you do? A snake sheds his skin, but he remains a serpent. Even if he tried to change, I don't think he could.'

'I have been so stupid,' Noelle murmured, sipping some of the hot, green tea.

'How is the baby?' Bonaventure said, over the strained silence that followed.

'I feel like a sweating lump of dough, Papa. I cannot sleep at night, my clothes are always soaked, and I cannot get out of a chair without preparing for the effort five minutes before.'

'It will be over soon.'

'And then what? Somehow I cannot see my Baptiste as a dedicated father.'

'Well, for myself, I was never the best.'

She stared hard at him. Her eyes appeared luminous in the green-grey light. 'You never behaved this way.'

'There was a war. It was more difficult then.'

'There is war here. It never slows Baptiste.'

Bonaventure sighed and passed a hand over his eyes. 'Oh, *ma petite*, what can I say to you?'

'I had better go home. I need to rest. I am always tired these days.'

'Of course. I'll have Tao Koo drive you home.'

He helped her out of the chair. For a moment he was close and she kissed him softly on the cheek. 'I should have listened to you.'

'Why? You never did before.'

She gave him a rueful smile and left.

* * *

After she had gone, Bonaventure lit a cigarette. *Ma petite Noelle!* Too late, you realise you should have listened to me! Baptiste is a fool. A man should keep his house in order. If he wants to sleep with his taxi girls, he should at least learn to be discreet.

Bonaventure loved his daughter and did not want to see her hurt. Of course, a man was still a man, but he would not have his daughter humiliated this way. He would talk to Baptiste, resolve this somehow. He himself had had mistresses, of course, while Noelle's mother was alive, but he had never flaunted them in her face, as Baptiste had done to Noelle.

But his anger was tempered with a dawning respect; while Baptiste was a less then ideal son-in-law, he had proved a very able lieutenant as well as a good pilot. In the last few months he had shown that he could negotiate with the Chinese traders and the Hmong, and knew how to charm the Americans.

In fact, Rocco Bonaventure grudgingly admitted to himself, Baptiste Crocé might yet prove a worthy heir.

Air Laos was now making hundreds of flights a month, dropping supplies to troops in the mountains, ferrying Lao and American officials between Vientiane and Luang Prabang, and of course trading in opium. Bonaventure ferried shipments to Rivelini in Bangkok, and had access to buyers in Saigon, through Tran van Li, which his competitors did not have. Demand was fuelling a revival in opium production from the tribes who grew it, and prospects looked bright.

There was every prospect that Noelle and his new grandchild would inherit a fortune, and they would need a strong man to caretake that inheritance after he was gone.

But Baptiste's fondness for women and drink might well prove a fatal weakness. Besides, to be accepted in the *milieu* required a certain toughness of character. *Un vrai monsieur* needed on occasion to do things that ordinary men shrank from, and he wondered if Baptiste Crocé had the stomach for it.

Perhaps they would soon find out.

30

Noelle was resting in her bedroom, the blinds drawn, when she heard the sound of an aircraft passing very low overhead. It banked and came around again. This time she thought it was going to land on the roof. She dragged herself up from the bed and went out on to the balcony.

The servants were in the garden staring up at the sky. Noelle, squinting against the glare, looked in the direction they were pointing. It was a twin-engined Beechcraft, one of her father's. As it banked over the Mekong, she saw the yellow and black tiger decal on the tailplane. A long banner streamed behind it, and in large red letters were the words:

'*Noelle, je t'aime. Pardonne-moi.*'

Noelle, I love you. Forgive me.

She put her knuckles to her mouth, angry and embarrassed. Typical of him. One lunatic gesture and he thinks everything is going to be all right.

The Beechcraft started to climb, silhouetted against the mountains and the lead-grey cumulus banking in the sky. The engines whined in protest as Baptiste brought the nose up. What's he doing? Noelle thought. If he's not careful he's going to stall.

A casual flip of the wings and the Beechcraft began to dive towards the ground. Her knuckles were white on the balcony rail. *Bastard!* You're showing off.

He cut power to the engines. Bring up the nose, she found herself praying. For the love of the Virgin, bring up the nose!

The Beechcraft dropped, the white banner streaming behind. He's not going to do it, she thought. He's left it too late.

Please, Baptiste. Don't do this.

The nose started to come up.

Too late.

He was out of sight below the coconut palms beyond Sri Chiangmai, on the other side of the river.

She waited for the explosion, the black mushroom cloud that would confirm what she already knew. She felt a keening sense of loss she had not expected. Yes, I do still love him, she thought. Bastard that he is, I still love him.

The Beechcraft appeared again, its silver belly flashing in the sun. The pitch of the engines had increased to a frantic mosquito whine, as Baptiste took her into a barrel roll. As he recovered from the manoeuvre he roared towards the villa, passing so low overhead that Noelle involuntarily ducked.

'Idiot!' she shouted at the retreating shadow of the Beechcraft. *'Idiot!'*

Jean-Marie was standing with a group of CAT pilots when Baptiste landed at Wattay. 'Crazy motherfucker,' one of the pilots breathed. Coming from one of the Air America men, that was high praise indeed, Jean-Marie thought. Bonaventure was there too, standing beside his black limousine, his face beet-red with rage.

'Does he know how much that machine is worth?' he shouted. 'That worthless bastard. *Espèce de con!'*

The Beechcraft splashed down and began to taxi across. But Bonaventure's temper would not wait. He marched across the mud to intercept. He pulled open the cockpit door while the Beechcraft was still moving. Baptiste braked to a halt and the two men continued their argument right there under the starboard wing.

A few minutes later Bonaventure jumped back in his car and roared away.

'He was really pissed off,' Baptiste said later, when he saw Jean-Marie. He gave a cheery wave to the American pilots sheltering under the eaves of their operations hut, smoking cigarettes. With the eye patch and the bottle of red wine he was reputed to take along on every flight, they thought he was as crazy as they were. They called him the Red Baron.

'Rocco thought you weren't coming out of the loop.'

'He was worried about me. I'm his favourite son-in-law.'

'He doesn't give a shit about you. Just his investment.' Jean-Marie shook his head and spat into the rain.

'I know what I'm doing.'

'You misjudged that roll. I didn't think you were going to get out of it. Anyway, what was that all about?'

'Just call me an incurable romantic.'

'The banner was romantic. Everything else was insane. Those things aren't built for acrobatic flying.'

'I wanted to show Noelle how much she would miss me if I wasn't around.'

'She'll never know how close she was to finding out.' The remains of the banner hung in tatters from the tailplane. It had been whipped to shreds by tree branches. 'That was nearly you.'

'Nearly is perfect. Nearly is touching death with your fingers, and moving out of reach before he can close his fist around your throat.' Baptiste gave him his go to hell smile, powder white teeth in a burned mahogany face. He pulled the Gitanes from his shirt pocket and lit one, slapping Jean-Marie on the shoulder. 'Want to give me a lift back into town?'

Oh, he looked so sure. But the hand that held the cigarette was trembling just a little, enough to make Jean-Marie wonder. Baptiste lost more than just an eye at Phong Savan, he thought. He lost his judgement also. A pilot with one eye had a diminished spatial awareness, Baptiste would never pass a medical for a legitimate airline. There was more than simply family ties between him and the Bonaventure family now. If he lost Noelle, Baptiste Crocé had no career, and no future.

Baptiste was disappointed. He had expected to find Noelle on the verandah waiting for him when he got back. Instead, the *boyesse* told him she was in the bedroom, resting. The weight of the baby had tired her, she said.

He found her lying on her back in the darkened room, in a thin cotton shift, her hands resting on her stomach. She appeared to be asleep.

'Noelle?'

She opened one eye. 'Is that you Baptiste?'

146

He felt a flowering of anger, frustration, bewilderment. It was not possible that she had not seen. He stood beside the bed and watched her go through the pantomime of waking.

'Yes, it's me,' he said.

'What are you doing home? Are the brothels all closed?'

For the love of God! 'How long have you been asleep?'

'I don't know. Why?'

'Half an hour? An hour? What?'

'Why all these questions? Is it important?' She frowned and sat up on one elbow. Her breasts were heavy and swollen under the straining cotton of the garment and for a moment he felt a familiar stirring. But she was right, she was as big as a whale.

'Have you been outside at all this morning?' he snapped.

She shook her head.

'The servants did not come to wake you?'

'I told Tao Koo I was not to be disturbed.'

He wanted to hit her. Instead he turned and went out again, slamming the door. All right then. If that was how she wanted to treat him, he would see if any of the taxi girls were working this morning.

Noelle heard the Packard scream out of the driveway towards Vientiane. She threw her pillow at the wall and sobbed with frustration. Could she not have relented just for a moment? Her stupid pride! Was it so hard to forgive him? Why did she have to punish him for all those qualities that had attracted her to him from the very beginning?

And why did he have to punish her for carrying his child?

Damn him. Let him crawl. If he really wanted her it would have to be on her terms.

31

Saigon

Sammy Chen lived in the north-west of the city, on a wide boulevard that linked Saigon to its ugly twin, Cholon. Behind the high, barbed wire-topped walls was a short concrete driveway lined with hibiscus bushes and pruned rose trees.

The house was substantial, solid brick with a red-tiled roof and upturned eaves. A pierced breeze-block screen shielded part of the verandah, in the current Saigon fashion.

This was the first time Rocco Bonaventure had met Sammy away from the Trung Mai Hotel, with its peeling paint and threadbare Chinese carpets. Logic and reputation had told him that Sammy Chen was not a poor man, but this was the first time the Chinese banker had allowed him a glimpse behind the mask. Traditional Chinese did not favour showy exhibitions of wealth. Money invited thieves and beggars.

A white-jacketed servant met Bonaventure at the door and led him inside. The interior of the house was cool, as expensive and tasteful as the Trung Mai was run-down and tawdry. There were silk carpets, fine lacquerware displayed in a walnut and glass cabinet, a table carved from Burmese teak and inlaid with mother of pearl.

Sammy appeared, wearing his usual uniform of crumpled white shirt and baggy, western-style suit trousers. He looked exactly as he did when emerging from his dingy office in his Cholon hotel, but in these surroundings he looked relaxed instead of shabby. The gold eye tooth flashed as he smiled.

'Welcome to my humble house, Mr Bon Van Chao.'

'My pleasure to meet you again, Monsieur Chen.'

'Please, come and sit.' Sammy led the way to a small room at the back of house. There was an antique wooden platform in the middle of the room, and Sammy and Bonaventure sat down on either side, their legs curled beneath them. Sammy clapped his hands for *yum cha*, and the servants poured them green tea and brought plates of candied fruits and lotus seed buns. From the open doors came the tonk-tonk of a goldbeater bird.

Bonaventure's business relationship with Sammy Chen went back to the days of French colonial rule. Despite his unprepossessing appearance, Sammy had become the leading opium trader in Cholon after the fall of the Binh Xuyen.

Sammy was a chiu chao from the Swatow region of southern China. The chiu chao spoke their own guttural dialect of Mandarin, and had the reputation of being ruthless and vicious. Wherever they went they quickly assumed a dominant position in local commerce. Some people called them the Jews of the East; except that, unlike the Jews, they brought muscle with them. The chiu chao triads were some of the most feared among Chinese communities the world over. To be pre-eminent among the chiu chao was to be both a great entrepreneur and a ruthless gangster.

Like the pleasant, plump little Chinese in front of him.

They made polite conversation as they sipped tea, and Sammy inquired politely after the health of Bonaventure's family. It was just after noon, and Sammy's houseboy brought *dim sum*; bowls of rice dumplings filled with shrimp and vegetables, and morsels of barbecued pork.

'The opium harvest is good this year?' Sammy asked him.

'I believe it is,' Bonaventure answered cautiously.

'I do not ask for myself. I have a brother in Hong Kong. He wishes perhaps to sell some opium for himself. But he has difficulty getting good supplies.'

'Hong Kong?' He must have triad connections there, Bonaventure thought. His brother might be an actual family member, or he might be referring obliquely to a colleague from his own triad.

'You think you can guarantee twenty ton, okay?'

Bonaventure tried to keep the excitement out of his voice. 'To Hong Kong? I cannot fly it there directly.'

149

'I have another cousin in Bangkok. One hundred per cent reliable. If you can deliver to him in Bangkok, he can deliver to Hong Kong.'

Bonaventure pretended to think about this. Bangkok! He already moved over a ton of base – equivalent to ten tons of raw opium – into Thailand for Rivelini, who transferred it to ocean freighters for members of a Corsican syndicate in Marseille.

'My cousin has trawler boat,' Sammy went on. 'Many. Maybe you prefer to make delivery to his boat in Gulf of Siam?'

Bonaventure experienced a frisson of alarm. What was Sammy trying to tell him? 'On the same terms, I assume?' he said.

Sammy Chen appeared to think about this. A little juice from the pork ran down his chin. 'I talk to Mittard. He says he can do for two thousand baht a ton less than you.'

Mittard! That was why he wanted the second plane, another pilot, he was trying to chip away at Bonaventure's market! He actually wanted to challenge him! Even if Bonaventure was able to fend him off, a price war would still bite deep into his profits. He imagined snapping Mittard's neck like a chicken, but instead he managed a cool smile, and a slight bow of his head. 'Sammy, I'm sure we can do better on price than Monsieur Mittard.'

Damn his soul to hell.

32

Vientiane

Bonaventure had summoned Baptiste immediately on his return
from Saigon, and now they sat alone on the balcony of his villa
with a bottle of pastis on the table between them.

The silence was strained. Bonaventure was almost taci-
turn and Baptiste wondered what the hell he wanted. He lit
one of his Gitanes and waited.

'How are things between you and Noelle?' Bonaventure asked
him, finally.

'Fine,' Baptiste said, wishing the old goat would mind his
own business.

'That is not what Noelle has told me.'

He tried to hide his annoyance. 'What happens in our home
should be our affair.'

'Not when your wife is the daughter of Rocco Bonaventure,
mon vieux. Now, do you want to tell me what is wrong?'

'There's nothing wrong! Nothing we cannot put right between ourselves. If we are left alone.'

Bonaventure raised one grey brush of an eyebrow and sipped
his pastis. 'Very well,' he said.

'How was Saigon?' Baptiste asked him, swiftly turning the
tide of the conversation.

'Worrying.'

Baptiste frowned. So this was why the old bear was in such
a lousy mood. 'What went wrong?'

'It's Mittard. He is starting to get on my nerves.'

'What can we do? The Americans don't care, and Mittard has
too many connections in the government here. But we still have

more planes, more resources. We'll have to squeeze him out.'

'That will take time, and it will cost me money. Something you have to learn, Baptiste. A good war doesn't last long, and you have to make the most of it. I don't intend to waste this opportunity, fighting off competitors by discounting to all my customers. Like I was a grocer or something.'

'Mittard's a minor irritation. Like a mosquito. He doesn't deserve our attention.'

'Mosquitoes carry fever. This mosquito we have to do something about. Permanently.'

Baptiste could feel Bonaventure's eyes on him. The rain stopped as suddenly as it had started. In the twilight of the storm Bonaventure's eyes assumed a strange luminosity.

Baptiste was uncomfortable with the direction the conversation had taken. He kept his silence.

'You know, I was wondering about you,' Bonaventure said.

'Wondering what?'

'Whether you have the guts for this business. I know you have courage. You have demonstrated that clearly enough. But that isn't what I'm talking about. In this business you need something quite different. There are men who can fight a tiger but won't wring a chicken's neck for their dinner. You know what I'm talking about?'

Baptiste felt sticky and hot, his own sweat mixing with the juice the monsoon squeezed out of him. 'We don't need to kill him.'

'You can think of a better way?'

He was silent.

'We can fix their plane,' Bonaventure was saying. 'A little *plastique* should do it.'

'Mittard will buy another one.'

'Not if he's inside it when it blows up.'

Baptiste lit a cigarette. The smoke tasted foul to his lungs and he suddenly had a headache. 'You can't just kill a man like that,' he said, and even as the words left his mouth he knew how ridiculous they would sound to *un vrai monsieur* like Rocco Bonaventure.

'Are you saying you can't do it?'

'He has a wife and child, for God's sake.' The previous year Mittard had married a Lao girl, a niece of Rattakone himself; another reason he had been able to operate so successfully in Laos.

'You're breaking my heart, Baptiste. If I collected all the tears I have seen in my lifetime, I would have enough to start my own ocean.'

Baptiste looked away. *Merde alors.* Oh, there were many things for which the devil would one day congratulate Baptiste Crocé, but murder wasn't yet one of them. He didn't think he could do it. He knew he didn't want to.

'Will you do it?'

'Why me, Rocco?'

'Because I want to see what you're made of. If you don't do it I shall encourage Noelle to seek a divorce. She will not need much persuasion right now. You really have made a big mess of things there, *mon vieux.*'

The rain began again. Baptiste stared at the garden. He felt like a man who had run down a blind alley with a pack of baying dogs at his heels. There was only one escape, and that was straight ahead, over a high wall topped with broken glass.

'All right,' he mumbled. But he promised himself that he would find some way out.

33

Noelle had Chao prepare a special dinner. There was carp and lemon grass soup with mushrooms, a freshwater stingray, chicken fried with ginger, yellow wheat noodles, spicy green papaya salad, and to finish sticky rice in coconut milk cooked in bamboo. The meal was washed down with cold bottles of Tiger beer that Bonaventure had had flown in from Singapore.

Afterwards they sat on the verandah with a bottle of Johnny Walker. Noelle mixed hers with soda water and lime juice.

Dinner had been a strained affair with Noelle and Jean-Marie making all the conversation while Baptiste sat in gloomy silence, getting slowly drunk. He had been acting strangely ever since her father had got back from Saigon. He seemed depressed, which was not like him at all. Baptiste Crocé was many things, good and bad, but he rarely surrendered to melancholy or introspection. She wondered if his mood had been inspired by their marital problems, or if it was something her father had said.

Jean-Marie was plainly embarrassed and had tried to paper over the long silences with nervous talk.

'That was a wonderful dinner,' he said, for the third time.

'It's good to see you back in Vientiane again. Isn't it, Baptiste?'

'Of course.'

Noelle heard the moment's hesitation in her husband's voice. But Jean-Marie shrugged it off. He turned to her and said lightly: 'I have begun to think he would be happier if I was flying for Air Laos and not the competition.'

Baptiste did not respond.

'You know, you shouldn't expect to have the field to yourself,

Baptiste. Everyone wants a piece of the action. That's natural. Besides, there's enough opium for everyone to get out with money in their pockets in the end.'

Baptiste gave Jean-Marie a pitying look, as if he was a particularly slow-witted child. 'Perhaps,' he said almost sulkily. 'But no one knows how long this is going to last.'

'Looks to me as if the Americans are here to stay. They won't let the communists take over here. They think they're fighting the Third World War.'

'He's right,' Noelle said, 'the Americans think they invented Laos.' Privately she despised them, aggressive people with loud shirts and too much money. They had created a minor boom in the local economy; the population had now swelled to seventy thousand people, her father no longer owned the only Mercedes Benz in the capital, and there was even Scotch whisky and French perfumes in the shops.

'I miss the old days, you and me, flying together,' Baptiste said to Jean-Marie, his mind obviously drifting elsewhere. 'Those days weren't as complicated.'

'Everything changes,' Jean-Marie said simply.

'Not always for the best.'

'You're so gloomy tonight,' Noelle said. 'Poor Jean-Marie. You invite him here for dinner and then make him depressed.'

Baptiste ignored her. 'Why don't you ask Rocco for a job?' he said to Jean-Marie.

Jean-Marie laughed, caught off guard by this unexpected proposal. 'Why would I want to do that?'

'It might be a good idea to try, that's all.'

'Mittard pays me well enough. I get twenty an hour. I happen to know Rocco only pays his guys fifteen.' He shook his head. 'Anyway, Rocco has enough pilots. If he wants more, he knows where to find me.'

'I could fix things for you.'

'Why?'

'Old time's sake.'

Jean-Marie shook his head. 'You're not making sense.'

'It's just you know what a bastard Rocco is. He might appreciate the gesture.'

'This is my father you're talking about,' Noelle said.

'Then you should know what a prick he can be better than any of us.'

There was an embarrassed silence. Baptiste lit a Gitane.

'You smoke too much,' said Noelle.

'And you remind me too much.'

Jean-Marie shifted uncomfortably. He finished his whisky and made a show of looking at his watch. 'I have to be going. I have an early flight to Pnom Penh in the morning.' He got up to leave.

'Think about what I said.'

'I've thought about it. The answer's still the same. Look, if you wanted me to be your partner again, Baptiste, that's different. But that's not what we're talking about, is it? It's nothing personal.'

'Yes, I know,' said Baptiste, and returned to a brooding silence.

Jean-Marie shot Noelle a look of bewilderment. She could only shrug her shoulders. Her husband's moods were a mystery to her as well.

'Goodbye, Baptiste. Thank you for dinner.'

Baptiste did not reply, did not even stand up. He continued to stare at the darkness, the whisky cradled in his lap.

It was Noelle who escorted Jean-Marie to the door. 'Is he okay?' he asked her at the front steps.

'How should I know? I'm only married to him.'

'I've never seen him like this.' He hesitated a moment. 'Is everything all right between you two?'

'We are going to have our first child any day. Why shouldn't we be deliriously happy?' She made no attempt to keep the bitterness from her voice.

'Don't give up with him. He's just a bit wild. Deep down he's a good guy.'

'How deep, Jean-Marie?'

'Keep digging,' he said, and gave her a rueful grin. 'I'm sure he loves you.'

'I feel like a barnacle. Just hanging on for the ride. Good night, Jean-Mar'. I'll keep you posted.'

'Good night, Noelle. And thank you for dinner.' He kissed

her hand and for a moment their eyes met and she saw the longing. Then he walked away into the dark.

Now why can't I fall in love with a man like that? she asked herself. Quiet, pleasant, courageous, honest. No. Within a week I would be bored to death. Me, I choose a bastard, and then hate him all along for being everything I knew he was when I met him.

C'est fou!

She put a hand to the roundness of her stomach and felt a kick inside. The child seemed to sense her moods and respond to them. Well, that's one good thing, she thought. You're not in the least like your father.

During the wet season the bonzes withdrew to their temples for a period of seclusion and meditation. The city no longer rang to the raucous din of the *bouns*. Today the wat was silent, the stoned courtyard glistened like a snake's back, wet with rain. The interior of the temple was cool, the golden Buddha statues glowed dully in the joss-heavy gloom.

The Blind Bonze was revered and celebrated across Laos. He had once placed his forecast of the winning number of the national lottery in a sealed envelope. When the envelope was opened, the forecast was found to be correct. Since then, he had adamantly refused to repeat the performance, even to augment the temple's funds.

The Blind Bonze knelt on a bamboo mat before a silver image of the Buddha, 'contemplating the Boddhi tree'. Chao, Noelle's *boyesse*, helped her to sit, her knees down to the side, and she bowed her head so that it was lower than the monk's, a gesture of respect. Then she waited for him to speak. She knew, from his reputation, that she might have to wait minutes or hours. Although he was blind, he would know she was there without her having to greet him.

His hands were held in front of him in a *wai*, a burning stick of incense gripped between the palms. Noelle was close enough to smell also the must of his saffron robe, the characteristic taint of the wet season. His eyes were white, sightless, the pupils turned back in his head, blind from birth.

157

The rain began again, pouring from the eaves in little waterfalls, flooding the courtyard. After a few minutes she felt herself growing impatient. She shifted uncomfortably. What are you doing here? she asked herself. You're a Catholic, a grown woman, a Westerner. Why are you bothering with all this superstitious nonsense? What is it you want to hear from this old monk? That Baptiste will change, that you will live happily ever after?

'Your son is growing big,' the bonze said suddenly in French. 'He will come soon.'

Noelle stared at him. How could he have known she was pregnant?

All she could think of to say was: 'The doctor says not for another month.'

The bonze inclined his head in respect to the doctor. The white sclera of his eyes returned their sightless gaze to the Buddha. 'You are angry,' he said softly.

'With my husband.'

'Yes. You are unsure what to do.'

Noelle experienced a prickle of fear. She was suddenly frightened and wanted to run away.

'There will be three men in your life,' the monk said. 'Two you will choose, one will choose you. Each will bring you a measure of pain, and a measure of joy. In the end you will have to choose between your blood and your heart.'

'And what should I do?' Noelle heard herself say.

'That is for you to decide.' The old monk started to shiver, as if he was very cold. 'There is only one way you can change your fate, as it is written on your forehead.'

Noelle stared at him. She was trembling now also. She had come here out of curiosity and desperation. But she had never expected this.

'One way?'

'If you abandon your baby son, a new fate will be written. That is the only way.'

Noelle tried to struggle to her feet. She didn't want to hear any more. But she couldn't rise without help, and called for Chao.

The bonze shuddered once more, and then he turned his head

towards her as if he could see her with the blank white moons of his eyes. 'Do not struggle,' he said.

Then he lowered his head and raised his hands in *wai* towards the silver Buddha.

Noelle took a handful of banknotes from her purse and dropped them on the bonze's mat. Then she looked around for Chao. 'Get me out of here,' she said.

She went home, feeling drained and damp and exhausted, and tried to sleep. But instead she stared into the dripping garden and heard the Blind Bonze whispering to her over and over again: '*If you abandon your baby son, a new fate will be written. That is the only way.*'

I will forget that I ever went there, she told herself. It's just superstition. One blind old man cannot know what lies in my future.

In the end you will have to choose between your blood and your heart.

34

Baptiste got to Wattay an hour after dawn. Already the clouds were piling up in the south-west, big white banks of vapour boiling up into the sky like steam from a volcano, building the thunderheads that would sweep over the city in the afternoon. The air was sticky warm, Baptiste's freshly ironed shirt already drenched with perspiration.

The Air America pilots were piling out of their bus, heading out to the STOLs and Cessnas that waited at one end of the pasture, or gathering in little groups outside the operations hut.

Baptiste's own Beechcraft was still outside its hangar, being loaded with the rice and ammunition Bonaventure had contracted to drop to a beleaguered Lao garrison in the mountains south of the Plain of Jars.

He parked the Packard under the trees. As he climbed out, he recognised Jean-Marie's ancient Buick a few yards away. He saw his blond hair by the old shed that served as a hangar for Mittard's Cessna.

He broke into a run. 'Jean-Marie!'

Jean-Marie was about to climb into the cockpit. He stopped and looked up. 'Baptiste?'

He was out of breath when he reached the Cessna and took a moment to recover.

'What's wrong?' Jean-Marie asked him.

'What are you doing?'

'What the fuck does it look like I'm doing?'

'Where's Mittard? I need to talk to him. I thought he was supposed to be flying to Pnom Penh this morning?'

'How do you know so much about our flight schedules?'

Baptiste shrugged, and Jean-Marie looked annoyed and puzzled.

'He's sick. Liver fluke. I told him he should be more careful what he eats.'

'*Putain!*'

'Look, what do you want, *ami*? I have to get going. If you want to see the boss, he's home in bed.' He slammed the cockpit door shut.

'Wait!' Baptiste shouted, and slapped on the perspex with the flat of his hand.

Jean-Marie waved him away. The Cessna's propellor turned slowly, then thrummed into life. Baptiste backed off.

'Well, fuck you, then!' he shouted, with sudden viciousness, and walked away.

The runway was still under several inches of water from the previous day's rains, and the Cessna threw a spray into the air behind it, like a speedboat. Finally it lifted into the air, the morning sun glinting on the fuselage. Baptiste shielded his eyes, watching it bank towards the south-east.

'I tried to warn you, Jean-Mar',' he said aloud.

There was a bright flash, a blossoming of orange flame, and the Cessna was gone. Baptiste watched a wing spiral into the Mekong through a cloud of trailing glycol vapour. The reverberation of the explosion washed through the trees with a sudden hot wind. There was silence over the aerodrome as the Air America pilots stopped their laughing chatter outside the operations hut to look up at the sky in deathly hush.

Baptiste turned and strode back to the Packard.

35

Baptiste avoided Amicu's. He did not want to mix with the *milieu* today, of all days, and he did not want to talk to Bonaventure.

The White Rose was in a side street off Vientiane's main strip, signposted with a wagon wheel. It was dank and dingy, even in the middle of the day, and its mainly American clientele – off-duty CAT pilots, spooks and diplomats, a few engineers – sat around in little booths or on wicker chairs, drinking *Bia Lao* or smoking pot. Upstairs were a few tiny cubicles furnished with nothing but single beds. At this time of the day there were no takers.

The girls in the White Rose were gentle and Baptiste found their efforts poignant in their lack of expertise. Any of them would perform an impromptu strip for one dollar. One of them – he knew her as Suzie – was desultorily trying to attract a little interest. 'You want to see show?' she said to him. She flipped off her bikini pants and took the Gitane out of his fingers. She placed it between the lips of her vagina and blew a smoke ring. She grinned up at him, inordinately pleased with her own performance.

Baptiste flipped a dollar note across the table and told her to go away. He returned his attention to the bottle of cognac on the table in front of him. He knew several of the men in the room, but they knew enough to leave him alone. There was an air of danger and disquiet in the bar, men talking in hushed voices, thinking about what had happened at Wattay that morning, brooding on their own mortality.

Thunder rolled around the mountains and through the open

door of the bar he saw the muted glimmer of sheet lightning behind the slate grey clouds.

He started when he saw Noelle. It was the last place he'd expected to see her. She moved awkwardly, the child sitting low in her stomach. Baptiste knew by her expression that she had heard the news.

She flopped on to the chair that Suzie had recently vacated. She was pale and exhausted, from grief, and from the journey on the *siclo* from the villa.

'Noelle. What are you doing here?'

'Tell me you didn't do it,' she whispered.

'All right. I didn't do it.'

He could not hold her eyes. He looked down at his glass, swallowed the powerful spirit, refilled it from the bottle, which was almost empty.

She sideswept his glass on to the floor. 'He was your friend!'

All conversation stopped and everyone in the bar turned and stared, even Suzie, and she couldn't understand a word.

'You're embarrassing me,' he said. 'Go home.'

'The mechanic who was working on his plane. Where is he?'

'I don't know.'

'How much did you pay him to put the *plastique* in Jean-Marie's plane?'

'You're not making any sense.'

'He was your friend, Baptiste!'

'Go home, Noelle.'

'I always knew you were a bastard. I never thought you were a murderer.'

'I said, go home!'

'What are you going to do? Hit me? Or perhaps you'll put some *plastique* under my bed tonight?'

He leaned towards her and whispered. 'You think it was all my idea?'

She searched his face. 'Papa?'

'Of course your precious papa! I'm just his lap dog! Isn't that what you always wanted? You told me we couldn't run away from him. Well, now you've got your way. I'm part of your cosy little family now!'

He watched her wilt. She must have worked this out by now. Had she really tried to convince herself that this was all his idea?

'You may be able to sleep with your conscience, but I can't,' she whispered. She stood up and looked around at the watching faces in the bar. 'A word of advice, boys. As soon as my husband leaves, you'd better check under your chairs for bombs.'

She ran outside. The monsoon had turned the streets to a slough of mud and garbage, chickens and water buffalo and pigs rooting in the drowned streets. There were splotches of red betel everywhere where the villagers hacked out their lungs in the steamy weather.

Baptiste ran after her, caught her arm and pulled her back. 'What the hell are you doing?'

'Let go of me!'

'Get in the car. You'll get soaked!'

'Let go!' She lashed out at him with her nails and he threw up a hand to protect his eyes. She slashed and kicked again, then pushed him with both hands. Off balance, groggy from too much cognac, he slipped in the mud and went down.

She stood over him, her hands on her hips, gasping from the effort. Her face was wet with tears. 'Stay away from me, Baptiste!'

'Crazy bitch!' he shouted. He staggered to his feet. Well, he had placed his bets, made his choices. Now he would have to live with them. Noelle struggled away from him through the cloying muddy street, with the curious waddling gait her pregnancy had imposed on her. For a moment he thought about going after her again, but his pride would not allow it. Inside he felt cold and barren. He went back into the White Rose and bought another bottle of cognac.

By the time Noelle reached her father's villa the rain was slamming down in sheets, the water ankle deep. Her hair was sodden and plastered over her face. She hammered on the door.

Tao Koo gaped at her. I must look a shocking sight, Noelle thought, my dress clinging around my swollen stomach, my feet covered in mud. Let them all be shocked, then. Let them all see. She brushed past him and stood in the middle of the entrance hall, water forming a little pool around her feet on the teak floorboards.

'Noelle!' Bonaventure ran down the stairs, his face white. 'Noelle, what's wrong? What has happened? My God, you are soaked through!'

'I've left him,' she said.

'Fetch towels,' he said to Tao Koo, who hurried off. Bonaventure came towards her and was about to take her in his arms when she backed away from him.

'I've left him,' she repeated.

'Baptiste?'

'He killed Jean-Marie. He was responsible.'

Bonaventure took a deep breath. 'I can't believe that,' he said.

'He said it was on your orders.'

Bonaventure raised his eyebrows in surprise.

Tao Koo returned with the towels. 'You'd better get out of those wet clothes,' Bonaventure said to his daughter. 'The baby...'

'It's true, isn't it?'

He returned his daughter's stare. 'I told him it was his responsibility to fix the problem. I didn't tell him how to do it.'

She wanted to believe him; all her life she had always believed him above the rumours she had heard.

Bonaventure took the towels from Tao Koo and sent him away with a nod of his head. When they were alone, he held out a hand towards her. 'Please, Noelle. You'll make yourself sick. You must get out of those wet clothes. You can use the bathroom upstairs.'

'I'm not going back to Baptiste.'

'We can talk about this later.'

'I mean it.'

'This is crazy talk. His child is waiting to be born.'

'It's no crazier than putting *plastique* on a friend's plane to get rid of competition.'

'Perhaps it was an accident. Who knows what happened out there this morning?'

He looked so calm, so reasonable, with his grey beard and his pressed white linen suit. Those concerned grey eyes. A rogue perhaps, but not a murderer. And yet...

'They say Mittard's mechanic is missing. They've looked for him all over Vientiane. The Cessna blew up in mid-air. In mid-air, Papa. Planes don't explode for no reason.'

'Of course they can. Mittard carried guns and grenades for the Americans and the Lao Army. Jean-Marie knew the risks.'

'Did he understand the risk of crossing Rocco Bonaventure?'

Suddenly he was angry. 'What do you take me for? A barbarian?' He threw the towels at her. 'I'm your father! How dare you talk to me this way!'

The pain hit her without warning. It was so sharp, so sudden, that it took her breath away. She collapsed against the wall and Bonaventure had to grab her to prevent her from falling. 'Noelle! What's wrong?'

For almost a minute she fought against the dizzying pain and could not answer him. Then the contraction passed, leaving her shocked and light-headed.

'Is it the baby?' he said.

The waters have not broken, she told herself. It couldn't be, not yet. 'I don't think so,' she said.

'Do you need a doctor?'

She shook her head. Her father's arms were around her, and she guiltily pushed herself away. 'I'll be all right.' The sudden pain had taken the fight and the anger out of her. She just felt tired and drained. When the baby comes, let it be a girl, she prayed. There's no man in the world worth a tinker's damn.

There were no more pains. She changed out of her wet clothes, and Bonaventure's *boyesse* brought her a dry blouse and a *pao sin*. She dried her hair but the ends still clung damply to her shoulders. Barefoot, and feeling ice calm, she padded along the hall and found her father in his study.

He was wearing the half moon spectacles that the doctor had prescribed for his failing eyesight. A thick leather bound ledger was open on the desk in front of him. He put down his pen and came around the desk as she entered.

'How are you feeling?'

'I'm all right,' she said, and ignored his fussing. She eased herself slowly into a chair.

He stood over her. 'That was a crazy thing to do.'

'I was angry.'

'You could have had the baby right there in the street!'

'Sit down, Papa. Please.'

Reluctantly he settled back behind his desk. 'You look terrible. I'm going to call the doctor.'

'I'm not made of porcelain. The local women have babies all the time and they don't have doctors fussing around them all the time.'

There was an uneasy silence.

'You are still angry with Baptiste?'

'A man is dead, Papa. Doesn't that matter to you?'

'I cannot afford to grow sentimental over someone I do not even know. Besides, one thing has nothing to do with the other. Do you really intend to leave Baptiste or are you just trying to frighten him?'

'I cannot stay married to a man like that.'

'Did he tell you he did it?'

'No.'

'There you are.'

'He said it was you.'

Bonaventure flinched. 'Little princess, I'm an old man. I don't care for money or material possessions no more. I just want to live to see my grandchildren play on my lawn. It was certainly no idea of mine to start causing trouble for myself in Vientiane by killing young pilots who are of no consequence to me anyway.'

She looked away, at the rain leaking down the verandah, drumming on the banana palms outside. Her eyes shone with tears, but she would not weep.

'If you leave him, where will you go?' Bonaventure asked her.

'Papa?'

'You think you can come and live here again, and everything will be as it was. I am afraid that is impossible. You married against my wishes. Even so, I am a good Catholic, and I do not believe in divorce. You will stay with your husband, and make the best of it. That is what marriage is.'

Noelle was silent for a long time. He wondered what she was thinking.

But finally, all she said was. 'Can you ask Tao Koo to drive me home, please?'

He kissed her on the forehead as she left, but she did not respond. He loved her, of course, but there was only so many ways that he would allow her to make a fool of him. Besides, Baptiste Crocé had proved his loyalty and he didn't want to lose him now.

36

Later, the doctor would tell her that it was the emotional stress, and not the physical exertion, that brought on such a violent and accelerated labour.

Noelle woke suddenly, the bed soaked. She felt between her legs, thought for a moment that she had wet herself. Then she realised what it was; her waters had broken. It was starting.

She felt beside her in the bed for Baptiste but he wasn't there.

She called for Chao, but realised it was later than she supposed and the servants had all gone to bed for the night. She lit the kerosene lantern beside her bed and struggled upright. And the first pain hit her.

It was bad, worse than the phantom that had struck her earlier in her father's house. It started as a crackling pain in her navel, like an electric shock, and stabbed around the small of her back, leaving her gasping and breathless. When it was over she lay helpless and panting for breath.

She had to get help.

She picked up the lantern and staggered outside. Cicadas that had somehow found their way inside the house from the garden banged into the light. A storm was raging around the house and somewhere a door crashed violently in the wind.

Noelle was terrified. Around and inside her the forces of nature were gathering, and she knew she had no control. There was nothing she could do to stop this now, nothing to prevent it tearing her apart if that was what it wanted.

Baptiste!

She remembered him standing on the bonnet of the Packard, holding the plastic roses. So beautiful, so irresistible, so dangerous. Our passions lead us to dark and lonely places, but then it's life that rushes us towards the consequences. I don't want his child any more, I don't want to endure this pain that's coming, and I don't want to be married any more to a murderer ...

Another contraction hit her and she cried aloud and sank on to the floor.

It was as if someone was prising her belly and her spine apart with a blunt lever. The pain racked her, a long wave of it, rising to a crest where she thought she would break, and she cried out again helpless and terrified. When she thought she could stand no more it set her down, fragile and trembling, on its far side. In her soul she could already feel the next trough forming.

She staggered to the back door, tumbled out into the black pitching night. Rain whipped her face. The servants' quarters were in darkness. She called for Chao but her voice was drowned by the hammering of the rain.

The palms and frangipani trees snapped like whipcord, black bats tumbled and flapped and darted in the teeth of the storm.

She beat on the door of the servants' quarters. Chao came out, wide-eyed with fear. She screamed for the others and dragged Noelle back inside the house.

Another pain, and Noelle sank to the floor and lay sobbing. She heard Chao shrieking instructions to the other servants. Rain hammered on the roof like a barrage of stones.

Chao picked up the phone, threw the receiver on the floor in frustration. Noelle knew what was wrong; the storm had knocked down the power lines. The Lao telephone system was never reliable even in the dry season.

She knew she did not have the strength to get back to her bedroom. She didn't care. She lay huddled on the floor and waited for the next pain.

Chao told the cook-boy to run to her father's house, nearly a mile away, and fetch help.

Baptiste should be here, she thought. He should be here.

The thought was snatched away in another snarling grab of pain.

*   *   *

170

When Baptiste woke up he was naked, sticky and hungover. He was on one of the narrow cots upstairs at the White Rose. His mouth was gummy and foul, and his head throbbed with pain from the cognac he had drunk through the day. For a long time he lay awake, listening to the rain, fighting back the familiar waves of guilt and sorrow, half-forming the justifications he would use to defend himself against the recriminations that came unbidden in the darkness.

Suzie – the smoker – lay naked across his belly. Another girl – he didn't know which one, it didn't really matter, he supposed – lay curled on the floor beside the bed. He didn't even know if he had paid them yet. Well, he would leave the money anyway. At two dollars a time there was no reason to be cheap.

It was Noelle's fault, he told himself. If she wasn't such an irascible bitch. He was only a man, after all. What was he supposed to do? He had to get his pleasures somewhere.

He eased out from underneath Suzie and fumbled for his clothes in the darkness. Memories of the previous day nagged at him like a toothache. He knew there was something he did not want to remember, pushed it aside in the fug of the hangover. He slipped on his clothes and stumbled outside.

There were still a few survivors downstairs in the bar, hunched over their drinks; even a taxi girl, smoking cigarettes in the fashion that the White Rose had made famous. As he came down the stairs she looked up hopefully. Baptiste's reputation for both stamina and generosity was well known.

'Smoking's bad for you,' he said to her.

'Want to light me up?' she said in French.

'All out of matches,' he told her.

She looked down at his clothes, and gave him a deprecating grin. His shirt and trousers were caked with dried mud. He remembered the fight with Noelle earlier in the day. *Merde alors!*

With that, the rest of it came tumbling back. Jean-Marie. Not guilty, he told himself. I just carried out her precious papa's orders. I didn't even put the bomb there myself. I was messenger and paymaster, that's all.

The headache had started again. There was a rhythm to the dull pain. Murderer, murderer . . .

He felt that even the drunks around the bar were staring at him with disgust.

'I have to go home,' he said to no one in particular. He felt as if he had fallen into a black pit. There was no way back up to the light.

Bonaventure took the front steps of the villa three at a time. As he burst through the door he found Noelle crouched on the floor, in a puddle of water, panting hard against the pain. Chao was half supporting her, clutching her arms.

'It's started, Papa.'

Chao had had two babies of her own so she knew what to expect. She had sent the servant boys out of the room and pulled Noelle's nightgown off. Her body was slick with sweat, and her breasts looked swollen and bruised. But it was her eyes that told the story; they were crazy with fear and pain.

'Where's Baptiste?' she shouted.

Bonaventure felt a rush of anger and helplessness. This was his little girl, his baby. 'I've sent Tao Koo to find the doctor,' he said to her.

'I want Baptiste! Why isn't he here?'

Bonaventure fell onto his knees beside his daughter, cradled her head in his arms. Please let nothing go wrong! Let the doctor get here soon. 'Everything will be all right,' he said. He felt her hand crush his fingers. 'Another pain?'

Noelle did not answer. She gave a long gasp, and then it was as if something had taken over her body. Her faced puffed to the colour of purple, until he thought the veins in her cheeks would burst.

Chao shouted a warning in her own language and made a quick examination. 'What's happening?' Bonaventure shouted, but he knew. The baby was about to come.

Tao Koo pulled up in the courtyard in the Mercedes, Doctor Leveque with him. Leveque had been with the army at Dien Bien Phu, had stayed behind in Vientiane after the armistice.

Inside the house, Noelle watched with detached interest as Chao dangled the slippery, squawking thing by the heels to clear its nose and throat, and then laid the child on

172

her belly. The umbilicus snaked between her legs to the child's stomach. It was still pulsing.

Then she heard Leveque say: 'She's haemorrhaging,' and looked up at the aghast faces of her father and the doctor but there was no fear left in her, just relief that it was all over.

'Put it to the breast,' Leveque told her, and Chao guided the child's mouth to her breast. Noelle felt the tugging of its gums at her nipple. Almost at once, the contractions started again but now it was a smaller, more bearable pain, and the spasms began to clamp off the blood supply to her torn vagina.

Relieved, Leveque slipped on rubber gloves and prepared to deliver the placenta. Bonaventure flopped on to his knees beside him. His face was grey with shock, his white hair plastered across his skull by the rain.

Noelle just wanted to sleep. She had never known anything so violent, so terrible. She felt like a piece of meat. She wished Baptiste were here.

'What is it?' Bonaventure whispered.

She looked down at the squirming, pink thing in her arms. 'It's a boy,' she said.

37

Baptiste climbed out of the Packard and stared at Bonaventure's Mercedes parked in front of the house, at the blaze of lights in the hall and the bedroom. The front door was open. What was going on?

The baby! Noelle!

He ran inside. Bonaventure was there with Leveque, the doctor. They stared at him as if he was a housebreaker. He realised how he must look, his suit muddied, his face heavy-lidded and worn by the day's sabbatical with the bottle of cognac and the taxi girls of the White Rose. *You should have been home*, their faces told him.

Another sin to add to the crimes of his life.

He heard a child's cry.

'She's in there,' Bonaventure said.

Chao had washed her and brushed her hair, tying it in a long pony tail behind her head. She looked pale and tired, but there was a stony resolution in her eyes. She sat on the bed, in a clean white nightgown, cradling the child in her arms. The baby's mouth was open, Noelle's swollen nipple still between its lips.

Baptiste felt soiled and ashamed. 'Noelle?'

'It's a boy,' she said.

He walked slowly across the room and held out his arms. She ignored him.

'Can I hold him?' he said.

Noelle stood up, staggered and almost fell. Leveque's stitches were like needles. Baptiste reached to steady her. She shook her arm free, and carried the child to the white cane bassinet in the corner of the room. She gently laid him down, pulled her gown closed, and tied the cord.

Then she crossed the room and slapped Baptiste's face as hard as she could. 'Get out,' she said.

'Noelle, please.'

'Espèce de con!'

'He's my son,' he said. Gentleness would have broken him. Instead her anger rekindled his defiance.

'Where were you tonight?' she hissed.

She knew from the look on his face.

'You spent the whole day and night there?'

'Jean-Marie's death hurt me too.' In a way it was true, he supposed.

'That is how you explain it?'

He did not answer her.

'A woman is more than just a receptacle for your sperm, Baptiste. You may see your son in the morning. I want to be alone.'

She staggered on her way back to the bed. Again he helped her, and again she shook herself free.

'I don't want you to touch me!'

'You can't stop me seeing my son,' he said. He walked over to the bassinet and picked up the child. It started to cry.

'See. An hour old and he knows what sort of a man you are.'

Baptiste tried to soothe the child, couldn't. He returned him to his bassinet.

'We'll call him Lucien,' he said, and walked out.

38

Hong Kong

The shark moved in, eyes bright, circling and watching. Douglas tried to kick his legs but they would not respond. The water sucked at his legs, leaving him helpless. The beast closed in, its mouth open, the serrated rows of teeth pink with blood.

He kicked again, desperately, and screamed.

The jaws closed around his leg, tearing at his flesh. He writhed like a worm on a hook. The pain coursed through his body and he scrabbled frantically at the air with his hands, trying desperately to be free.

But it dragged him down into the darkness and when it finally tore away he saw a part of himself was in its mouth, and it swallowed it in a gulp, like a pig at a trough.

Still it wouldn't leave him. It rushed in again, he felt the teeth clamp on to his leg once more, tearing at it like a dog, he saw more of his flesh, raw and pink, in the creature's maw. The water clouded with the red mist of his own blood.

He sat bolt upright.

His heart pounded in his chest like a jackhammer. He felt as if he was going to vomit. His body ran with sweat and the thin cotton sheets of his bed were screwed into knots on the floor. His chest worked like bellows, as he gulped in the fetid air of the room and tried to calm himself.

It was all so real.

Every night since they had pulled him from the water it had been the same dream. Of the actual night he could remember so very little, and nothing after the shark had first attacked. The patrolboat, the journey in the Royal Navy helicopter, the casualty room of the Queen Elizabeth Hospital, all misty and unreal. It was the dreams that were vivid and close, and they would not leave him; it was always the same, the shark in the water, circling, then leisurely moving in for the kill. Only, in the way of dreams, it would never end. The pain and terror would just go on and on until he awoke. The dream never faded, never changed.

Sometimes he wondered if he would ever be free of it.

Eyrie of the Dragon Fist

The blue and white tail of the Pan Am 707 passed so low overhead that the walls trembled as if it was an earthquake. Douglas imagined that if he leaned out from the balcony he would be able to touch the wings. For a moment the black shadow blotted out all light from the window and then it roared on, another great silver bird about to settle on the concrete lake of Kai Tak.

Dragon Fist was sitting at the table counting Hong Kong dollars and arranging them into piles. He would then wrap a thick rubber band around them and place them in a large black briefcase. There was a cigarette in one corner of his mouth.

'I want him dead, Sharkfin,' he said to Douglas.

The attack on Dragon Fist in Half Dog Street was almost a year ago, but it had not been forgotten, by Dragon Fist himself, or the triad soldiers, or any of the inhabitants of the Walled City. It remained a slur to be corrected, a stain against Dragon Fist's reputation, even though he had escaped the attack uninjured. They had learned that the black-jacketed man who led the attack was a 14K Red Pole by the name of Ma Shen-fu – better known as Tiger Claw Ma, because he sometimes fought with barbed wire wrapped around his knuckles. Dragon Fist's spies had told him that it was Tiger Claw who had conceived and planned the attack. Afterwards he had mysteriously disappeared from the Walled City, his 14K bosses no doubt aware that his presence invited another gang war. But now he was back, had even ventured into

Half Dog Street, swaggering and arrogant as ever.

Douglas was now part of Dragon Fist's personal bodyguard inside the Walled City. He slept separately from the other 49s here in the Dragon's Eyrie, and went everywhere with his uncle whenever he came to Hak Nam. It was his reward for the wounds he had taken on his uncle's behalf, and for the skill he had shown in the fight. After the battle, he had spent just over a week in Queen Elizabeth Hospital. Now, a year later, the hair had grown back over the wounds in his scalp, but there were still raw, pink cicatrices on his left forearm, where Tiger Claw's soldiers had slashed him with their cleavers.

There were other changes, too. The whores no longer teased the limping teenager. He was called Sharkfin, as a sign of respect for his fighting prowess, and because of his mutilation by the shark in Mirs Bay. He even wore a shark's tooth on a gold chain around his neck, as a constant reminder to others that he had already been in the jaws of death once and so was no longer afraid.

Dragon Fist threw another bundle of Hong Kong dollars – five thousand, Douglas estimated – into the briefcase with a careless flick of his wrist.

'You want me to do it?' Douglas said.

Dragon Fist laughed. 'You? What makes you think you can do it, little shark?'

Douglas pointed to the scars on his arm. 'Someone has to pay for this.'

The money was counted, the final bundle thrown in the briefcase and the locks clipped shut. Dragon Fist pushed his chair away from the table and folded his arms, examining Douglas as if he was something he wanted to buy. 'I wonder if you could, little Sharkfin. I wonder if you could.'

'I know I can. Let me do it.'

Dragon Fist speculated for a moment. His *sai lo*, his little brother, had earned him enormous face. Perhaps the gods intended a good future for the boy. He stood up. 'Come with me,' he said. 'I want to show you something.'

39

It was a humid July morning, and after two days of monsoon rains the air was like clear steam. Connaught Road was a chaos of traffic and people. Douglas saw old Chinese launch themselves in front of buses and cars, missing death by inches but ensuring that any evil dragons that were following them were destroyed by the onrushing traffic. There were garish crimson rickshaws, pulled along by scarecrow coolies with muscles like knotted rope, hauling their loads of fruit or chickens, shouting a whining barrage of invective at anyone who got in their way. Old women in black pyjamas and oyster hats shouldered panniers of ducks, plastic flowers, rice and stones on bamboo poles that bowed across their shoulders; their children scrabbled for a few meagre coins, selling newspapers, unloading lorries, cleaning shoes. That's what you are running from, Douglas reminded himself. Any price is worth escaping life in the street.

As they drove up to the Midlevels, the timeless flag of China appeared at the windows and balconies of the tenements and the shophouses that lined the streets; hundreds of bamboo poles, lined with laundry.

The Porsche left the fug of the city behind, Douglas and his uncle cocooned in the plush, air-conditioned interior. Its tail wound around the curves of the Peak, the twin exhausts barking like a dragon. Up the mountain, where the poor never go.

Dragon Fist owned an apartment in the Midlevels, a true eyrie from which he could gaze down on the squabbling mass of humanity below and congratulate himself on his joss and his choices.

The apartment was all polished chrome and leather with full-length windows and smoked glass. There were two girls in short silk dressing gowns sitting on a sofa, staring at a television. When they saw Dragon Fist, one of them got up and switched it off.

Douglas stared. They were beautiful, truly beautiful, not like the scarred and hard-faced whores in the Walled City. They were soft and rounded, and they wore jewellery, and he could smell their perfume. Their lips shone with carmine lipstick. There were no needle marks on the backs of their hands.

'You want to have them?' Dragon Fist asked him. 'You can have them both at once if you want, or one at a time. I don't care.'

Douglas didn't answer.

'Or maybe you just like to watch.' He gave an imperceptible nod of his head. The two girls peeled off their silk robes. They knelt side by side on the leather sofa and haltingly began to touch and kiss each other. Douglas watched, transfixed. Sex was nothing new to him. He had lost his virginity soon after his arrival in the Walled City, when he and some of his uncle's soldiers had raped a fourteen-year-old girl, on Dragon Fist's orders. And he had seen plenty of yellow films in the Walled City.

But this was different. This was perfumed and sophisticated, and it was a private show.

'You see. I can make people do whatever I want,' Dragon Fist whispered in his ear.

He turned his back on the women and walked away, indicating that Douglas should follow. It was a massive room, split-level. There was a huge mahogany desk at the end of the room, and behind it a window looked out over the harbour. Along one wall was a bar, carved from polished rosewood. Dragon Fist poured two glasses of Dewar's whisky and gave one to Douglas.

He was amused by his nephew's open-mouthed amazement. Where did he think I lived? In a shack in the Typhoon Shelter?

He threw himself into a soft leather chair behind the desk, swivelled it around so he could gaze at the harbour, spread out below, fleets of junks with patched and tattered canvas sails wallowing in the wash of the armada of smaller motor boats, the walla-wallas and the sampans. In the gage roads were the merchant vessels, huge P&O liners, Blue Funnel and Jardine Matheson freighters, small Pacific Island merchantmen. A US warship, sleek and grey, was anchored at Wanchai.

'How much have you learned about the society of the Hung Mun, little Sharkfin?'

'I've learned there's no other way to live.'

Dragon Fist went on as if Douglas had not spoken. 'As you know, all the ranks have a numerical code. At the moment you're just a *sze kau*, a 49, a foot soldier. But you have potential. But perhaps one day you will become a 426, a Red Pole, like me.'

The girls had dressed and had once again returned their attention to the television. For some reason it angered him. He would like to have shouted at them, made them do what he wanted like Dragon Fist had done.

'Come with me,' Dragon Fist said.

Dragon Fist showed him another miracle, a bathroom and toilet, with gleaming marble tiles on the floor. Water came when you turned a tap, the toilet flushed, there were no sewer spiders coming out of the hole in the ground.

Through another door there was a bedroom big enough to sleep five families inside the Walled City. There were red silk sheets on the bed.

Then Dragon Fist led Douglas on to the balcony. It was late-afternoon and the sun hung above the hills of Kowloon like a gold coin. Soon it would retreat behind the violet mists into China.

The air was clean, much cooler than below near the harbour. This was where the gods would come to live, Douglas thought.

'You can breathe up here. Not breathing in someone else's stink, eh, Douglas. Isn't that what you want?'

'I'll do anything,' he whispered.

His uncle grinned. 'I know.' He was silent a long time. 'Well, have you been sending the money you've been making back to Swatow like a dutiful son?'

Douglas wasn't sure how to answer.

'Of course you haven't. Why bother, Sharkfin? If they're too stupid and helpless to help themselves, why must they drag you down for the rest of your life? It's just superstition. The old ways have nothing to do with the new Hong Kong.'

'I want to have this too.'

'Perhaps one day. If you are loyal. I can help you.'

'Let me prove I can do it. Let me kill Tiger Claw.'

'You won't beat him in a proper fight, Sharkfin. He's too quick, perhaps quicker even than me, and he has two good legs. You'll have to use your brain.'

'I'll find a way.'

Dragon Fist pointed across the bay. A jet hovered over the Walled City, its red and green navigation lights blinking against the darkening backdrop of the hills. 'See, that jet is just passing over Hak Nam now. That's your prize and your kingdom, Douglas. If you chop Tiger Claw.'

40

Tiger Claw was young, no more than twenty-one years old. He had been born in the Walled City, had started work in a factory making plastic flowers when he was nine years old. His father was an opium addict, and both his older sisters had been sold into a brothel. By the time he was sixteen he was sick of working in a cramped, furnace-hot room for a few cents a day. Like so many others, he decided that the triads were the only road out of his misery. He dreamed of becoming a triad fighter, and with joss, perhaps even a Red Pole.

He began running errands for the 14K, became a look-see boy for the opium den, then volunteered to do a little *pin-mun* – illegal business. He started selling packets of number three heroin in Temple Street. His activities brought him into contact with other triad youngsters, and he quickly learned to fight. Tiger Claw was blessed with snake-quick reactions and silky co-ordination.

He also possessed a great talent for viciousness. His childhood in the squalor and darkness of Hak Nam left him with no more conscience than an animal. Survival, and his place in the pecking order, were the only two priorities he knew. Wrapping barbed wire around his knuckles as a fighting tool was just one of his many inventions, and his fighting skills quickly brought him to the attention of the 14K. He was initiated as a 49, a soldier. Finally he was promoted to a Red Pole; the weapons and martial arts expert, its enforcer, toecutter, general to the soldiers.

But Tiger Claw had one weakness. Like so many of the triads, he was addicted to heroin. It was addiction, and not fear of retribution, that had driven him from the streets of Hak

Nam after the fight in Half Dog Street. He had spent a period of rehabilitation in a Christian mission run by a Carmelite nun. It had ended when he killed the nun's chaplain one night in an argument over a wristwatch that had been stolen from one of the other inmates. Tiger Claw had settled the discussion by slitting the man's throat with a kitchen knife.

Back in Hak Nam Tiger Claw had disposed of the man who had taken his place in the 14K with a meat cleaver. He had sliced through the muscles on the man's back and shoulders. The man would live, but he would never be able to move his arms again. Tiger Claw had doomed him to a life as a shuffling, bowed cripple, a permanent reminder to all those who wished to usurp his authority in the future.

He had since been disgusted to learn that he was tainted by the accusation that he had fled the Walled City because of the attack on Dragon Fist. The only way he could eradicate this stain on his reputation was to confront the Fei Lung once again across their own borders.

Now he ordered his soldiers to venture into Fei Lung territory and demand protection from the den managers and the brothel keepers on their side.

The challenge had been thrown down. Dragon Fist would have to answer it.

The shadow of the BOAC Constellation passed in front of the windows, its engines drowning out the last of Douglas' words to anyone standing outside the room. When he had finished Dragon Fist threw back his head and laughed.

'It might work!'

'It will work,' Douglas said.

One of the other triads frowned. 'How do you know he will be where you say?'

'Our spies,' Dragon Fist answered for his nephew. 'We know where he is every minute of the day, same as he knows where I am.'

'It would be easier to take him on his way back to Kowloon.'

'And easier to get caught. Besides, this is for the people of Hak Nam to see.'

'By tomorrow night Tiger Claw will be dead,' Douglas promised.

Dragon Fist laughed and nodded. 'We'll see, Sharkfin, we'll see!'

They were known as the Night Soil Women. Every morning they were a common sight in the Walled City, dragging the slopping buckets of excrement through the alleys in large rattan baskets, their scarves wrapped around their noses, their heads down, calling a warning as they dragged their loads. They were old, nut-brown women with wizened faces and dirt-encrusted claws, harridans who were treated like lepers by even the prostitutes and the heroin addicts.

Today there were half a dozen of them, attacking the stone steps of the tenement in Indian file, dragging their noxious loads up to the roof overlooking Beggar Street. It was a long journey, and a hard one, and several times they had to stop to catch their breath; but they were diligent with their slopping loads.

Today they had a special chore to perform, and they were intent on doing it well. After all, they had been well paid.

The clatter of machinery echoed down the alley from the one-room factory where sweating men in dusky white vests made the meat balls that would go into the stews of the street hawkers on the streets outside Hak Nam. In the adjoining shop a dozen women worked in a windowless room, bowed over wooden benches, feeding shirts into cotton bobbins in the grimy yellow light of a single bulb. An open watercourse flowed along the centre of the alley, a dribble of greasy water trickling down the slope. Years of rubbish, thrown from above, mixed with the leaking water to form a grey and matted mess on either side of the drain.

Douglas wrinkled his nose against the stench. Since his visit to the Midlevels such sights and smells had become repellent to him. Before, he had almost accepted them as part of his life.

There were four other men with him; Half Ear Louie, Freddy Yang, Fishball Tak and Jimmy Wong. They were all tense, tight with adrenalin. Three of them held meat cleavers, the choppers that most of the triad fighters favoured. Douglas and

Freddy Yang also had sharpened bicycle chains. Freddy had his wrapped around the knuckles of his right fist.

A man walked out of Beggar Street and came towards them. He was wearing a red T-shirt. As he passed them he stopped for a moment, and held his right fist in front of his chest.

It was their signal. Tiger Claw was there.

Douglas led them down the alley and they ran around the corner into Beggar Street.

Tiger Claw was taking money from the *pang jue* and stuffing it into his pockets. He was wearing a black leather jacket and black sunglasses, as he had been the day of the attack in Half Dog Street. He saw Douglas and grinned.

'The Fei Lung sends cripples out to fight now, they are so desperate.'

'It only takes cripples to fight old women like you.'

Tiger Claw stopped smiling, stung by the insult. His 49s pulled cleavers and chains from the backs of their jeans and from their jackets.

There were six of them. Outnumbered by just one, Douglas thought.

He looked up at the narrow blackness above and shouted: 'Let the fragrant rains come!'

It took several seconds. Tiger Claw was momentarily bewildered; then he and his *sze kau* were drenched in excrement as the nightsoil women released their loads. It hit the ground with the force of a monsoon. Tiger Claw and his men shouted out in astonishment.

The battle lasted less than one minute. Douglas rushed forward, the other triads right with him. Their opponents were soiled with filth, staggering in outrage and disgust. Douglas and his companions hit them then, in those precious few seconds of surprise. Choppers flashed briefly, there were a few muted screams, blood spurting from wounds.

Douglas headed straight for Tiger Claw.

Unlike his less experienced soldiers, the 14K Red Pole had not been distracted by the unexpected drenching. He had kept his attention focused on his enemy and moved quickly into his fighting stance, a long knife held ready in his right hand. Douglas moved in quickly, slashing wide with his own cleaver, forcing him back. But Tiger Claw was too canny a fighter to be cornered, and kept moving to his left, circling, keeping his back from the wall, trying to close in.

From the edge of his vision Douglas saw that the battle was already breaking up. Bodies littered the alleyway, blood and ordure in appalling pools. He realised with satisfaction that in less than a minute they had taken out half a dozen of Tiger Claw's best fighters. But now more 14K were rushing from the other end of the alley to join the battle. He shouted at his own *sze kau* to retreat.

At that moment Tiger Claw stepped inside his guard and slashed at him, the edge of the blade tearing through his sports jacket and lacerating his forearm. Douglas cut down with his own weapon, forcing Tiger Claw back, then turned and ran from the alley.

Tiger Claw was surprised by Douglas' sudden retreat, but by the tradition of triad fights in the Walled City, the battle was now over.

But then Douglas stopped at the corner of Half Dog Street, turned and shouted to Tiger Claw: 'Ma Shen-fu, that's my shit on your head!'

Tiger Claw bellowed with rage and ran after him.

Douglas disappeared along Half Dog Street. His fellow *sze kau* had already fled into the gloomy maze of alleys on their side of the border. Douglas twisted down a concrete tunnel, threw himself on his hands and knees, crawled for five yards, then staggered to his feet and limped on.

When he looked around he saw Tiger Claw had closed on him. Douglas, with his crippled left leg, was no match for him in a race. He remembered what his uncle had told him.

He's too quick, perhaps quicker even than me, and he has two good legs. You'll have to use your brain.

Tiger Claw was running at full speed down the tunnel. Douglas turned to face him.

Suddenly Tiger Claw was flat on his back. It was as if an invisible hand had chopped him in the throat. The piano wire that had been strung across the tunnel had taken him across the bridge of the nose.

He lay spreadeagled on his back, stunned. A red line

appeared across his face, level with the eyes, and it started to fill with blood, blinding him. His knife had been jarred from his wrist by the impact and lay yards away in the filth of the watercourse.

Douglas stood over him, grinning, saw Tiger Claw's arms and legs jerk as he tried to recover.

He did not hesitate. He plunged down with his cleaver into Tiger Claw's stomach. The other man roared, the agony bubbling up in his throat, his legs jerking at the air. He twisted on to his side, both hands clutching at his stomach, the grey-green of his intestines spilling through the slash.

Douglas stepped back and watched Tiger Claw writhe and kick. But there was no time for much play. He moved in again and with great deliberation chopped down at the other man's neck, twice, three times. Blood from the carotid artery sprayed over his white T-shirt.

He looked up. Two of Tiger Claw's *sze kau* had followed to the end of the tunnel. Douglas wiped Tiger Claw's blood from his face with his hand, held it up and showed it to them.

Then he turned his back on them contemptuously and walked away.

It was his moment of sweetest victory. Within hours everyone in the Walled City would know of it. This place might be hell, but at least he was master of it.

41

Laos, March 1964

The Packard was at the side of the road with its hood up. Jonathan Dale slowed the jeep for a closer look. He saw a young woman sitting in the shade of a pipal tree, a few yards from the car, a small child on her lap.

It was getting late. The rice fields had turned platinum under a falling sun. From a nearby wat the booming of a drum summoned the monks to prayer. The sun glinted on the gilded spire of a stupa.

Well, he couldn't just drive past. He stopped the jeep and got out.

Noelle buttoned her blouse and stood up. The big American saw what she was doing and looked away embarrassed. He was tall and lean, in his early-thirties she guessed, with fair hair and cornflower blue eyes. His skin was tanned dark, so she assumed he was not new to the tropics.

Lucien was tired and clung to her shoulder, crying.

'Can I help you, ma'am?' the American said to her in English.

'I don't know,' she said, appraising him candidly.

He indicated the Packard, unsettled by her attitude. 'I thought perhaps you had a problem here, ma'am.'

She had not much liked any of the Americans she had met in Laos, and she wasn't sure if she was going to like this one any better. But he wasn't loud, his voice was rich and gentle, and his face suggested intelligence.

She hitched Lucien on her hip. 'My car. She is broken.'

'Well, you can't stay here.'

189

'Yes,' she said, and her tone indicated that this much was obvious. 'But Lucien, he is upset. So I must attend to him first. He still takes the breast, you see.' To her amazement, the American actually blushed. 'Now he is fed I shall wait for a taxi. This heap, she is my husband's problem now.'

'I can give you a ride into town.'

'Thank you.'

He hesitated, and jerked a thumb at the Packard. 'Want me to take a look first?'

'You understand machines?'

'A little.'

She shrugged.

He looked under the bonnet. His hand accidentally brushed the radiator. 'Shit! Excuse me, ma'am.'

'I am not offended, monsieur,' she said. Indeed, she was intrigued. He behaved like an awkward schoolboy, yet he was the size of a mountain.

'Fan belt's broke,' he said.

'This is bad?'

'Well, it's not major.'

She realised that he was looking at her legs. She felt a sudden glow of pleasure and alarm. 'You like my legs, monsieur?'

He couldn't look at her. 'No. Well, yeah. They're great legs.'

'I am married, monsieur.'

She found confusion charming in such a good-looking man. She wasn't used to it, had certainly not encountered it often in Asia.

'Are you wearing stockings?'

The question threw her off balance. A fetishist, perhaps. She felt a thrill of fear and held Lucien tighter in her arms. The boy sensed her fear and started to cry again. They were four kilometres from the city. Perhaps I should throw him my underwear now, or do I bluff him out? Nearby some children were attempting to shoot down coconuts with a slingshot, and two village women were returning from market, their baskets of pumpkin and sweet potato slung across their shoulders on poles. They were within shouting distance. But would they help her against this giant American if she screamed?

190

He was still staring at her. 'I mean, if you're wearing stockings I could fix your fan belt. Nylon's very strong. You just wind it around the pulleys on the pump and the alternator. Kind of makeshift, but it will get you back home.'

She laughed, relieved, and he looked even more uncomfortable.

Lucien was still crying. She thrust him into the man's arms. 'Here. Hold him please.' Incredibly, Lucien quietened immediately. He would not do that even for his father. 'What a talent,' she said, and hitched up her skirt.

Dale was still staring at her.

'Sorry, ma'am,' he said and turned around.

She unhitched one of her stockings and handed it to him. She took Lucien back and he went over to the Packard and bent over the engine.

She watched him work. He was wearing an olive drab shirt and drill trousers. There were knotted muscles in his forearms and his body looked powerful and hard. It did not quite match the face, which suggested he was more than just brawn.

'You are a soldier?' she asked him.

'No, ma'am. I'm attached to the United States Embassy. Agricultural adviser.'

'Ah, you are a spy then.'

He looked up, nearly banged his head against the open bonnet. He looked stricken. 'Hell, no. Who told you that?'

She laughed. 'How long have you been in Vientiane, monsieur?'

'Two weeks.'

'Some advice, then. If you do not want people to think you are a spy, you should tell them you are a journalist.'

He seemed bewildered. He finished hitching the nylon around the pulleys. There was grease on his hands, which he wiped on the legs of his trousers. 'Just need to top up that radiator. Got some water in the back of the jeep.' He came back with a large plastic container. 'Are you on your way back to Vientiane, ma'am?'

'I went out to Tha Deua. They have a market there. I wanted to buy some bear.'

'Excuse me?'

'Lucien has the cough. Every night he barks like a seal. I

191

have tried everything the doctor gives me. Then one of my housegirls tells me she can make me some medicine, but she needs special oil they make from bear fat.'

'I think if I was Lucien I'd hang tough with the cough.' He finished refilling the radiator and stood back. 'Should be okay now.'

'Thank you, monsieur. You are very kind.'

'It's okay,' he mumbled.

She put Lucien in the car and jumped behind the wheel. The engine coughed back to life. 'I don't even know your name,' she said to him.

He slammed the bonnet down. 'Dale. Jonathan Dale.'

'Thank you again, Monsieur Dale.' She reached out of the car, took his hand and shook it. It was huge, twice the size of her own.

'My pleasure ma'am.'

She gave him her best smile. She would remember him. Powerful, polite, good with children. What a discovery.

Perhaps there was hope for America yet.

42

Baptiste watched Noelle from the verandah as she sat in the garden, a leather bound book in her lap, Lucien playing at her feet among the fallen mangoes. Her face was serene, and the swell of her breasts was accentuated by the V-neck of her cotton smock. She toyed distractedly with a curl at her cheek. Adorable, innocent. He longed for her now, as much as he had longed for her before he first lured her into his bed. He was tired of the taxi girls and the desultory affairs with the bored wives of French and American diplomats. Suddenly the most exotic and unattainable creature in Vientiane was his own wife.

A large beetle with metallic green wings slowly climbed the white verandah post. He drew back viciously and smashed it with his fist.

They ate in silence; rice, serpent-fish, *laap* – vegetables tossed with lime juice, garlic, green onions and chillies – and fresh mangos. There was a pitcher of *citron pressé* in the middle of the table.

Lucien ate some of the mango, but there was more rubbed into his red cheeks than had gone into his mouth. Halfway through the meal he started to cry. Noelle took him out of his chair to nurse him.

'He's a fussy eater,' said Baptiste. 'You encourage him.'

Noelle ignored him. He lit a cigarette and tapped impatiently on the edge of the table with the box while she tried to quieten Lucien.

'You're choking him,' she said.

'It's my home. I'll smoke if I want to.'

She bit her lip and returned her attention to her son. 'You have to fix the car,' she said.

'Why? What's wrong with it?'

'The fan belt's broken.'

He almost smiled. 'The fan belt? You wouldn't know a fan belt if it crawled out of the car and bit you on the bottom.'

'Don't be crude. Because I'm a woman doesn't mean I'm useless.'

He shrugged it off. 'I'll have a look at it.'

'Papa came by this morning. He's talking about having a big party next week.'

'Special occasion?'

'It's his birthday. He'll be sixty years old.'

'Is that all the old goat is?'

'We have to go.'

'I wouldn't miss it for anything.' He shifted his leg. It ached incessantly. During the wet season it was almost unbearable. He could feel the black dog on his back, the beginning of one of the dark moods that had begun to settle on him with increasing frequency. Perhaps tonight he would go back to The Green Latrine or the Suck and Soda and buy a taxi girl to try and take away the mood of depression that had fallen over him. Or perhaps he would get drunk and drive his Packard down the main street blindfolded with Gilbert Pépé and Marius Nicoli shouting directions, as he had done on his thirtieth birthday.

But the thought of a woman or a bottle of cognac did nothing to lighten his mood.

That night Baptiste climbed into bed beside his wife. His lovemaking was uncharacteristically rough, almost desperate, but she did not respond. He was making love to a ghost.

Without her passion, be it her love or hate, he had nothing. She had defined the borders of his character, and he realised that somehow he had come to need her.

43

Bonaventure was on the verandah with a group that included General Rattakone and Phoui Nosovan, the two most powerful men in Laos. Well, apart from me, Gates thought with satisfaction. They were conversing in French, all smiles. But that could mean anything with the Laos. They might have just told a joke, or threatened to kill each other. It was the one thing he really admired about them, their inscrutability, although he knew that for them a poker face was simply good manners.

'Happy Birthday, Rocco,' said Gates.

Bonaventure turned and beamed at him. 'Gerry.' He excused himself from the group and moved away.

'You're looking well, Rocky. What is it today? Fifty-five?'

Bonaventure laughed. 'Sixty today. But you know this. You are just trying to flatter an old man.'

'You're looking good for it.'

'When the hair turns white it doesn't matter a damn any more about the numbers. Old is old.' He took Gates by the elbow and led him to a corner. 'So, how was Saigon, *mon vieux*?'

'Interesting. Want to talk about this now?'

'Why not?'

The afternoon was hot, but it was pleasantly cool under the verandah. Gates detected the musty smell of uniforms and rotting fruit from the garden. There was a shout of laughter from a group of Americans from the embassy. Several of the Laos looked over, and for a moment their eyes registered disapproval.

Gates continued in the same monotone delivery. 'Now that Diem has gone the Vietnamese are thinking of ending some of his more puritanical restrictions on trade through Saigon port.'

195

Bonaventure nodded. Diem had been murdered in a bloody coup the previous year. The war there was escalating, despite America's best efforts – or perhaps because of them – and the Vietnamese needed more money to sustain it. Instead of just collecting rake-offs from the chiu chao who ran the opium dens in Cholon, they were going to allow them to expand the business and export through Saigon port as well.

'I had a meeting with Tran van Li. He thought you might want to talk to him about it. He feels Saigon might be able to offer you better facilities than Bangkok. For anything you might like to export.'

'Perhaps,' Bonaventure said.

'I said I'd mention it to you.'

'I appreciate your concern,' Bonaventure said, deadpan. 'Perhaps there is another favour you can do for your old friend.'

'Shoot.'

'It's about that fat pig Rattakone.' And he smiled and raised his glass to the Lao Commander of Armed Forces on the other side of the verandah, who smiled back. 'I would trust him only as far as I could propel him with my foot, and with his weight and my gout, that distance is not great.'

'What's the problem, Rocky?'

'I think he has plans to take over my business.'

'Can he afford the goodwill?'

'There is no goodwill in South East Asia,' Bonaventure said, pretending not to understand the joke. 'Perhaps I am mistaken, but I believe he thinks his Air Force can do the job.'

Gates shrugged. This wasn't his problem.

'I would like to speak to you in private about the possibility of leasing cargo space on your aircraft should our position in Laos become ... unpredictable.'

Gates raised an eyebrow. 'Sure, Rocky. It doesn't hurt to talk. But not here. Drop by the embassy tomorrow. Right now there's someone I'd like you to meet.'

Bonaventure was right, of course. Gates had already learned through his own sources that Rattakone wanted the entire opium harvest for himself. All he had to do was withdraw the *réquisitions militaires* and Air Opium would no longer be able to fly.

But Gates also knew he was sitting on a keg of powder: *the possibility of leasing cargo space on United States planes*. Air America aircraft were already carrying KMT opium out of the Shan states and Northern Thailand to pay for arms. If Rattakone threw the Corsicans out of Laos, they could perhaps earn a little extra cash for the Company's military efforts. The opium had to come out, to keep the Meo happy, to allow them to continue as a functional force. How else were they going to pay for the M-16s?

In the end what the hell did it matter who did the carrying? That was the way he saw it anyway. Someone had to get their hands dirty for America. And it wasn't going to be any of those idiots and bleeding hearts in Congress.

A strange place to stage World War Three, Dale thought, as he looked around the faces on the verandah. A comic opera kingdom, *Lan Xan*, the Laos called it, the Land of a Million Elephants. Most Americans would never be able to find the country on a map. It was the last place the United States and Russia would have anticipated having to face each other down, but it was here among the rice *paddis*, the snake-roofed temples, and the bamboo and thatch stilt houses that the battle was about to be joined.

Dale had been in Laos less than two weeks, and he was still bewildered by the internecine politics of the country. High society in Laos was an exotic blend. As he looked around the room he saw Lao generals, Corsican gangsters, British diplomats and Swedish engineers as well as others like himself, Americans in civilian clothes seconded from other branches of the military for special operations. They all mingled on the verandah, holding glasses of imported French champagne, while pretty Lao girls in bright silk *pao sin* brought delicacies such as prawns and pâté, especially flown in from Bangkok for the Westerners in Bonaventure's own planes; while the high-born Laos enjoyed pig's blood and bat wings and roasted sparrow.

He spotted Gerry Gates coming towards him. Gates was

Dale's immediate superior, about ten years older; a lot of experience in South East Asian affairs, they had told him in Saigon. A good Company man. He had searching, quick eyes, that seemed to appraise a man instantly.

At his side was a massive, grey-bearded man in a white tropical suit. Their host. Dale knew him only by reputation, one of the Corsican *milieu*, *un vrai monsieur*, one of their biggest gangsters. An opium smuggler.

'Jack,' Gates was saying, 'someone I'd like you to meet. This is Rocco Bonaventure, one of Vientiane's leading citizens. Rocky, this is Jack Dale. I was telling you about him. He's going to be helping me teach the locals how to develop their agriculture.'

They both laughed at that.

Someone called to Gates from across the room. 'Tomorrow,' he said cryptically in Bonaventure's direction, and moved away, smiling.

Bonaventure turned to Dale. 'So, how do you enjoy Laos, Monsieur Dale?'

'I haven't seen much so far,' he answered cautiously.

'You come here from America?'

'I've spent a little time in Manila and Saigon.'

'For myself I have been a long time in *Indochine*. Nearly twenty years. No doubt you have seen already that we do things here a little different. *L'argent sous la table* is not a crime here, yes? It is just a way of doing the business. It is a Buddhist country. The philosophy is not the same. You understand?'

Dale had the impression he was being lectured. He decided it was time to turn the conversation around. 'How's the airline business?' he said.

'I am not so big as my American rivals, but I survive.'

Dale knew he was referring to CAT – Civil Air Transport – or Air America as the locals called it. They had a fleet of Dakotas and Cessnas and Helios and Pipers out at Wattay. Everyone in the embassy believed CAT was a wholly owned subsidiary of the CIA.

'In Laos, aviation is a growing business,' Bonaventure was saying. 'Without the aeroplane, no one goes anywhere, especially in the monsoon. Only two jeeps in all of northern Laos. Last year they collide, head on, boom! Can you believe?' Bonaventure was amused by this notion and gave a raucous laugh. 'We carry rice, ferry engineers and diplomats, the Laos as well.' He lowered his voice. 'Sometimes we carry a little hard rice also.'

'Hard rice?'

'You have not heard this expression yet? Hard rice, Monsieur Dale: guns. It is hard to fight a war without them.'

'What about opium?'

Bonaventure's eyes flashed. 'Some more champagne?' he said, and took two glasses from a tray held by a diminutive Lao hostess. 'You have no idea how much trouble I have to get a few bottles of Veuve Clicquot.' Someone placed another record on the gramophone inside the house and he held up a hand. '*Écoute!* "*La Vie en Rose*". This song reminds me so much of Paris.'

It's deliberate, Dale thought. He's just trying to throw you off balance. It's a little power game that he likes to play.

'Do you like Piaf?'

'She has a fine set of lungs. But we were talking about opium?'

'You are not going to lecture me about the opium, Monsieur Dale? When you Americans do everything but collect the sap yourselves.'

'Because we look the other way does not mean the United States government approves.'

Bonaventure was enjoying himself now. 'Look the other way? Without you there would be no opium business in all Indochine! We will have no airfields to fly the opium out of Laos and no one in Saigon to sell to! And you tell me that all you do is hide your faces in your hands and count to ten.'

'It's a question of priorities.'

'Of course.' Bonaventure sipped the champagne.

'We are engaged in a battle between good and evil in Indochina, between freedom and the darkest, most oppressive regime the world has ever known. We have a choice between fighting that evil and stopping a little opium smuggling. I think that choice is obvious. It still doesn't mean we approve.'

'I can live without your approval, Monsieur Dale. But if

you think this evil you fight is so terrible, why don't you Americans fight the war properly, and not just send us agricultural advisers? I do not criticise you, of course. But it is against my interest to see you lose.'

'We can't run a full-scale war in Laos. It's logistically impossible.'

'Then if you will learn to compromise, you must learn also to live with me. It is a pleasure to meet you, Monsieur Dale. I hope your stay in Laos is a big success.'

He had hoped to see her again. And there she was, on the other side of the verandah, making conversation with a Lao diplomat and an American engineer. She was smiling, but her eyes were fixed on the middle distance. She looked bored.

She looked very different from the day he had met her by the river. She was *en tenue de soir*. There was no child on her hip, and instead of the pony tail her hair fell in curls around her shoulders. She was wearing make-up, there was a high gloss on her lips, and her eyes as they turned in his direction were coal and sapphire. That day by the river she had seemed hot, weary, vulnerable, if a little belligerent. In these surroundings she looked like a princess.

He felt his pulse quicken. She's married, he reminded himself. You shouldn't be thinking about her this way.

And now she was smiling back at him with genuine pleasure. He watched her excuse herself, with infinite charm, and cross the verandah towards him. 'Monsieur Dale.'

'Ma'am.'

'Please call me Noelle. When you say ma'am, I feel like I am a hundred years old.'

He felt a stirring of genuine alarm. He had heard of her, of course, from Gates, from everyone. 'Noelle Crocé? You are Rocco Bonaventure's daughter?'

'I am sorry, this offends you?'

'Of course not. It's just that ... I've heard of you.'

'Only good things, I hope,' she said, her voice sharp. 'So – what are you doing here, Monsieur Dale?' She lowered her voice theatrically. 'Are you representing the spooks?'

'Gerry Gates brought me along as his guest.'

'I do not know him. What does he do? Wait, let me guess. He advises on the agriculture also.'

'Yeah. He's an expert on hard rice.'

'Excuse me?'

'It's a new American invention.' He could smell her perfume, roses and mousse de bain, was uncomfortably aware of how close she was standing. As a woman she could only mean trouble. As Noelle Crocé he suspected she could be disastrous. 'How's the car? Did you get your stocking back?'

'You would like to keep?' She was smiling, watching him from under lidded eyes. She's flirting with me, he realised with mounting excitement and panic.

'Your stocking?'

'Perhaps you will like him as a souvenir?'

'I don't think it would be appropriate.'

There was a soft pulse at her throat. Her lips glistened with champagne. 'It is good the engine she does not blow up. Maybe you will undress me completely for this.'

He tried to shut out the image she had presented to him. It was as if there was an iron band around his chest. He again reminded himself that she was another man's wife and Rocco Bonaventure's daughter. A lethal cocktail. He had to defuse this somehow. 'I don't know where you'd get a fan belt for a Packard in this part of the world,' he heard himself say.

She bit her lip, amused. 'What sort of ... what is it, fan belt ... do you use on your jeep?'

'I've never had to replace one yet.'

'Well then, you must be careful, Monsieur Dale. You know how it is. There's never a girl around when you need one.'

He did not know what to say to that.

She looked over his shoulder and her eyes widened. 'Merde alors. My husband he watches me daggers. I must be boring again. Au revoir, Monsieur Dale.'

'Ma'am ... Noelle.'

As she walked away she turned around and gave him a frank and brilliant smile. Before he knew what he was doing, he blurted out: 'If you do find the stocking ... I'm staying at the bungalow just down the road. Maybe you could drop it in.'

'You can put him on the end of your bed.' She leaned towards him and whispered. 'Maybe Papa Noël will fill him for you.'

She moved away through the crowd towards one of the most startling-looking men Dale had ever seen. He had a bronzed face with sharp Gallic features, and long jet black hair that hung over his collar. Over one eye he wore a black eyepatch. It made him look both sinister and dissolute, a brigand in a white silk shirt. The other eye was staring straight at Dale and there was no mistaking the expression there. At that moment Baptiste Crocé very clearly wished him dead.

'Who was that?' Baptiste murmured.

Noelle tried to sound indifferent. 'He stopped to help me the other day when the car broke down.'

'You never told me about that.'

'I thought I had,' she answered, deliberately vague. 'Yes, you remember. You told me I didn't know what a fan belt was.'

'He's an American?'

Noelle shrugged. 'Yes. A friend of Monsieur Gates.' She held up her empty glass, trying to distract him. 'Will you get me another glass of champagne, *chéri*?'

'You've had enough already.'

'There is nothing worse than a reformed drunk, is there, Baptiste? I'll get it myself.'

She moved off through the crowd. Anyone who did not know her would not have realised that she was already a little drunk.

She is a remarkable woman, thought Baptiste.

And a lying little bitch.

202

44

There was a group of Air America pilots sitting at the bar.
One of them had found a mimeographed sheet of English and
Lao phrases and they were making up a conversation between
themselves, for the benefit of the taxi girls who were listening.
They had little knowledge of the tonal and phonetic subtleties
of the language, so the results were appalling. Both the pilots
and the hostesses found the dialogue hysterical, but probably
for very different reasons, Baptiste decided.

'*Sa bai dii*,' one of the Americans drawled. '*Sa bai dii baw?*'
Greetings. How are you?

'*Khawy sa bai dii. Jao seu nyang?*' his partner replied.
I'm fine, what's your name?

'*Khawy seu Chuck. Kao paak phaa-saalao dai baw. Khawy
bao dai.*'

I'm Chuck. Can you speak Lao? I can't.

Rocco was in a sour mood, a glass and a bottle of pastis on
the table in front of him. A taxi girl sat on his lap, whispering
hackneyed endearments in his ear, which he ignored. She
picked up his hand and placed it on her crotch, but he
snatched it back again, irritated.

When he saw Baptiste he pushed her on to the floor. She got
up and flounced away.

Baptiste sat down. He poured himself a glass of pastis and
lit one of his Gitanes. 'What's up?' he said.

'Heard the news?'

He shook his head.

'The communists. They have massacred an entire Meo
village in Sam Neua province.'

Baptiste was shocked, in spite of himself. Not that he

203

gave a damn about the Meo. But until recently the war had been a quaint affair, predictable like the monsoon. The Pathet Lao held the Plain of Jars during the dry season, the royalists took it back again in the monsoon. There was almost a sense of ritual about it.

In battle Laotians traditionally aimed high, and expected their enemy to do the same. Sometimes the government forces would send a message to the Pathet Lao that it was about to attack a certain village and the communists would retreat. A few days later the communists would send a message that they were ready to counter-attack, and the Lao Army would fall back. Occasionally a few soldiers would be killed, but this was largely through accidents or overexuberance.

But now the conflict had taken a sinister turn. The slaughter of the Meo village was just one more indication of the Pathet Lao's new commitment. It had become, in many ways, a real war.

'It had to happen eventually,' Croce said.

'We should make plans for the future.'

'The Americans will not allow the communists to take over in Laos.'

'The Americans will fight as long as it suits them, and as long as it doesn't cost them too much. Indochina is just a chessboard to them.'

'Don't let Dale and his friends hear you say that. They think they're fighting for freedom.'

'There's no such thing as freedom. Only power.'

Baptiste smiled. Bonaventure was becoming more irascible every day. Old age, perhaps. Old age and the tropics. They never mixed well.

The American pilots had reached new heights of hysteria with their improvised Lao conversation. The taxi girls had controlled their giggles long enough to help them in their intonation.

'*Thao dai?*' one of the pilots said.

How much?

'*Laa-khaa jet phan kip*,' his buddy said, batting his eyelids in a coquettish imitation of a taxi girl and raising his voice an octave.

The price is 7000 *kip.*

'Nii nyai maen baw. Phaa-saa lao oen an-naii waa nyang?'

This is big, isn't it? What do you call this in Lao?

His buddy shook his head. *'Khawy kin muu baw dai?'*

I can't eat pork.

One of the pilots was laughing so hard he fell off his chair.

Idiots.

Bonaventure turned to Baptiste. 'How are things at home?'

'Better.'

'You don't seem sure.'

'It's just the child. You know.' It was a lie. For the last two years they had lived a tense and fragile truce. Many times he had tried to bridge the gap between them without success. Noelle's moods veered between long, brooding silences and flashes of quick and venomous temper.

'You must think I'm blind,' Bonaventure said.

Baptiste stared sulkily into his glass.

'What are you going to do?'

'I don't know.'

'You must try harder. Stay home more. Look after her properly.'

'She knew what I was like when she married me.'

Bonaventure leaned forward, placed a hand on the younger man's arm. 'Baptiste, I like you. And you have done well in the business. You have a talent for this, you know? But you must learn tactics. It is okay to be so passionate, so spontaneous, when you are young. When you are older it becomes a weakness.'

Baptiste jerked his arm away and blew a long stream of smoke towards the ceiling. He did not like being lectured by anyone.

'Noelle is my daughter,' Bonaventure went on, his voice sterner. 'I'm getting old and Indochina is going to shit. Perhaps I'll retire.'

'What are you telling me?'

'I'm telling you, I'm losing patience. If you can't work things out between the two of you, then I shall.'

'It has nothing to do with you.'

205

'It has everything to do with me. She's my only daughter. Don't forget that.'

'We'll work it out.'

'I hope so.'

Baptiste felt a jolt of fear. Without the Bonaventure family, what would happen to him? He would be left with hardly any money of his own, Bonaventure had made sure of that. All the assets were still in his name. If he and Noelle were divorced before the old buzzard died, he would have nothing. And with only one eye he would not get a licence to fly for any other airline.

'*Tawng kaan pha set toh,*' the pilot with the high voice was saying.

I need a towel.

'*Tawng kaan maw,*' his partner groaned.

I need a doctor.

Baptiste slammed his glass on the table. The Americans and their puerile jokes were getting on his nerves.

'Go home,' Bonaventure told him. 'Go home and be with your wife.'

Baptiste left the bar. Two taxi girls were chatting with one of the *siclo* drivers. They cat-called to him as he came out. For once he ignored them. He felt as if he had stones in his chest.

Noelle lay under the mosquito netting, listening to the rise and fall of the cicadas. Tonight it was hot, too hot to sleep, and she tossed restlessly from side to side. There was a cold ache in the pit of her stomach, the physical presence of loneliness and regret.

She found herself thinking yet again about the American. She was embarrassed at the way she had thrown herself at him at her father's party, and felt her cheeks blush hot in the darkness. She had drunk too much champagne that afternoon.

Shame. Another ingredient to throw into the heady mix of emotions that she lived with every day; confusion, despair, frustration, loneliness, longing and anger. If she simply hated Baptiste it might be simpler. But sometimes when they were together, she still found herself falling under his spell.

His looks and his charm could mesmerise her even now, make her forget the poison in him.

And he *was* the father of her child; Lucien was the bond that tied them together. Baptiste was her husband, for life, that was what the Holy Church had told her.

But often she just wished him dead; it would be the easy way to be free of him. The temptation of forgetting everything he had done would not be there. But this way, every time she relented and made love with him, she felt as if she had traded with the devil. Staying with such a man, or leaving him, both were wrong.

All right then, even if she could not leave him, she would not allow him to imprison her. There was another way, a choice dark and rich with sin, revenge, justice and need. If you can't be good, Noelle, be as bad as you want.

She dressed quickly. The servants were all in bed. She went downstairs and fetched Chao. 'I have to go out. You will sleep in Lucien's room and be there in case he wakes. I will be back soon.'

And she ran out into the night.

45

Dale had been drinking with Gerry Gates and an attaché from the United States Embassy at the Hotel Constellation. When he got back the bungalow was in darkness. He felt tired, more tired tonight than he had ever felt in all his years overseas. There had been too many nights when he had come home alone to empty rented houses or sparse hotel rooms.

Now it was only his burning sense of destiny that kept him going. No one had said that it would be easy to be on the side of the angels. In any crusade there were sacrifices that had to be made.

He lit a small paraffin lantern and carried it into the bedroom. As he placed it on the table beside his bed, he saw the silhouette of a human form in the rattan chair by the window. His whole body jerked with adrenalin, as if he had touched a live wire.

He threw himself on to the floor away from the light, reached inside his jacket for his revolver with his right hand, and lay face down in a firing position, both hands holding the weapon in front of him. His thumb clicked off the safety.

Whoever was in the chair uttered a sob of alarm.

'Noelle,' Dale said.

He climbed slowly to his feet, holstered the revolver, feeling foolish. He picked up the lamp and brought it over to the chair.

They stared at each other, frozen.

'I think you are going to shoot me,' she whispered.

'Sorry. Old habits die hard.'

For a long time, just the hissing of the lamp. If she had been an assassin he would not have been as surprised – or as terrified. He sensed he was about to cross a border into no man's land.

'I know I must not come here. A hundred times I am to leave and a hundred times I sit down again.'

When he did not answer her she said: 'You think I am a tramp.'

He shook his head. His arms and legs felt like lead. 'I'm just surprised, that's all.' His voice didn't sound like his own.

'Do something,' she said.

He put the lamp on the floor. He knelt down in front of the chair and they continued to stare at each other, the lamp throwing flickering shadows over their faces.

Noelle got to her feet. 'I am wrong to come.'

He grabbed her arm and pulled her back into the chair. He pulled her face towards him and kissed her roughly on the mouth. Immediately her arms went around his neck, clinging to him as if she were drowning. Her tongue explored his mouth with an abandon that shocked him. He heard the buttons of his shirt rip.

Like being caught in the open in a hurricane, he thought. Too late to run for shelter now.

They lay naked side by side on the bed. He felt the sweat cool on his body. There was a syrupy stickiness on his groin, and his heart was hammering in his chest. He could scarcely believe what had happened to him. Guilt nudged at him, faint but irritating, like the buzzing of a mosquito in a darkened room. He tried to ignore it, just wanted to lose himself in this shocking, impossible dream.

He felt her fingers trace the contours of the muscles in his chest and shoulders, find the scar just below the collarbone and circle it questioningly.

'Bullet,' he whispered.

'Where?'

'The Philippines. I was an adviser to Magsaysay.'

'Agriculture?'

He detected the playfulness in her voice. 'Something like that.'

She wrapped her leg across his thigh, he felt her breath on his cheek. It was hot, and smelled of mint. Noelle was not like any European woman he had ever known. She did not appear to be embarrassed, did not try to hide herself under the sheet. He could not imagine any American woman coming to a man's room like this, pursuing him so . . . well, shamelessly. Why had she done it? he wondered.

Perhaps she sensed the direction of his thoughts. She sat up. 'You think I'm a whore,' she said.

'No.'

'Of course you do.' She said it as if it was irrefutable fact. She pushed the mosquito net aside and went to the window. Her breasts looked swollen; even in the yellow glow of the lamp he could make out the dark pattern of milk veins in her breasts. He remembered when she had climaxed how a little milk had spurted from her nipple on to his cheek.

Her mood had changed abruptly. She crossed her arms protectively across her breasts. 'You must not feel bad. I did this to get revenge on my husband.'

What am I supposed to say to that? he wondered.

'Did you hear me?'

'Don't be angry.'

'Why shall I be angry. Because I do everything wrong in my life?'

'Is that all this is for you? Revenge?'

She turned away, and did not answer.

'Why don't you leave him?'

'And go where?' She started to snatch her clothes from the floor.

'What's wrong?'

'I must go home now.' She threw her dress over her head and hopped across the room trying to fumble into her underwear. She collided with the chair and sat down heavily. '*Merde!*'

The sudden shift in her mood bewildered him. He had never been reckless like this, he realised, had always needed to convince himself a hundred times that he was right before he did anything. He had never acted so spontaneously, had certainly never instigated anything without thought to consequences. So how could he hope to understand this woman?

She found her leather sandals on the floor and sat on the edge of the bed to put them on. 'I find my way in, I will find my way out. Just leave the money on the dresser.'

He reached out and put a hand on her shoulder. 'It wasn't wrong,' he whispered.

'Of course it is wrong! What is the matter with you? You don't have no morals?' She sounded as petulant as a schoolgirl and he didn't know how to answer her.

He heard her stamp away down the front steps. He lay back and stared at the ceiling. Already the last hour was receding like a half-remembered dream.

As soon as Noelle reached the house, she heard the sound of a child crying. She had been gone longer than she intended. Poor Lucien.

Then she saw the Packard in the driveway and stopped, shocked and afraid. Baptiste spent almost every night in one of the bars or nightclubs, but tonight of all nights he had returned early. Well, Noelle, not only is your revenge complete, it is out in the open. Dale's seed was still damp between her legs and her cheeks blushed with shame. Perhaps she deserved Baptiste. If she took into account all the things she had done in her life maybe she was the perfect match for him after all.

Chao was walking the child up and down the long hall, her bare feet padding on the teak. Her eyes were sullen, accusing.

'*Un cauchemar,*' she said, patting Lucien's back. A nightmare.

Noelle took Lucien from her and at once he stopped crying. She carried him back to his bedroom. There was no sign of Baptiste. Perhaps he had been too drunk to notice she was gone.

She sat down on the edge of Lucien's bed. He immediately demanded her breast. She was tender after the lovemaking, and winced at the pain.

'Where have you been?'

She looked up. Baptiste was standing in the bedroom doorway, his hands on his hips. Lucien started crying again.

'Wait until he's settled,' she said.

'I said: Where have you been?'

'I was out. Now stop shouting! You're upsetting Lucien!'

'Out where?'

'When have you ever been concerned where I was before midnight?'

'You have a child, Noelle!'

'So do you!'

'You should have been here with Lucien! What sort of a mother are you?'

The accusation took her breath away. Unbidden, the memory of her first glimpse of him returned to her, the night he had driven into the lobby of The Constellation. Whatever had made her think a man like that would be a model husband and father? 'I won't win any prizes for motherhood. As you don't, for being a husband.'

Three steps into the room and he was standing over her. Lucien wriggled and shrieked. She tried to quieten him. From the periphery of her vision she saw Baptiste's fist open and close. She heard his breathing, fierce and quick in his chest.

'Don't try and threaten me, Baptiste. Hit me and I'll take a knife to you, I swear it. And if I miss, my father won't.'

She glared up at him.

'I would never hurt you,' he whispered. 'You're my wife.'

'I wish I wasn't.'

'Just tell me where you have been!'

'You never tell me where you go when you come in late at night. Why should I tell you?'

He bent down so that his face was inches from hers. 'You whore!' he hissed.

'Everything I am, I owe to you.'

Now she was sure he was going to hit her. But instead he backed away and slumped against the lintel of the door. 'I love you, Noelle. I love you more than anything in my life.'

His voice sounded broken. She had expected anything but that. Hot tears streaked her face. Why was it that he had been unfaithful a score of times and had never shown a moment's remorse; she had cheated him once and her chest felt like a barrel of stones? Perhaps that was the difference between Baptiste and her.

'I will try and change,' she heard him say. 'I promise. You're everything to me. Everything.'

He stumbled back to his own bedroom. Lucien quietened, and she rocked him back to sleep. He was getting too long for her to hold in her arms now. Perhaps Baptiste is right, I have babied him too long. Is it because I want to protect him from his father?

Or because I want to make him utterly different?

She started to tremble. What had happened with Dale – how could she explain or excuse it? She did not understand herself any more.

She could have absorbed all of Baptiste's anger. But now she felt herself wither with the force of his regret.

46

Xiengkhouang Province

Beyond the lines of sandbags and barbed wire the dark green mountains rose into a washed blue sky. A corporal brought their breakfast onto the verandah, *foy* rice noodle in a soup of vegetables and meat.

It was almost eight o'clock. Dale watched a soldier run to the middle of the beaten earth parade ground to sound the seven o'clock reveille.

Colonel Kaysone grinned as he bent over his bowl and began to scoop the noodles into his mouth. 'Late again!' he chuckled.

It was at times like these that Dale's hopes turned to dust and despair. It seemed impossible that these cheerful, lazy people had been committed to hold back the Pathet Lao and their Chinese overlords.

Kaysone gave a high-pitched giggle. 'What do you think? Can we win this war?'

Dale looked at Gates. 'Trust us, Colonel,' Gates answered. 'The United States won't let you lose.'

He giggled again, and returned to his breakfast.

Dale turned his attention to the town below the garrison. The Hmong were down from the hills for the market. They were distinctive in their black pyjamas, edged with dark blue, their hair long, straggling over their collars. They looked Chinese but their skin was a smoky bronze. Several of them had slingshots hanging around their necks.

The irony was inescapable. Because they dared not use their atomic weapons against the Russians and Chinese they would fight their proxy war here, using people who still thought the earth was flat and hunted with Stone Age weapons.

The colonel must have divined what he was thinking. 'You think perhaps these *Meo* can beat the Pathet Lao?'

Dale did not know. He would soon have a better idea. He and Gates would spend the next weeks and months deep in the mountain jungles with these people, living with them, eating their food, sleeping in their huts, training them for the guerilla war against Pathet Lao.

But right now the war was not the only thing on his mind. He had not seen Noelle again before he left Vientiane to come north. The memory of that one night stayed with him, a bewildering enigma. Why had she come to him? Why hadn't she come back? Was that all there would ever be?

He pushed his breakfast away.

'Are you all right, Jack?' Gates asked him.

Dale shrugged. 'I'm just not hungry this morning,' he said.

'You'll be okay,' Gates said and slapped him on the shoulder, thinking it was just pre-combat nerves.

But Dale doubted that he would be okay. In fact Jonathan Dale wondered if he would ever be quite the same again.

47

Kowloon Tong

In this part of Hong Kong there were no high rises; there were miniature Indian palaces and English Tudor country homes, all with their own gardens, all astonishingly expensive. Kowloon Tong was Hong Kong's equivalent to Beverley Hills.

At the end of one of the more secluded streets was a high wall topped with broken glass and barbed wire, and two huge wrought iron gates with mounted close circuit television cameras. A man in dark glasses watched them drive through, holding a Dobermann on a short chain leash.

The winding driveway was flanked by cypress pines and manicured lawns tended by Hakka gardeners. It led to a white two storey house built entirely of concrete and glass.

As they parked the Porsche, Dragon Fist explained what was happening. 'There's a big meeting, tonight. A lot of big shots will be here. The house belongs to the 489 of the Fei Lung. He took over six months ago when his brother died, even though he still lives some of the time in Saigon. You have to be very respectful, okay?'

Douglas nodded. He was excited. He was getting close to the heart of power now. He could feel its pulse.

A white-jacketed servant led the way through an echoing marble foyer to two great carved doors, guarded by gilt dragons. They were ushered into a long rectangular room, dominated by a mahogany table with ball and claw feet. Douglas could see his reflection in the polished marble floors. There was little other furniture in the room; a chair, upholstered in tiger skin, a spirit altar, a ceramic spitoon decorated with hand-painted pink flowers, a photograph of the Queen.

There were eight of them, all middle-aged chiu chao Chinese, playing mah-jong. Douglas was disappointed. They were dressed much alike, most of them in shirtsleeves and trousers with high belts; some of the leading triads in Hong Kong and they looked like the old men who practised tai chi in the park.

'Sit down,' the 489 said, indicating two straight-backed chairs, and then he turned back to the game and ignored them. A servant brought them *yum cha* and they sipped the scalding tea and waited. A goldfish with huge winged fins watched them through the thick glass of its aquarium.

Finally, when the game was finished, Sammy Chen stood up and came to sit in the tiger skin chair.

'I have a job for you,' he said.

Dragon Fist nodded eagerly, Douglas noticed, like a child asked to run an errand.

'I need someone washed. Someone very big, very important. His name is Chen Jia-guo.'

'Of course, Kee Lung.' Kee Lung – Fearless Dragon. This kind of respect was only given to a triad leader.

'It will not be easy. Since my brother's death he has been hiding himself at the Mongkok Typhoon Shelter. No one can go there without being seen. When I sent our Grass Sandal to talk to him, he fled by sampan across the water.'

'I will do it,' Douglas said. 'I will wash him for you.'

Sammy studied him with elaborate care. 'You are the one they call Sharkfin? I have heard great reports about you from your uncle.'

Douglas nodded eagerly. 'I can wash him. I can wash anyone you want.'

Sammy gave Douglas a small, chill smile. He reached into his shirt pocket and handed Dragon Fist several prints. 'Photographs of my cousin,' he said.

Dragon Fist was staring at Douglas, his face pale. Then he bowed once more to Sammy Chen. 'I understand, Kee Lung. I will see that it is done.'

'Good.'

217

Sammy got up and went back to the mah-jong game. Dragon Fist bowed to their backs. Douglas did the same, and followed him out.

'Don't ever do that again!' Dragon Fist shouted when they got back into the car.

'Why are you angry, *tai lo*?'

'You do not say, "I can do this, I can do that"! I brought you here tonight to learn. But you don't learn anything, do you? *I can wash anyone*. Maybe it's you who needs to be taught a lesson!'

Douglas was bewildered by his uncle's fury. 'A thousand times a thousand apologies, *tai lo*.'

'You ever take away my face like that again, you're the one who gets washed!'

Douglas bit his lip and said nothing. He was too impetuous, he realised. It had always been his fault; too eager to impress.

They drove through the gates and made their way back to the Walled City in silence. Finally Dragon Fist said: 'You think you can do it, then?'

'If there is a secret way in, I will find it.'

Dragon Fist nodded. He hawked and spat out of the window. After a while he seemed to overcome his anger. 'All right, then.'

'Why does Kee Lung want this man dead?'

'Chen Jia-guo is his cousin. When Kee Lung's brother died, he thought he should be the new 489. He said Sammy came up too fast, he called him an eye-eye, an illegal immigrant. This is because he has never lived in Hong Kong, only Saigon.'

'If it's true, why didn't the other bosses support him?'

'Because Sammy Chen and his brother had organised the opium traffic together for so long. Only Sammy can control it. He has the contacts, knows the supply routes. Everyone is getting richer, and Sammy is the one who gets the credit. Who cares if Chen Jia-guo is right or wrong? He's a fool. He tried to have Sammy chopped. Now he has to hide out in Mongkok like a water rat.'

The Walled City appeared ahead of them in the night,

the lights of the great tenement blocks blazed against the black backdrop of the mountains. Douglas ached to escape. He was sick of living in the squalor of the Walled City, and sick of being his uncle's lap-dog. He wanted a house in Kent Road, like Sammy Chen.

Perhaps, with the washing of Chen Jia-guo, they would finally set him on the road.

48

Douglas sat in Dragon Fist's sports car on Ferry Street and stared across the water at the ramshackle city of huts that spread over the mud and oil-streaked water. Dragon Fist lowered the Zeiss binoculars and passed them to Douglas.

'Here,' he said.

The Mongkok typhoon shelter was a conglomeration of wooden huts that ventured into the harbour from the sea wall. The huts were built on bamboo stilts, a maze of seemingly fragile structures linked by springy wooden catwalks that could be laid or removed in seconds. The only other access was by sampan. It was impossible to get inside quickly as every entrance was guarded by look-see boys with an electronic bell push to sound the alarm if they were attacked. The sampan girls who plied the waters of the Shelter were often paid to give a secret signal if their passengers were police or from a rival triad.

'You see?' Dragon Fist was saying. 'He's safe in there. No one can get in, day or night, without him being alerted. Meanwhile he still has his income from his opium den and a place to keep his soldiers.'

Douglas thought about the problem for a long time. Finally he said: 'We could try and get in underneath.'

'Underneath?'

'No one would see us.'

'It's impossible. Anyway, who would want to drag themselves through that filth?'

'I would,' Douglas said.

Dragon Fist snatched back the binoculars and studied the typhoon shelter once more. 'Perhaps,' he said grudgingly. 'At low tide. But you would have to know where he was in advance, or you would just stumble around in the mud all night.'

'Perhaps we just need to bribe the addicts who live there. Give them some money to buy more opium. It's all they ever think about anyway.'

'You also need a plan of escape. Or his soldiers will cut you to pieces.'

'We'll start a fire, create a diversion. Then have a sampan come and pick us up. That way we can bring back Chen Jia-guo alive if you want.'

Dragon Fist considered the plan for a long time. He took a manila envelope from under the seat and passed his nephew the black and white photographs of Chen Jia-guo that Sammy Chen had given him. 'This is him. It will be dark so you'll have to remember his face better than your own mother's.'

'I've forgotten my mother,' Douglas said.

For ten Hong Kong dollars their spy, a sampan girl, moored her boat next to the hut that Chen Jia-guo used as his headquarters. She painted a yellow cross on the underside of the hull, clearly visible from the shore side. At low tide, Douglas, Freddy Yang and a dozen *sze kau* waded into the mud from the shore and started the long journey.

The underside of the Mongkok Typhoon Shelter was a hellish swamp of squelching mud thickened and greasy with human ordure, rubbish, and mountains of discarded shellfish. Water rats rustled and squabbled in the shadows.

They struggled through this fetid swamp for almost an hour before they detected the sweet, treacle smell of opium from above, and the droning murmur of voices from the smokers drawing the dream smoke into their lungs. Douglas searched the darkness with the narrow beam of a pencil torch. It settled on the emaciated corpse of an opium addict, his face set in a death's head grin, the rats feeding on his corpse.

They moved on. At one stage, Freddy Yang spat a muffled curse as a rain of urine trickled on his head from the darkness above.

Finally, knee deep in mud, they reached the sampan, and waited there for long minutes to make sure they were unobserved. Douglas carried a rope on his right shoulder, a grappling hook attached to the end. He threw it onto the bamboo decking above and pulled himself up.

He crept towards the entrance of the nearest hut. The look-see boy was asleep. Douglas took a handful of hair and jerked his head back. The boy's eye blinked open and he saw Douglas standing over him with a meat cleaver in his right fist. He had no time to react before it slashed into his throat, the scream cut off before it began. He lay on his back, bubbling and writhing. After a few seconds he subsided and was still.

Douglas ran inside. There were three men, all asleep on simple wooden cots. One of them shouted an alarm. Douglas silenced him by bringing the handle of the cleaver down on his skull. By now several of his own triads had joined him, pinning the two other men onto their beds, knives glinting in the torchlight.

Douglas shone the torch in their faces.

The third man was Chen Jia-guo.

'Wash the others,' Douglas said.

Their throats were expertly slashed with razors.

'Let's get out of here,' Douglas said.

Chen was bound hand and feet and pulled outside. Two triads dragged him to the edge of the platform and tipped him over into the mud below. There was a wet sound as his body hit the mud, his scream of pain muffled by the gag in his mouth.

Freddy Yang doused the bamboo floors with petrol from a can and scampered down the rope. Douglas tossed a lighted match inside and jumped clear. He felt the rush of heat as the hut exploded into flames. They scrambled through the sickly mud, dragging Chen between them. Above them they heard the panicked screams of the look-see boys and the shouts of alarm as the sleeping villagers woke to the smell of smoke and flames.

Douglas, Freddy Yang and two others bundled Chen Jia-guo into the boot of an old Austin they had parked on the waterfront and drove north to the Kowloon reservoirs under Beacon Hill. Their bodies and faces were caked with reeking mud and filth. Even hardened as they were to the stench of Hak Nam, they had to drive with the windows down.

Pitch black.

The Austin's headlamps were the only lights out here at this time of night. Freddy Yang stopped the car and Douglas jumped out and threw open the boot. Chen Jia-guo was pulled out, still trussed like a fowl, and between them they kicked him down the slope towards the edge of the reservoir.

Douglas handed the torch to Freddy Yang, went back to the car and took the pistol Dragon Fist had given him from the glove compartment. He unwrapped it from its oilcloth and followed the others down the slope.

Chen Jia-guo lay at the water's edge squirming like a beached fish. Freddy Yang shone the torchbeam full in his face and put his foot on his throat. Douglas bent down and whispered in his ear: 'I must never cause harm or bring trouble to my sworn brothers. If I do, so I will shed blood from the five holes of my body.'

He cocked the pistol, placed the muzzle against Chen Jia-guo's ear and pulled the trigger. He fired again into the corpse's left ear, then the two eyes, and then the mouth.

By the time he was finished there was little left that was recognisable as a human being.

They walked away and left the body where it was. The police would find it and identify the remains from fingerprints. That was all that was needed. It would serve as a warning to others, that they should not underestimate the new 489 of the Fei Lung triad.

49

Vientiane, June 1964

At sunset the women went down to the river to wash, their
children playing and splashing in the water around them. Noelle
walked along the high river bank, watched a pirogue with a
high-curled prow glide past below, its reflection mirrored in
the lavender water. The river twitched, choked from the recent
rains. Fish sucked pits from the water below.

She loved coming here in the evening. Lucien was a demand-
ing child, and at this time of the day she left him in the care of
Chao so that she could have this hour to herself by the river.

He was still a hundred yards away when she saw him. He was
standing on the riverbank, staring into the milky brown water,
hands thrust deep into his pockets. When he saw her he took
his hands out of his pockets and turned around. It occurred
to her that he had been waiting for her.

'Noelle,' he said.

She knew she should walk straight back to the house. Instead
she went to join him under the eucalyptus tree.

'How long have you been back in Vientiane?' she said.

'I got back last night. I thought I'd take a walk out here. I
was hoping I'd see you.'

She wondered what he wanted with her. Had he come sniffing
around for more sex? Perhaps he thought she was an easy lay,
someone to help while away the long Vientiane nights when
he got bored with the taxi girls at the White Rose.

'I am a married woman, Monsieur Dale. No one must see us
talk like this.'

'The last three months there hasn't been a minute I haven't spent thinking about you.'

The unexpected declaration made her feel suddenly vulnerable, as if she would like to put her head on this man's shoulder and weep, pour out all her sins and her regrets.

My God, she thought. I am in imminent danger of making a complete fool of myself. So she turned the subject away from herself. 'And where have you been all this time, Monsieur Dale?'

'I don't think I can tell you that.'

'Top secret agriculture?'

He gave her a lop-sided grin. 'That's right. Classified rice.'

'No more scars?'

'I try to stay out of trouble.'

'If you want to stay out of trouble, you will not have come here.'

They walked for a while in silence, away from the house.

'What do you want, Monsieur Dale?'

'You. I want you.'

'You forget. I am another man's wife.'

'Are you?'

'Of course.'

'That's not how I see it. I think you're desperately unhappy, trapped in a life you don't want with a guy you don't love.'

She started to walk faster. It hurt to hear herself so accurately described. 'So not only do you fix cars and advise on agriculture, also you read palms. You are truly a man of many talents.' She had not meant to sound so truculent, and her own belligerence surprised her. He had wounded her more deeply than she thought.

'I didn't mean to offend you,' he said.

'I am not offended.' She wanted to rage, wanted to weep. It was not just that she was married, she had Lucien. Besides, she hardly knew this man. After Baptiste, she no longer trusted her judgment of character.

She whirled around to face him. 'Please. Just go away.'

'I think I love you.'

Damn him. She didn't want to hear this. Not now. 'Then I am sorry for you.'

'Sorry?'

'That night – I should not have come. It was wrong.'

'It was the rightest thing I've ever done.'

'Please. Please go away.'

He stared at her, shock and disbelief etched into his face. Americans! Everything was so simple for them. Was that it? You can walk in, take another man's wife, just because you want her?

She reached up and touched his cheek, with sudden tenderness. 'It was a beautiful night. You are a wonderful lover and a very gentle man. But I have a son and a husband.'

He was about to say something else but she put her finger to his lips.

'Please, do not say anything,' she said, and walked quickly away. 'I cannot see you no more.'

She hurried away. She looked back just once, saw the glow of his cigarette in the dusk. When she reached the bend in the river, she ran all the way back to the house.

The sun had dropped down the sky, turning the surface of the Mekong to pools of gold and throwing a sudden dusk over the valley. Noelle was surprised to hear shouts and laughter on the back verandah. Baptiste was home, playing in the garden with Lucien in the gathering gloom. The boy was perched on his shoulders and Baptiste was pretending to be an aeroplane.

'No more,' he shouted. 'It is too dark to fly! I have no landing lights!'

'Please!' Lucien was bobbing up and down. 'Just once more!'

Baptiste relented. 'All right, all right. Are you ready for take off? Full throttle. Release the brakes. Away we go!'

He launched himself off the verandah steps and leaped into the garden. Noelle's heart was in her mouth. If Baptiste fell, the boy would be thrown headlong. But of course he did not slip, he landed on both feet, Lucien shrieking and giggling.

'Bank twenty degrees to port!' Baptiste shouted, and whirled around the mango tree at the bottom of the garden. The servants stood around laughing and clapping.

Baptiste almost ran into a badminton net strung between two lime trees. 'Mountains!' he shouted, and sidestepped left at full tilt, leaping over a rattan basket of weeds. 'Turbulence!'

The boy bounced on his shoulders, laughter hiccoughing out of him.

'Ready to land?' He swept up towards the verandah steps, saw Noelle and stopped, breathing hard. '*Chérie.*'

She felt something squirm inside her. Oh, how she had loved this man. Still did sometimes, damn him. 'Teaching him to fly already?'

Lucien clenched handfuls of his father's thick black hair to steady himself. Baptiste grinned sheepishly. 'He's a little heavy on the controls,' he said.

Seeing their faces so close together Noelle had time to take in the similarity; the same thick black hair and deep blue eyes, accentuated by thick lashes and eyebrows. Put an eyepatch on little Lucien and he would be a miniature version of this man. She hoped he had not also been blessed with his father's temperament.

'Almost time for his supper,' she said. 'Or do you plan to teach him night flying?'

'No night flights allowed in Laos,' said Baptiste. He lifted Lucien off his shoulders. 'Time for you to eat, *mon petit chou.*' He kissed the child as he lowered him to the ground. But Lucien wanted more and howled.

Chao shushed him and led him inside. The gardener and the cookboy melted away into the shadows.

Noelle and Baptiste stared at each other in awkward silence.

'Did you enjoy your walk?'

'It was pleasant.'

There was the old fire in his eyes tonight. 'You look wonderful,' he said.

She felt her resolve weaken. She almost hated herself for her stubbornness. She took one step towards him. If I throw myself down those steps into his arms it will be over. Perhaps we can leave this misery behind. But what about all those nights I was alone while he got drunk and played with the taxi girls? Even the night Lucien was born, God damn him to hell! And do I really believe he knew nothing about the plan to murder his best friend? Can I really ever trust this man again?

'I thought we might dismiss the servants early and have dinner alone tonight.'

Noelle shook her head. 'I am very tired, Baptiste. Perhaps another night.'

He swore harshly under his breath and stormed past her up the stairs and through the house. She heard doors slam and the Packard's tyres squealing as he drove back into Vientiane.

Dale heard the creaking of the timbers on the verandah and was instantly awake. He turned on the kerosene lantern beside the bed and listened. A door rattling in its frame, gentle footsteps padding across the floor. He was about to reach for the revolver that he kept in the drawer beside the bed, then changed his mind.

She stood in the doorway, both her hands raised in the air. 'No gun this time?' she whispered.

'I mined the floor before I came to bed.'

She lowered her hands, crossed her arms and leaned against the lintel.

'A few hours ago you said you never wanted to see me again.'

'I lied.'

She pulled her dress over her head. She was naked underneath. She pulled the braids from her hair, and tossed her head to shake it loose. She held her hair back with her hands, her elbows almost touching in front of her chin.

'You like what you see?' Her voice was torchy, hoarse with excitement.

'I liked what I saw from the very first time,' he said.

'It is very bad I am here, Dale.' Dale. Easier to pronounce than Jonathan, he supposed, and it kept him at arm's length. She crawled towards him across the bed, until she was kneeling over him.

He reached up and touched her cheek. 'I think I'm in love with you,' he whispered.

She put her finger to his lips. 'I am going to hell for you, I think.' She leaned across him to turn off the lamp. He gripped her hips, holding his face between her breasts, breathing in the sweet perfume and the softness of her skin. She moaned softly and he threw her on to her back and desire overtook them both with the suddenness and violence of a wild monsoon storm.

50

The early-morning mist shrouded the road, muffled the cackle of the geese waddling in front of an old farmer, and the soft ringing of the *siclo*'s bell as its driver ferried an old wife to market.

Bonaventure took a bite from his croissant and chewed slowly, reflectively. Noelle toyed with her coffee.

'What brings you here so early, *chérie*?'

'I need to talk to you.'

He knew what this was about. 'Where's Baptiste?'

'He had to fly to Ban Me Thuot. He took off at dawn.'

He nodded. Six hundred kilos of opium, part of the consignment for Sammy Chen.

'So, how are things between you?'

'The same.'

'The same,' he repeated. Noelle pushed a curl from her eyes, and regarded him evenly. *Merde. Ce qu'elle est belle!* he thought. Even on this chill December morning, dressed impeccably in her long black leather coat and red woollen suit, she somehow managed to look half-naked. What was it? The way she moved, the way she spoke? There was this aura of sensuality she carried with her. Like her mother.

If only I had an ugly daughter.

'I'm going to leave him, Papa,' she was saying.

'We have had this conversation before.'

'And I have always given in to you before. This time I mean it.'

The sun rose and the haze began to lift. A flotilla of ducks flew over, a perfect V formation. Two boy bonzes walked along the road, holding the begging bowls with which they had earlier collected their breakfasts.

'I will not permit you to leave him,' he said.

'I don't care what you will permit any more, Papa. You do not have to take me back. You can always let your daughter and your grandson starve on the street.'

'Don't try me too far.'

'That is exactly what I intend to do. Only now I am so desperate that I think this time my will is stronger than yours.'

Impossible girl! He should never have had her educated! She was too smart by half. He pushed his breakfast away. He had quite lost his appetite.

'You must try again,' he said.

'Papa, why should I stay with Baptiste? He has been unfaithful to me countless times. I cannot trust him, and I cannot forgive him.'

'In the eyes of the Church you're married to this man for life.'

'Don't be such a hypocrite, you old goat! You don't give a damn what the Church thinks! You never have. You wear the Church like an old medal, you dust it off whenever it suits you!'

'You will not talk to me this way!'

'Papa, you lost the right to my respect when Jean-Marie Pepin died. Don't dictate to me any more. I am leaving Baptiste and I am taking my son!'

Bonaventure was rattled. She meant it, the little minx. She was right, he would not let her starve for even an hour, even to teach her a lesson. It would be a stain on his own pride.

The rhythmic clacking of wood on wood, as a Chinese soup cart stopped on the road outside and tried to attract customers. Steam from the shimmering brass pot rose into the still morning air. Bonaventure watched the hawker, thinking how much simpler the little coolie's life was than his.

'Give me a few days to think about this,' he said.

'Think about it all you want. I'm leaving.'

'And go where? What will you do, how will you live when I am no longer here to take care of you?' His fist slammed on the table.

Noelle did not even blink. 'I can take care of myself.'

'And what about the business?' Oh, what was the point of arguing with her? She never thought about the future. He sat back in his chair and gave a long sigh. 'You will have your way, Noelle, you always do. You do not have to leave him. I will make sure Baptiste is no longer a problem in your life.'

'I don't want him hurt.'

'What do you think I would do? I'm not a barbarian.'

Noelle raised one eyebrow, eloquent testimony to her opinion on that. Outrageous. He would have liked to put her over his knee. I have been too soft with her. As a child I indulged her too much, thought it was funny when she showed spirit. Now there is nothing I can do with her.

He threw down his napkin and stood up. 'Just leave it to me. I will arrange it,' he said and stormed out.

Why did God curse him with such a headstrong child?

Vientiane was changing rapidly. Two-storey brick buildings were sprouting in the town centre, wreathed in bamboo scaffolding. Enormous two-tone US cars with big fins now shared the roads with the oxcarts and water buffaloes.

Since the crisis, the United States Legation had been promoted to an Embassy. It was located in the same street as the national bank, and as Dale drove past he saw the manager's laundry fluttering on a line next to his reception room. He passed the Russian and North Vietnamese Embassies and waved cheerily to the guards outside.

Crazy place.

Buzzards roosted in the trees next to the embassy, waiting for scraps from the abattoir next door. Dale parked the car and walked inside, under the chinoiserie of dragons that no one had ever thought to remove.

He found Gates in his office studying a survey map of Laos on the wall behind his desk. It was dotted with coloured flags and markers that showed the relative positions of the Hmong, the Royal Lao Army and the Pathet Lao, as well as Air America landing strips. Once again the red flags had been pushed off the Plain of Jars. In another few months, when the monsoon ended, they would return.

Gates looked around as Dale entered, tapped his finger on

the top right hand corner of the map. 'Sam Neua,' he said, without preamble. 'That's where we go next. They're taking heavy losses, and Vang Pao wants us to train more recruits.'

Dale nodded and sat down.

'Coffee?' Gates asked him.

Dale shook his head.

'What's the problem?'

Dale had thought about this all night. It was now obvious to him that he couldn't stay on in Laos. He didn't particularly like Gerry Gates, but he was the only one in the embassy in a position to help.

'I want you to get me back to Saigon.'

Gates made a sour face. 'What the fuck for?'

'I just need to get out of Laos.'

Gates sat down, took out a packet of Lucky Strike, offered one to Dale, who shook his head. Gates took his time lighting up, giving himself time to think. 'Okay, what's this about?'

'Can you get me back to Saigon?'

'Maybe. But this is where the action is, Jack. You're not going anywhere until you tell me what's going on.'

Dale leaned forward, his elbows on his knees. 'It's kind of personal.'

'No such fucking beast in the Company, Jack. You can't have anything personal. Everything is business.'

Dale stared at the floor.

'What the fuck is it, Jack? If you got a clap, we can fix it right here.'

'If I had the clap, I wouldn't be telling you, Gerry.'

'So what is it? You getting blackmailed by the Russians? They find you in bed with your cook-boy or something?'

'Gerry, just get me out of Saigon.'

Gates groaned. 'Wait a minute. It's a fucking woman, right?'

Dale's silence affirmed his guess.

'It's not a taxi girl, because they don't count, and anyway, I never seen you with a taxi girl. Somebody's wife? Who? Not the Ambassador's, she's bigger than a B-52. Christ, Jack, none of them are worth...' The pieces suddenly fell into place. 'Not Noelle Crocé? Oh, Jack, not her. Tell me it ain't true.'

'So can you get me to Saigon?'

Gates rubbed his temples. Migraine coming on. 'If you've upset the Bonaventure family, Saigon is not going to make much difference. We don't want to start a vendetta with the Corsicans. How far has this thing gone?'

'Far enough.'

'Jesus H. You been screwing her, Jack?'

Dale gave him a look of such dangerous intensity that Gates looked away. He thought about it for a long time. 'Forget I asked you that. Leave it with me, okay. I'll see what I can do.'

Dale got up and went to the door.

'Jack.'

Dale turned.

'Be careful.'

51

There was a handful of journalists in the corner of the bar of the Constellation drinking through the colours. They had started with milky Pernod and water, and were noisily working their way towards black byrrh rum. They had survived the yellow pastis and green creme de menthe, but were stuck on blue.

One of them wondered aloud what colour lighter fluid was.

Gates arrived on time for his rendezvous with Rocco Bonaventure. He, exercising a lifetime's habit, was five minutes early.

Gates saw him, nodded a greeting, and sat down. Bonaventure raised one finger from the arm of his rattan chair, and a Lao barman hurried over with a cognac and soda, and another pastis for the monsieur.

'Hello, Rocky. Quiet in here tonight.'

'You cannot blame these gentlemen for that,' he said, indicating the group of French and British journalists.

'Well, all in the spirit of international goodwill.'

'There's no such thing,' Bonaventure grunted. He took out a pack of Gauloises and offered one to Gates, who shook his head.

'Trying to cut down, Rocky.'

'You don't think you're going to live a long and happy life?'

'I guess not. But no anyway.' He took a long swallow of his cognac.

'You look nervous,' Bonaventure observed.

'Maybe.'

'You said on the telephone that you had something important to discuss.'

'Important, but not pleasant.'

Bonaventure's face darkened. 'Rattakone?'

'No. It's personal.'

The Corsican passed a hand over his eyes. 'It's my son-in-law, isn't it?' He said it like a man telling a doctor that his gout was worse.

'Sort of.' Gates leaned forward and lowered his voice. A theatrical gesture, Bonaventure thought, as no one could hear them with the racket the journalists were making in the corner. Or perhaps it was just a mark of respect. 'It's Noelle. Did you know she was having an affair?'

Bonaventure felt the blood drain out of his face. So this was why she wanted to leave her husband. Daughters, he decided, were a curse. The devil's invention, to stop a man enjoying the serenity of old age. There were a thousand questions. 'Who?' was all he could manage.

'Jonathan Dale.'

Bonaventure drained his pastis and hammered the empty glass on the table. A Lao scurried over from the bar with a replacement. The old Corsican smoked and drank for a little while, as he tried to refocus the world through this new perspective. 'How long has this been going on?' he said at last.

Gates shook his head.

'When did you find out?'

'Today.'

Bonaventure took a series of deep breaths like a man preparing to dive off a cliff. 'Why are you telling me this?'

'Because I want you to help me resolve this. I'll make sure it doesn't continue. Dale will be out of here by the end of the week. I'll get him back upcountry where he can't do any more harm. But I thought maybe you'd care to explain the realities of this situation to Noelle.'

'Perhaps I might also like to have a word with this Dale.'

'You take care of yours, I'll take care of mine. The important thing is to make sure Crocé doesn't find out. I don't want anything to happen here that might embarrass me at the embassy.'

'You mean like Baptiste blowing your Monsieur Dale's brains out.'

'Something like that.'

Bonaventure felt the rage building inside him. First she had defied him and married a man he had warned her would only cause her heartache. Then, when she tired of him, she had humiliated him in front of everyone by whoring herself with an American. Did she have no shame, no respect? If Gates knew, how many other people in Vientiane knew? Perhaps tomorrow it would be on the front pages of *Lao Presse*: ROCCO BONAVENTURE'S DAUGHTER IS A WHORE.

'Thank you for your information,' he said, and got up suddenly, spilling his pastis.

'Just take it easy, Rocky,' Gates said.

'If God had wanted me to take it easy, he would not have given me a daughter. *Bordel de merde!*'

Noelle sat by the window and watched the moon rise over the Mekong behind a bank of ominous black cloud. The night was cool and she had slipped on one of Dale's olive drab woollens. The fibre was rough against her bare skin.

He was sprawled on his back across the bed. So like an American, she thought, they just lounge everywhere and expect people to make space for them. Even when they are asleep. But it amused her rather than irritated her. She watched him as he slept. Next to her, he was a giant, his chest and arms layered with muscle, yet when he was asleep, his face half-hidden by shadow and his hair tousled, he looked like a small boy.

He stirred, and rolled dreamily on to his side. His eyes blinked open. 'How long have you been awake?' he drawled, his voice husky from sleep.

'A long time.'

'What are you doing?'

'Just staring at the moon. Thinking.'

'What were you thinking about?'

'I am wondering what I am doing here. I am crazy I think.'

'I planned the whole thing. Crawled up to your house one

night and sawed through the fan belt on that monster you drive around in.'

'This is what they teach you in agricultural school.'

She heard him laugh. 'I got a confession, Noelle. I don't know a whole lot about agriculture.'

'I am so shocked.'

'I guess you saw straight through me, huh?'

'What is it you really do when you go up into the mountains?'

'We meet with the Hmong mostly. Give them advice.'

'What advice? How to fight wars?'

'Well, everyone has to know how to fight. If they want to stay free.'

'So you are a soldier?'

'Kind of.' He hesitated: she knew he was deciding whether to tell her the truth or give her his cover story. 'End of the Pacific War, I was a green lieutenant in the Marines. Came back with a Silver Star and a Purple Heart.'

'Very colourful.'

'Purple Heart's a citation you get when you take a wound for the Old Glory.'

'Another scar you do not tell me about?'

'This one's a little more private. Grenade fragment in the butt. Want to feel it?'

'I bet you say that to all the girls. If this scar is so bad, I'm sure I would have noticed by now.'

'I got a cosmetic surgeon on to it. It's my best feature.'

'Second best.'

He laughed at that. 'Anyway, after that I got a desk job for a while. Guess it was kind of a novelty sitting down again. But I soon figured I could be in the Army a long time before I went up the scale. The Air Force was a younger service, there was more opportunity. I took some written tests, then got myself transferred to Air Force Intelligence.'

'What kind of tests?'

'Two and two plus spelling your own name right two times out of three. I just slipped in.'

'And then?'

'Then that's all I'm allowed to tell you, ma'am. The rest of my life is classified.'

237

'Except for when Magsaysay shot you in the shoulder.'

'He didn't do that. I was just working for him at the time.'

'You drive his car, take dictation, what?'

'Classified.'

Even in the darkness she could see he was grinning at her. Hard not to smile back. She often found herself laughing when she was with him. She tried to imagine spending twenty-four hours a day with this man. What would it be like? She felt something squirming in her like a litter of new kittens. Don't be an idiot and fall in love with him, she told herself. This is revenge, this is indulgence, an end to loneliness. Don't make the same mistake you made before.

Don't fall in love with him.

The rain began again, slapping on the leaves outside the window, a soothing backdrop to the murmur of their conversation.

'Your turn,' he said.

'My turn?'

'To tell me all about you.'

'I am born in Moscow. I am sent here by Stalin to prise secrets from lonely American spies. The rest is classified.'

'Three things. One: I'm not a spy. Two: Stalin's dead. And three: I didn't realise I was lonely until I met you.'

'See. I'd make a rotten spy.'

'I really want to know about you,' he said, suddenly serious.

'What do you want to know?'

'Well, for instance – how do you get on with your father?'

A loaded question. 'Why?'

'Just something that puzzles me about you. I mean, you know how he makes his money, right?'

'Every businessman trades in a little opium in South East Asia. No one thinks it is bad. In Laos, the opium is like the motor car to Detroit.' Strange how she felt the need to defend him when someone else spoke aloud the same accusations she levelled at him herself. 'He is perhaps a *mauvaise caractère*. But he is not bad.'

'A loveable rogue? Like your husband?'

238

'Yes, like Baptiste.'

'Only you don't love him.'

She did not answer.

'What are you going to do, Noelle?'

'About what?'

'About us.'

'Nothing,' she said. All right, she knew that tonight, tomorrow night, soon, she would be discovered and it would be over. She dared not even think of the consequences of what she was doing. And although she wanted to get away from Baptiste, she was just as terrified of landing in another nightmare with this unknown American.

A loose shutter rattled somewhere in the house.

'I want you to come with me,' he said.

'Come with you? Where?'

'To Saigon. I've requested a transfer. You can get away from Baptiste and your father.'

'No.'

'Why not?'

She shook her head.

'But you don't love him. You can't stay with a man you don't love. It makes a mockery of everything.'

'But how do I know I love you?'

'I'm offering you a way out.'

'I do not want your favours!'

'I didn't mean it that way ...'

'Anyway, I have a son!'

He sat up in bed. 'Please, Noelle. Think about it.'

'No! It is easy for you. You come to a foreign country, you help people you don't really care about shoot at people you don't know, and you fall in love with women you can't have. For myself, my life is much more complicated.'

'I can't live without you now.'

'Living is easy. You just breathe in and out and remember to eat.' She did not understand what had suddenly made her so angry. She threw off his jersey and scrambled in the darkness for her clothes. She could almost feel his hurt and bewilderment.

She left without another word.

Papa had always told her she was reckless. Perhaps he was right. But this time she would try and learn from her mistakes. She would take stock and think. She would not be made a fool of twice.

52

The perfect solution had come unbidden to Rocco Bonaventure.

The first problem had been what to do about the American. It had occurred to him that Dale posed a real threat if his daughter had it in mind to form a permanent attachment. The idea made him wince.

The second problem was Baptiste. The Church did not sanction divorce, and arranging an annulment was traditionally a long and expensive business. The prelates in Saigon might let themselves be persuaded, but by the time they had finished they would have squeezed enough out of him to build themselves another cathedral. And even then Baptiste could still make himself difficult. He would probably demand to see Lucien occasionally, might even try and take him.

There had to be a cheaper, more effective answer.

It was a pity Baptiste had been unable to manage his daughter a little better. He had a lot of potential in the business. But he was now clearly a liability; the trick was how to get rid of him without offending his daughter's sensibilities.

Now he thought he knew.

The servants and their families were playing badminton in the front yard when Baptiste arrived. Bonaventure was sitting on the verandah, drinking *un sundowner*.

Baptiste shouted a greeting and ran up the steps two at a time. He looked relaxed and confident. His linen suit was pressed and freshly laundered, there was a cigarette held between fingers filled with chunky gold rings. A lot of style but little substance, Bonaventure thought. *Quel dommage*.

Baptiste sat down, and Bonaventure poured some Pernod into

his glass. Baptiste scooped some ice from the silver bucket with his fingers and dropped it in, the yellow spirit immediately transformed to the colour of milk.

They talked for a while, as they often did, about opium shipments, new orders, problems with the Beechcraft. I will miss him, Bonaventure thought with genuine regret. He has taken over many of the irksome details of the business, and proven himself a capable manager. What am I going to do without him? Perhaps it is time to retire, after all.

'There's something I have to talk to you about,' he said, at last. 'It's Noelle.'

Baptiste's face immediately became sulky.

'Please, Rocco. We have been through this before. This is my problem.'

You're so arrogant, Bonaventure thought. It will be a real pleasure to prick your balloon. 'She's having an affair.'

That wonderful olive skin actually turned a little pale. He saw the Adam's apple bobbing in his throat as he tried to swallow. Poor bastard. He wondered if this was how he had looked when Gates had told him.

'You can hardly blame her. You have not exactly been the model husband.'

'She's my wife,' he managed, in a strangled voice.

'I warned you about this. You should have taken better care of things at home.'

'Don't lecture me!'

'I don't intend to,' Bonaventure went on remorselessly. 'It's a little late for that.'

Baptiste stood up, his hands balled into fists on the verandah rail, now helpless in the grip of his own rage. 'Who is it?'

'It's an American. His name is Dale, Jonathan Dale. He's one of their agricultural advisers.'

'An American?' Baptiste said with disgust. She really knew how to rub salt into a wound.

'I want you to take care of this,' Bonaventure said.

'Take care of it?'

'The Corsican way.'

'I'll cut off his balls!'

'That's the spirit,' Bonaventure said cheerfully.

242

'It was Pepin! She never forgave me for that. But it was your idea!'

'Don't blame other people for your own messes, Baptiste. That should be your first lesson in life.'

Baptiste turned away, and stamped down the front steps. But halfway down he wheeled around and came back. 'I never wanted him dead!'

Bonaventure sipped his Pernod. 'But you did it. You're soft, Baptiste, that's your trouble. I wonder if you even have the guts to deal with Dale. Or do you want me to do it for you?'

'Damn you,' he hissed and stalked away.

Bonaventure smiled. Baptiste would take care of Dale. Then Gates would come to Bonaventure. And he, with regret, would pass the problem back to Gates. He could hear himself now: *I'm sorry. He acted without my consent. Do what you have to do. He has gone beyond my protection.*

Yes, Baptiste would solve the problem of Jonathan Dale. And Gates would solve the problem of Baptiste Crocé.

Perfect.

Noelle was in the garden with Lucien, throwing a ball. She heard a door slam inside the house, heard Baptiste shout at Chao. He burst on to the back verandah. She knew as soon as she saw him that the secret was out.

Lucien ran across the grass to meet him. Baptiste scooped him up in his arms but kept his eyes on Noelle and his expression did not change.

'Was it revenge?' he said.

Noelle felt suddenly calm. She had wondered if she might deny, threaten, justify. But instead she felt very calm and she knew that she would just tell him the truth.

'Was it revenge?' he repeated.

'At first,' she said. 'Then it was something more.'

'You won't take Lucien.'

She stared him down.

'Did you hear me? I won't ever let you go, either of you. I don't care what you do, if you run away to the end of the world, you'll never get away from me.'

'It's over between us, Baptiste.'

243

'It will never be over! Not until I say so!'

He kissed Lucien and put him back on the grass. She thought that now he would rage, would perhaps even hit her. Instead he turned on his heel and slammed back out of the house.

She had never been to Dale's bungalow in daylight. It was part of their pretence, a fragile belief in the sanctuary of darkness. There was no more need to hide. Now she had to warn him.

His jeep was gone.

She ran up the steps on to the verandah, banged on the door with her fist, ran past Dale's startled houseboy.

'Dale!'

'Monsieur Jean n'est pas ici,' he told her.

On an impulse she went into his bedroom.

A bachelor's homely sprawl. A shirt thrown across a chair, a pair of hiking boots, caked with orange mud, a Princeton beer jacket hanging on a door handle. The familiar smells of his cologne.

It looked utterly different in the daylight, its geography familiar but lurid. The bed had been made, military fashion, the room bare except for the rattan chair by the window and a teak chest of drawers next to the bed. She found a bottle of Johnny Walker beside an abandoned letter. She picked it up.

Dear Susan,
I don't know where to start. There's so much I have to tell you ...

My God.

Dear Susan?

She opened the drawer on the bedside table very slowly, as if she feared there might be a live snake inside. There was a paperback biography, dog eared, of Kennedy, another of Tom Paine. She threw them on the bed. Underneath the books was a pile of letters, tied with a rubber band. She snapped it off, and a photograph fell out of one of the envelopes.

She held it in trembling fingers: a beach, somewhere. A smiling woman, smiling children, in the middle a man in bathing trunks. Jonathan Dale. Family man.

Dear Susan.

The photograph slipped from her fingers on to the floor. Her whole body shook. Strange, because she felt nothing, nothing at all. After all, she was not in love with him. She had been lonely, and she had wanted to make Baptiste bleed. Dale had meant nothing to her. She turned and walked slowly out of the house with the regal bearing of a queen.

53

Baptiste walked into the Constellation holding a loaded revolver. It was a Smith & Wesson with six rounds in the chamber. He appeared to be drunk but in fact he was ice cold with rage and deadly sober. He looked around the bar and fired one shot over the barman's head, shattering a bottle of byrrh. It exploded and rum and shards of glass sprayed across the room.

Now he had everyone's attention.

He took three paces into the bar. 'Where's Dale?'

Gerry Gates was sitting with two crew-cut men in short sleeved shirts, near the door. He nodded and they casually rose to their feet and walked out.

'I thought Buffalo Bill was dead,' Gates said.

Baptiste swung around and pointed the gun at Gates' head. 'Where is he?'

'Why don't you put the gun down and we'll talk about this?'

'Just tell me where he is.'

'So you can blow his head off?'

'I intend to start much lower down.'

Gates folded his hands on his belly, looking relaxed. Men had pointed guns at him before. 'I got a feeling you don't understand the Big Picture, Baptiste. Let's go somewhere else and we'll talk about this.'

Baptiste did not move. 'Just tell me where he is.'

Gates shook his head. 'If you're gonna shoot me, it will have to be in the back.' He stood up and walked out.

Baptiste let him go. The revolver moved in an arc around the circle of shocked and silent faces. He knew most of them.

One of them, a French journalist, managed a sheepish grin.

But no Jonathan Dale.

He swore, lowered the gun, and followed Gates into the dark and rain-slick street.

The Americans were waiting for him. They each grabbed an arm, and Gates swung out of the shadows and hammered his fist into Baptiste's stomach. The air went out of him and he sank to his knees, the revolver dropping into the mud.

Gates picked it up, emptied the bullets out of the chamber and signalled to his colleagues that they were to bring Baptiste with them. He swung open the back door of a Chevrolet that was parked a few yards away and Baptiste was bundled in between the two men, still doubled over and gasping for breath.

Gates got behind the wheel and drove away.

They parked by the river, at the southern end of the town, out of sight of the road.

Gates swung around in the front seat. 'I'm going to do you a favour,' he said.

Baptiste was pinned between the two Americans. He had recovered from the blow he had taken, and his eyes were now black and ferocious, like a cornered animal's. If he gets smart this boy is going to be dangerous one day, Gates decided.

'I do not need any favours.'

'Shit, sure you do. You just been set up, boy.'

Gates saw a flicker of doubt in the other man's face.

'Who told you about Dale?' he went on.

Baptiste just stared at him.

'Okay, let's do this your way. You don't have to say nothing 'til I've finished. That square with you? Okay, then try this for size. It was your daddy-in-law, wasn't it? Old Rocky himself. He told you. And you know why he told you? Because he wanted you to do just what you're doing now. Think a minute. What if that bottle of rum you took out back there happened to be Jack Dale? What do you think we would have done? Wrung our hands and taken up a collection for the funeral?'

Baptiste didn't answer. But Gates could see he was getting through.

'It *was* Rocky, wasn't it?'

'It was Rocco,' he agreed.

'Right.' Gates smiled, pleased with his own perspicacity. 'Let me read it to you how I see it. He wants you out. Only he doesn't want to do it himself. He wants us to do it for him. He's a smart man. You don't get to be *un vrai monsieur* doing charity work, right? The guy plays hardball, Baptiste. You should have worked that out by now.'

He nodded, and the anger in his face was now replaced by frustration and embarrassment. 'He knows I have always been reckless,' he said.

'Reckless is one thing. Suicidal is another. He played you for a sucker, boy. You don't want to start a vendetta with us. You'll find yourself without a friend in the world. And the first guy who'll cut you off is Rocco.' He tossed the revolver back at Baptiste who caught it in both hands, staring at it as if it was an incriminating photograph. He tucked it into the jacket pocket of his suit.

'You want to test my theory, you go fire that thing at a member of the United States mission in Laos. Jack Dale is a coming guy in agriculture in our country. We don't want to lose him.'

Baptiste's one good eye met his, black and angry once more. But he understood.

'Jack Dale won't be giving you any more problems. He'll be gone by the end of the week.'

Baptiste nodded.

'Now I'm sorry for the punch. It's not my usual style. Maybe one day you'll thank me for it. You want a lift back to town?'

'I think I want to walk. I need time to think.'

Gates nodded at one of the crew-cut men who opened the door and let Baptiste out of the car. The Corsican leaned in the passenger window. 'Are you married, Monsieur Gates?'

'No, son. Never had the time.'

'You do not know what you're missing.'

'You want my advice? Watch your ass. I do believe Rocky intends to hang it on the line to dry.'

Gates reversed on to the road and the Americans drove back to Vientiane.

* * *

248

It was a long walk back to town, but Baptiste had a lot to think about. He felt like a chess player who had nearly been checkmated in his third move, to be rescued by a spectator who shouted out a warning just in time. He had been stupid. What had Gates called him? A sucker.

Well, it would be the last time anyone made him a sucker. And certainly the last time for Rocco Bonaventure.

54

Tao Koo was flustered. He whispered urgently in the monsieur's ear. Bonaventure flushed and threw a piercing glance over the top of his pince nez.

'Monsieur Dale. He's here?'

'He says he wants to see Madame Crocé,' Tao Koo answered, in French. 'I told him she is not here, but he says he will not leave until he has seen her.'

Bonaventure uttered a growl of indignation and got to his feet. He huffed down the steps from his study and threw open the door.

Dale towered over him. The first time Bonaventure had met him, at his birthday party, Dale's height had made him seen angular and ill at ease. Angry, he made a far more arresting figure.

'You are not welcome here,' Bonaventure said, in English.

'I have to see Noelle.'

'She is not here.'

At that moment Noelle walked out on to the verandah from the dining room. Both men turned to stare at her. She looked pale, but resolute.

'Noelle,' Dale said.

She stopped a few feet from him, completely ignoring her father. She looked up at the big American, searching his face as if he was a friend from school whose name she had long since forgotten.

'I have only one thing I must ask you. Are you married?'

'It's not as simple as that,' he said, and his destiny was decided.

'Just tell me. Please. The truth.'

'I wanted to tell you. Let me explain.'

She drew back and hit him. Bonaventure was sure the sound of the slap must have echoed right across the Mekong into Thailand. Dale didn't flinch.

Noelle turned and went back into the house.

Bonaventure felt a glow of satisfaction, but his face remained stern. 'You have your answer,' he said. 'Please leave now.'

'If I had some time I could have worked this out,' Dale said to him, as if he could have understood or sympathised. He walked slowly away and slumped behind the wheel of his jeep. It seemed as much as he could do to start the engine.

Bonaventure watched the jeep splash back through the orange mud in the direction of the city.

The hold of the DC-3 was crowded; boy bonzes in their orange robes; mothers with betel-blackened teeth nursing squalling infants; Lao government officials; an army captain asleep on some piles of grain. The CAT warhorse had been fitted out for any transfiguration, there was an overhead wire for paratroops leading to the door, stretchers secured against the bulkheads, and outlets marked 'troop oxygen' on the ceiling. There were even some ancient bullet holes in the fuselage, partly concealed with typhoon tape.

Gates and Dale squatted side by side near the rear, in combat fatigues. They had to shout to make themselves heard over the din of the engines as the DC-3 taxied to take off across Wattay field. 'This is your last trip, Jack,' Gates yelled, over the din of the engines.

'My last trip?'

'After Sam Neua, you go back to Saigon.'

Dale closed his eyes and swore softly under his breath.

'It's what you wanted, isn't it?'

'I thought I did.'

'Well, you can't stay here, for Christ's sake.'

'I changed my mind. I'm not going!'

'The fuck you're not! This may have started out as a request, Major, but now it's an order. You don't have any choice.'

Dale felt an ache growing inside him, almost a physical thing, deep in his chest, anger and recrimination and frustration. He had known from the start that he could not make this work, that he had been a fool to try. What hurt him was that he had never had the chance to explain himself. He had hurt her and had never been able to soften it with his reasons, his mislaid plans. She was Bonaventure's daughter and there was no escaping that.

Besides it was a little late in life to fall in love with a woman for the first time.

55

Bonaventure was asleep on the verandah, his head lolling over the back of the rattan chair. He looks so old, thought Baptiste, the tobacco-coloured skin etched with deep lines, the thinning white hair revealing little patches of white scalp.

I'm doing you a favour, he decided.

He fetched a brocade pillow from the living room, then took a broad belt from his jacket pocket. He laid it gently over the old man's chest, slipped the free end through the buckle behind the chair, and snapped it tight with his left hand. Bonaventure's eyes blinked open and he stared at Baptiste in bewilderment. He tried to move his arms but the belt held them fast to the sides of the chair. Before he could cry out, Baptiste pushed the pillow over his face with his free hand, and held it there.

PART TWO

Chasing the Dragon

'If you want to go into the subversion business, collect intelligence and move arms, you deal with the drug movers.'

— General Paul F. Gorman,
former Head of US Southern Command.

56

Hong Kong, 1967

Sammy Chen was skimming the *South China Morning Post* in the back of his air-conditioned Mercedes when a huge crowd spilled on to Queen's Road in front of them, and the traffic came to a stop in a deafening cacophony of horns.

Sammy leaned forward and tapped his driver on the shoulder. 'What's the hold-up?'

'The communists again, Kee Lung. See. Here they come.'

Now Sammy could see them too. Many of the crowd were holding little red books which they held in the air above their heads as they marched. Some of them were armed, knives and crowbars, clubs and bike chains. A thin line of police blocked their way and this was enough to incite the ones at the front of the mob. They began hurling bricks and stones taken from a nearby building site, the police falling back, sheltering from the barrage behind their wicker shields. The plate glass window of The Hilton's coffee shop crumpled inwards and shattered.

'Drive around the block if you can,' Sammy said mildly.

As much as he hated the communists, Sammy was delighted with recent events. Mao Tse Tung's Cultural Revolution in mainland China had spilled over the border into the New Territories and Hong Kong. A lot of people were afraid, but not Sammy Chen. He considered it fortuitous in many ways, double lucky.

The reason he was so sanguine had to do with another upheaval taking place in his adopted country, Vietnam, which synchronised perfectly with recent events in Hong Kong. The Americans had committed hundreds of thousands of soldiers to the escalating war there, and many of these men came to Hong Kong for R&R. They had plenty of money and were eager to spend it all quickly on every vice that the triads could provide, because in a week they would be back in the deadly jungles of the Mekong and the DMZ and this might be the last chance they would ever have to love a woman or get drunk. For others, drugs helped them forget the loneliness and their fear.

Meanwhile, just a few miles away, Mao's People's Guard were massing on the borders. Rumours of invasion were rife, but Sammy Chen did not think that Mao would be so stupid as to make good on the threat. Hong Kong brought in too much capital to Red China, and even communist countries like China needed capital.

What it meant was that the Army and the police were fully occupied with the communists, who were stirring up trouble in the colony, spreading insurrection and planting bombs. They no longer had the resources to expend searching for narcotics and Sammy had been able to import huge quantities of opium and morphine without interference.

Thanks to Vietnam and Mao, the Fei Lung would grow strong, and Sammy Chen would carve himself a notch as the greatest opium runner in Asian history.

57

July 1967 was a vaporous cauldron, miserably hot even for Hong Kong. The daytime temperature did not fall below 92°F for two months, the humidity consistently hovering close to one hundred per cent. The asphalt melted in downtown Victoria, and the colony prayed for a typhoon. There had been no rain for eight months and the reservoirs were baked pits.

The authorities enforced water rationing by closing the valves on the mains. Once every four days for just two hours the taps yielded up brackish trickles. But the water pressure was too low to carry water above the sixth floor of most of the jerry-built high rises, and in the Walled City the inmates of that stinking hell had to queue for hours at a public tap to refill their slopping paraffin tins, then labour up the concrete stairwells with their precious cargoes.

Even the triads suffered. To make heroin they needed water, and the rationing slowed production in the Fei Lung's heroin factory in Kowloon, just outside the Walled City. When opium boils, it stinks like rotting garbage, so the factory had been situated in an apartment on the very top floor of one of the teeming tenements, where the wind would help to partly disperse the stink.

The heat made life miserable for Chiu Ah Fung and his assistants. Chiu – better known as White Powder Chiu – had been hired by Dragon Fist as a 'cook', as the triads referred to the master chemists who managed the heroin refining process.

When Douglas went to the apartment that morning to check on progress the temperature was already hovering around a hundred degrees, after an overnight low of eighty eight. It was so hot in the tiny room that Chiu had to keep removing his spectacles to wipe them. Douglas wondered how he endured it. An electric fan laboured in the corner without making the slightest difference to the furnace-like heat in the apartment.

Chiu was young, younger even than Douglas, with bad teeth and a pockmarked face, now almost hidden behind a gas mask. He looked like a camera salesman from Nathan Road. The only remarkable thing about him was a talent for chemistry, especially the complex and difficult process of converting opium to number four heroin.

This morning he was busy with the new batch of opium that had been smuggled in. He had heated some water in a large drum and now he tested its temperature with a finger. Watching him, Douglas still marvelled at how much of the process relied on the chemist's intuition.

As assistant dumped a sack of raw opium into the drum and Chiu stirred the solution with a wooden stick. When it was dissolved he would add lime fertiliser to the mixture and scoop out the frothing white layer at the top of the drum. It would be filtered, reheated, and this time, instead of fertiliser, he would add concentrated ammonia, and the morphine would solidify into chunks at the bottom of the drum. It required great precision on the part of Chiu, because if the solution was allowed to heat too long all the morphine would be destroyed.

At the end of the process the ten kilos of opium would be converted into one kilogram of morphine.

Douglas was fascinated by the process, not because of any innate interest in chemistry, but at how so much money could be created from the simple product of a flower.

The raw opium arrived on Thai or Vietnamese fishing trawlers which chugged into the waters off Hong Kong, where it was transferred to oceangoing junks. Once inside colony waters the opium was passed to one of the thousands of sampans that fished offshore. The harbours were so crowded it was virtually impossible for the authorities to detect smugglers.

Now Mao's Revolution was under way the Royal Navy had more pressing concerns than the smugglers. The triad cooks in the illicit laboratories of Kowloon and the New Territories were now producing as much 'brown sugar' or China White as Hong Kong needed.

*　　*　　*

Douglas could not stand the heat inside the apartment factory
any longer. He left Chiu to his work. He knew that after the
chemist had produced a sufficient quantity of morphine,
he would mix it with an equal amount of acetic anhydride.
It would then be boiled for six hours at exactly 85°, and when
the impurities were filtered out, the granular heroin crystals –
brown sugar – formed at the bottom.

Douglas certainly did not want to be around when the rarer
white number four heroin was being produced. The 'brown
sugar' was placed in a large flask, alcohol and ether and
hydrochloric acid were added, and if the process was done
expertly, the white flakes of the ninety-nine per cent pure
China White heroin were filtered out under pressure.

If the process was bungled, the ether exploded, and the
factory and everyone in it were reduced to vapour.

But the value of the heroin made the risks worthwhile. The
Americans on leave from Vietnam did not like to 'chase the
dragon', the traditional Chinese method of smoking the crude
number three brown sugar; they wanted to use a needle and
put it directly into their blood stream, and for that they
needed the pure white powder.

And they were paying enormous prices.

The heroin business was now so lucrative it brought in
more money than even the traditional triad fiefdoms of prostitution and extortion. Douglas had learned that whatever was
illegal was valuable, and heroin now had the potential to
make a few brave and intelligent men wealthy beyond the
wildest dreams of mere mortals.

Women for prostitution were cheap and readily available
everywhere. Heroin was white gold.

Sammy Chen was a genius, Douglas decided. He had anticipated what would happen in Saigon and Hong Kong and had
met the demand. It was pure capitalism at work.

The 489 of the Fei Lung was an inspiration to Douglas Ho,
who was sick to the stomach with the Walled City, its filth and
its stench. He wanted to live on the Peak, have other people do
his bidding for him. Let someone else fight the wars and collect
the money and beat the whores and the petty thieves.

Sammy Chen had helped him realise that his own greatest weapon was not his crippled body, but his brain.

With it, he could still claw his way out of the City of Darkness.

The oppressive heat had thrown Douglas Ho into a black mood as he contemplated his life. As his uncle's first lieutenant, Douglas was entrusted with the task of overseeing all the triad ventures inside the Walled City, as well as supervising White Powder Chiu's heroin factory. It now seemed to him that he did all the dirty work, while his uncle sat in the Mid-levels with his women and his drugs enjoying the profits. Three years ago, when he kidnapped Chen Jia-guo from the Mongkok typhoon shelter and washed him, it was his uncle who had taken all the credit.

He had finally decided it was time his contributions to the triad were properly rewarded. He would instigate his plan during the weekly police raid on the Walled City.

Fishball Tak led Sergeant Tan and his five constables – all Chinese – through the maze of alleys into the heart of the Walled City. When they reached the coffee shop in Rat's Piss Alley he ushered them inside, and pulled up stools for them around a chipped Formica table.

Douglas emerged from a back room to join them, and slipped a brown manila envelope across the table to Tan, who immediately ripped it open and started counting the notes inside. There was no need for discretion. Besides, Sergeant Tan was not the sort of man who was able to put a rein on his greed, and ten years of service in the Hong Kong Police Force had hardly taught him otherwise.

The shop owner brought them all Cokes and sweet cakes and at Douglas' instruction Fishball Tak scurried away again.

While they were waiting for him to return, the talk was of the communist riots and the stifling heat. Even in the coffee shop, with an ancient air conditioner wheezing and dripping in one corner, the heat was a tangible thing, every breath stale and fetid. The room smelled of sweat and sour milk.

The men drank their Cokes and called for more. As they were finishing Fishball Tak returned with two addicts he had hauled from the opium den in Half Dog Street. They were volunteers and hardened addicts by the look of them, Douglas decided, with shrunken cheeks and the tell-tale grey-green pallor to their skin. They were wearing only stained vests and khaki shorts.

A constable put them in handcuffs and the two waited patiently outside while the police finished their morning repast. They would be arrested and imprisoned in Tai Lam on narcotics charges. But they knew they would be provided with opium in prison, and receive compensation from the triad for their trouble; the police would have two arrests for their charge sheets, and the triads were left to run business as they saw fit in the Walled City.

It was a long-standing and mutually beneficial arrangement.

The police got up to leave without providing compensation for the Cokes and the cakes, as was the usual custom. But this time, as the constables filed outside, Douglas took Sergeant Tan aside. He laid out his proposition in urgent whispers.

It was the audacity of the idea that had appealed to Douglas. Tan had mentioned casually one day that his brother was a sergeant on one of the police launches that patrolled the waters around Hong Kong, similar to the one that had rescued Douglas from the water in Mirs Bay. The full complement of each craft was twelve men; two British officers in command, one of the sergeants and the rest of the crew were Chinese constables.

Just a few weeks ago some Chinese had shot their two commanding officers in their bunks while they slept, and then sailed up the Pearl River to deliver the boat to the communists at Canton.

And that was what gave Douglas the idea.

What if Tan's brother could organise a similar hijack while his police boat was on patrol? What if he was able to bring it to the pier in Aberdeen, where Douglas and Tan would be waiting?

Tan reacted with horror. 'Impossible!' He turned away.

But Douglas gripped his arm and whispered to him about the fortune that was at stake ... the biggest delivery of opiates that had ever reached Hong Kong. 'I know when and I know where,' Douglas said. 'Enough to make a few brave men wealthy beyond their dreams!'

'It can't be done!'

Douglas ignored him. 'We bury the opium on one of the islands, and head back for Hong Kong. I can arrange false passports and airline tickets for Taiwan. You and I will not be implicated. When the fuss has died down, we can sell it quietly, you can arrange to send your brother and his friends their share.'

Tan was accustomed to petty graft, but the idea of stealing from the triads appalled him. 'We'll get caught,' he stammered.

'No. It will work,' Douglas said. 'And you will earn more in a night than you can make in ten years in the police force.'

Tan hesitated, torn between greed and terror. 'If they see the police uniforms...'

'We will be dressed as Chinese. There are hundreds of sweat-shops inside the Walled City. How difficult do you think it is for me to have six Chinese uniforms made? Some cheap rough green cloth with red stars, that's all. It will be night, and the people we will be dealing with are terrified fishermen. They'll go running back to Dragon Fist crying that Uncle Mao has stolen all their drugs!'

Tan shook his head. 'It's crazy!'

Douglas leaned closer. 'There's four hundred kilos of opium, two hundred of black and sixty kilos of number four heroin. The heroin alone is worth three quarters of a million US dollars.'

'Let me talk to my brother,' he said.

Douglas shrugged again. 'It's one chance in a lifetime for him. For me, there are other opportunities.'

'This is a big risk, Sharkfin.'

'If you don't risk, you never win. It will make us rich, richer than you can ever imagine.'

'I said I'll talk to him.'

'The shipment is due next Monday night. You have to be ready by then.'

'It's madness.'

Douglas shrugged, nonchalant, as if it was something he did all the time. 'It's up to you. I'm giving you your big chance.'

Tan nodded and went outside to join his constables. One of the addicts was sweating and shivering, going into withdrawal. He couldn't wait for them to get him to prison.

'I need your answer by tomorrow,' Douglas called to Tan.

He nodded, and Fishball Tak led the police and their manacled evil-doers back through the stinking furnace of the Walled City.

The next day there was another police raid on Hak Nam. Because it had not been previously arranged Sergeant Tan and his men had to linger for almost ten minutes in the street while the look-see boy ran to fetch Fishball Tak.

Tak returned them to the coffee shop in Rat's Piss Street where they drank Cokes until Douglas Ho could be brought from the Dragon's Eyrie.

Sergeant Tan left his constables inside the coffee shop and the two men conferred in urgent whispers in the alley.

'My brother says he'll do it.'

Douglas nodded. He'd thought so.

'When do we do this?'

'Monday. We have to leave the dock at Aberdeen by midnight.'

Tan was so nervous and excited his voice trembled. 'We'll be there.'

As he walked away, Douglas smiled. Ordinary men had such small minds. If a man thought three-quarters of a million dollars was a lot of money, he would never be rich.

58

Police 53 pulled in to the jetty at Aberdeen Harbour at three minutes past eleven on the Monday night. Tan and Douglas waited together, speaking in monosyllables, smoking cigarettes. As the launch bumped against the pier, the two men jumped aboard and the launch immediately sped away again.

The weather was perfect, Douglas decided; fog wreathed the bay, reducing visibility to less than fifty metres. The second watch piloted their way through the sea lanes using the radar. The first watch – including a British inspector – were tied hand and foot and locked in the for'ard crew quarters.

Tan's brother, Louie, was in command. He was younger than Tan, but taller, with the hard knotted muscles of a mariner. A Chinese constable was at the wheel, another in the radio room, and a Chinese sergeant in the engine room. Two other constables from their watch that Louie had not trusted had been tied up at gunpoint with the others.

'Where to?' Louie asked Douglas.

'Nam Mo Chan island,' Douglas told him. 'The rendezvous is for one o'clock. We have to get to her first.'

Louie nodded. 'Just time enough to bury the opium and get back to Hong Kong.'

Douglas said a small prayer to the gods, and to Kuan Yin, the Goddess of Mercy who had pulled him from the mouth of the shark seven years before. He touched the tooth at his throat for luck. He could not fail tonight. It was too big a gamble.

Louie found her on the radar long before they saw her; the green shadow on the screen the only shipping in the vicinity of the island. Douglas had brought the uniforms with him in a holdall. Tan and the others changed quickly, then hoisted the red star-patterned communist Chinese pennants at the stern and masthead.

Louie ordered the engines reduced to idle. The motor throbbed in the water, the exhaust drifting into the blanketing fog.

'A hundred yards,' barked Louie.

The *Fu Kwok* loomed ahead of them, through a sudden break in the fog. Tan snapped on the searchlight, catching the fishing boat in the silver phosphorescence of its beam.

It was a high-pooped junk, with forward-leaning fore and mizzen masts and a patched copper-brown batwing sail. It was unlit, just two pale green lamps on the main mast. Even from this distance he could smell the waft of fish and bilge from the holds.

Tan picked up the loud hailer and barked out a string of orders in Cantonese: 'This is Lieutenant Chi Chong-po. You have illegally entered the waters of the People's Republic of China. Weigh anchor immediately, we are coming aboard! If you resist we shall fire upon you.'

Douglas could see men and women running frantically across the decks, caught in the silver finger of the spot beam. He allowed himself a tight smile. They would be shitting in their drawers.

He remained in the wheelhouse with Louie, while Tan and two of the crew prepared to board the junk. Tan had a Smith & Wesson revolver strapped to his hip. The other two crewmen had Chinese made AK-47s from the ship's weapons locker.

Douglas helped the engineer load the Browning. If the captain did anything stupid, the belt-fed fifty-calibre gun would rake the decks of the *Fu Kwok*.

The police boat hove to alongside the junk, and Tan and the two constables clambered aboard. Douglas listened. Tan's voice carried clearly to him on the fog.

He was really very good.

The captain of the junk was on his knees on the deck begging the captain not to arrest him. It was an honest mistake, he said. They were, after all, just humble fishermen.

'Perhaps you were paid by the Americans as a spy,' Tan said.

That was enough to send the captain's wife and most of the crew into paroxysms of terror. They howled their innocence. Meanwhile Tan sent one of his men below decks. The howling ended abruptly, and there was an expectant silence. Minutes later they came up to report they had found sacks of opium in the holds.

'Opium!' Tan shouted.

'See! We're not spies!' the trawler captain shouted. 'We're just poor opium smugglers!'

'That's worse,' Tan told them. 'Opium is the beast of the capitalist running dogs. They have used opium for all our history to exploit the people! I should shoot you down right now!'

The family and crew grovelled on the decks, begging for their lives. Tan continued to berate them. Don't enjoy yourself too much, Douglas thought. We don't have all night.

Finally Tan told them he would show them mercy. He would let them live, to demonstrate the beneficence of the enlightened government of Chairman Mao. But the opium would be confiscated and used for medicine in the People's Republic.

He nodded to his two men and they began to haul the sacks of opium from below and throw them down on to the deck of the *Police 53*. Douglas and the engineer left the Browning to help drag the sacks into the stern.

The unloading took a further ten minutes while the junk master and his family moaned and babbled and begged to be allowed to keep some of their opium. Tan quietened them by playing with his revolver in front of their faces.

Finally the job was done. Tan's colleagues clambered back into the launch. Tan paused for one further tirade in the name of Chairman Mao and then climbed aboard also. He grinned broadly at Douglas as he came back into the wheelhouse.

'Idiots,' he said.

268

59

They anchored the launch a hundred metres off Joss House Island on the lee side of the island. The radar showed a wide bay and a shallow beach. It remained invisible through the fog.

Louie and the engineer stayed on the boat with Douglas while Tan and two of the constables went ashore in the dory. Louie glanced anxiously at the luminous dial of his watch.

'This is taking too long,' he said.

The dory disappeared through the fog, sitting dangerously low in the water, heavy with the opium sacks.

'Plenty of time,' said Douglas.

It was almost three a.m. when they heard the dory chugging back through the fog. Louie had just relayed another false position report and now he was hunched over the wheel, drinking black coffee from an enamel cup. His face was etched with strain.

Again he looked at his watch.

'At last,' he said.

Douglas checked his watch also, then took the type 54 pistol from his sports jacket, cocked it, put the barrel against the base of Louie's skull and fired.

In the confines of the wheelhouse, it sounded like a cannonshot. The engineer launched himself up the companionway from the radio room, startled. He stared into the black muzzle of the pistol, bewildered.

Douglas fired again and a dark hole appeared in the centre of the man's forehead. He fell, leaving a spray of blood and tissue splattered on the bulkhead. Douglas peered down the companionway. The man lay sprawled across the deck floor, his legs crumpled underneath him, scalding coffee spilled across his shirt.

He won't feel a thing now, thought Douglas.

The pitch of the dory's motor changed as Tan and his men slowed the boat in response to the sound of the gunshots. They would be hesitating, confused and uncertain. Douglas ran out of the deckhouse and took up position behind the for'ard Browning.

'Louie?'

It was Tan's voice, coming to him through the fog.

'Louie? Sharkfin?'

The dory's motor died. Its silhouette broke through the curtain of fog. One of the men, Tan probably, was at the bow, crouched over, peering ahead at the lighted wheelhouse of the launch.

An easy target.

The Browning was heavy, it usually took two men to fire it, but the belt had already been fed into the magazine. He pressed the trigger.

The machine gun was armed with one-and-a-half ounce bullets that could penetrate light armour and chop a wooden-hulled boat like the dory into matchwood. The gun slid easily on its mountings. Douglas aimed and fired. He heard screams.

Douglas went to the spotlight, turned it on, then walked unhurriedly back to the Browning to survey the damage. The front of the dory had disintegrated as if it had run through an invisible bandsaw, and wallowed in the water, hull up. Two survivors flapped at the water. Douglas lowered the Browning and fired another burst.

Silence.

The dory sunk below the surface. He counted two bodies, floating face down among the debris, one streaming a grey glob of intestine behind, like a trawler's net. There were stains on the oily water. They slowly drifted away into the fog.

Then he heard it. Someone gasping, splashing in the water. He left the Browning, took the pistol out of the waistband of his trousers and went to the bow to wait.

There.

270

It was Tan. He was rolling in the water, paddling frantically with one arm. His head was barely above the surface, the current dragging him towards the bow.

Douglas waited.

Ten yards away.

He waited, took careful aim, and fired the rest of the clip. Tan floated past on his back. The stain spread in the water behind him like oil from an old sampan.

Douglas threw the weapon in the water after him, then collected the holdall from the wheelhouse and went down the companionway to the engine room. He took a water-proof halogen torch and watertight bag containing plastic explosives out of the kit bag. He moulded the explosives to the hull, attached a home-made detonator, and set the timer using an old-fashioned alarm clock.

Armed only with the torch now, he went back up to the deck, and stood at the starboard rail. One of the men locked in the hold had broken free and was beating on the bulwark door with his fists. Douglas ignored his screams. He was remembering the shark that had taken him that night in Mirs Bay. Tonight again there was blood in the water, and they might already be sniffing it out like rutting pigs. He imagined their terrible snouts racing up from the deeps.

Steeling himself against the fear, he dived in and began to swim.

The beach was utterly alien at night; there was not one landmark he recognised from the previous day. But he had anticipated that.

The fog cleared for a moment and he could make out the silhouette of the *Police 53* two hundred metres away. He thought he heard the sound of a splash and shone his torch across the water. He could see nothing, but imagined the sharks helping themselves to the spoils.

He walked back along the beach, keeping the sea on his right hand side. After ten minutes the sand gave way to rocks that led out to a headland. He walked up the strand, found the dinghy among the brush where he had left it. Inside was another zippered holdall with two changes of clothes, one the black peasant pyjamas of a coolie, the other the jeans, sneakers and sports jacket that were the badge of the triad.

Well, I'm not going anywhere in this fog, he thought, and settled down to wait, shivering in the chill morning air, confident in the knowledge that at the other end of the beach he had over a million dollars worth of Sammy Chen's narcotics.

Now he just had to cash in his chips.

A hollow boom rolled across the bay, followed by the shock waves of the explosion as the police launch went down. With joss the authorities might never find the wreckage, and there was no one left to reveal the mystery of the missing gunboat. They would blame the disappearance on the Chinese, another casualty of Mao's Revolution.

There was absolutely no connection anyone could make between the *Police 53* and Douglas Ho.

60

Aberdeen

The press of junks and sampans in Aberdeen harbour is home to thousands of families, who cook and eat and sleep and mate among the rigging and the nets. Wing Fat-hei was just one of them. His life was poor but simple, lived out among the stench of fish and the filth of the harbour.

But for the past few days the crushing monotony of poverty had been replaced by the vivid colours of terror. After that night off Nam Mo Chau, he had not had one moment's peace. He had babbled out an explanation to his contact in Aberdeen. The man had raged at him, threatening him and calling him a liar. Wing Fat-hei did not know what he was going to do. None of it had been his fault, yet now he expected to be punished. Fate had brought this misfortune upon him, and there was nothing he could do now but wait and pray.

He had spent all that afternoon in the temple of Kuan Li, had lit incense for her and left a small offering of rice and flowers. He hoped it would be enough to buy her favour.

He returned later that evening just as the pearl necklaces of the electric light bulbs were flickering on along the piers. The lights of the sampans ferrying tourists between the waterfront and the Jumbo restaurant bobbed on the darkening water.

When his own sampan bumped alongside the *Fu Kwok* he looked up and saw three men in dark zippered jackets standing on the poop. He could have told the sampan girl to turn around and take him back to the harbour but he knew that would only buy him a few hours. He could not escape the triad. And besides, there was his family to think of.

273

He recognised one of the men, his contact for previous opium shipments. He was known only by his nickname, Fishball Tak. He was smiling. Fishball Tak never smiled, so Wing knew he was in big trouble.

'We've been waiting for you,' Fishball Tak said. 'We have some unfinished business.'

Lockhart Road was ablaze with neon·signs: Pussy Galore Bar, Happy Boy, Lucky Place, Americana. Girls in tight silk cheongsams slit to mid-thigh touted at the doors, American sailors tottered drunkenly along the sidewalk, music pulsed into the street and the tangle of traffic. Wanchai was filled with GIs looking for sex and drugs and drink. All their needs were catered for in Wanchai, individual territory carved out block by block between Hong Kong's triads.

Dragon Fist had an office over a bar called The Candy Store. One of his *sze kau* escorted Douglas up the stairs. He went in. The room was heavy with smoke, the air stale and hot, despite the air conditioner that laboured in the corner against a blacked-out window.

He was in conference and looked displeased at the interruption. He looks prosperous, thought Douglas. He was wearing a black sharkskin suit and had a gold Rolex Oyster on his wrist. Two of his protectors, Freddy Yang and Half Ear Wang, were with him.

Douglas was disgusted by his uncle's physical appearance. There were dark shadows under his eyes and his cheeks were hollows. Without his fancy clothes he would look like any other street addict in Hak Nam.

'I got a message that you wanted to see me,' Dragon Fist said.

Douglas bowed in respect. 'It's about the *Fu Kwok*,' he said.

He had his attention. 'What do you know about the *Fu Kwok*?' Dragon Fist hissed.

'I know one of our shipments has gone missing.'

'So?'

'There was a policeman called Sergeant Tan who made regular visits to Hak Nam.'

'I remember him' Dragon Fist said.

'The day after the opium went missing, Sergeant Tan failed to appear for duty. I made some enquiries. His brother was crew on a police patrol boat that disappeared from its dock that night.'

Dragon Fist drew on a cigarette. 'The captain of the *Fu Kwok* thinks he strayed into communist waters. He says a communist gunboat stopped and boarded him and confiscated the cargo.'

'He's lying.'

'Why are you so sure, Sharkfin?'

'Because I found this Sergeant Tan. He told me the whole thing was arranged between him and the captain of the fishing boat.'

Dragon Fist made a noise like the hissing of a snake. He leaned forward. 'Where is Sergeant Tan now?'

'The strain of answering questions was too much for him. He had a weak heart.'

'That was stupid, Nephew. You should have left the questions to me.'

His addiction has made him testy, Douglas thought. 'A thousand apologies, *tai lo*.'

'Kee Lung wants his opium back very badly.'

'If you like I can take the *Fu Kwok's* captain back to the Walled City and wring the truth out of him.'

'No, leave it to us,' Dragon Fist told him, and smiled, without humour. 'He might have a weak heart.'

'Is there anything else Sergeant Tan told you before your questions became too difficult?'

Douglas told him everything he knew about the plan to hijack the *Fu Kwok*; everything, of course, except his own part in it.

'You can go,' his uncle told him when he had finished.

'Yes, *tai lo*,' Douglas said. Dismissed like a coolie! Perhaps you would like me to kow-tow? You deserve everything that is coming to you!

But he did not allow these thoughts to show on his face. Instead he bowed and left.

*   *   *

That night Freddy Yang and Jamie Wong went to Aberdeen to find Wing Fat-hei, the master of the *Fu Kwok*, but he and his whole family were already gone.

Dragon Fist was in a dilemma. If he reported what Douglas had told him without having Wing in his possession, and without knowing the exact location of the missing shipment, he would lose face. He decided he would wait until he had tracked down the fisherman. It shouldn't take long.

61

Walled City

Wing Fat-hei was forced up a steep bamboo ladder into a tiny loft. There were bamboo cages around the room, and at first Wing thought they were for fowl. But as his eyes grew accustomed to the light he realised that the occupants of the cages were human.

His wife was almost doubled over inside one of the cages, trussed up like a duck. His four-year-old daughter lay on her side, shivering with terror. His son, barely a year old, was screaming, snot-nosed and filthy.

Three triads stood in the middle of the loft. One of them was boiling water in a pot over a kerosene stove.

One of the triads, wearing a black nylon jacket and denim jeans, limped towards him. He was smiling, but his eyes were cold, the coldest eyes he had ever seen.

Wing looked away, terrified.

'My name is Douglas Ho,' the man said. 'I am the worst future you ever imagined. I am the dragon you awakened unintentionally, the evil spirit that has waited in the shadows for you since the day you were born. Do you understand?'

'Please,' Wing moaned, 'I have told you the truth about the opium. Please let us go!'

He fell on his knees in front of Douglas and kow-towed, his forehead on the filthy floor. Douglas pulled him to his feet and shoved him towards the cages.

'Do you see this?' he asked.

He picked up the pot of boiling water and carried it over

to the cage where Wing's wife was imprisoned. 'I tip a little of the water...'

He heard the scalding hiss and his wife shrieked, twisting and jerking in agony, but unable to move inside her terrible bamboo prison.

Douglas carried the pot of water to Wing's son's cage.

'Don't!' Wing begged. 'Please! I am telling you the truth! I did not steal the opium! Oh, please!'

Douglas smiled and returned the pot to the stove. Wing could not take his eyes off it. What other tortures did this monster have in store?

Goddess of Mercy, Kuan Li, please!

The man with the cold eyes and the limp was speaking again, his voice soft and hypnotic. 'I want you to understand something, Wing Fat-hei. I own you. You are going to do everything I tell you to do because I alone own you now. Do you understand?'

Wing did not understand. But he nodded his head, knowing only that he had to protect his family from the terrible tortures this monster would inflict if he did not do what he was asked. If there was hope, any hope at all, he had to take it.

'I'll do anything, anything,' he sobbed.

'Good,' Douglas said. 'You are a wise man.'

Sammy Chen sat at the end of an enormous dining table of polished walnut, perhaps fifteen paces long. He was the only person at the table. He was in his shirtsleeves, and his braces hung around his hips. He was eating a bowl of goose intestines and cold crab meat with silver chopsticks.

'Douglas Ho,' he said, and it might have been a benediction or a curse.

'Fearless Dragon,' said Douglas, bowing.

'Why are you here?' The mildness of his tone was deceptive, Douglas knew.

'There is something for your ears only, Kee Lung.'

'Oh?'

'It is about the missing shipment.'

Sammy Chen nodded and feigned only mild interest.

Douglas went to the door and brought Wing Fat-hei into

278

the room. Sammy Chen's nostrils twitched at the offence. 'The fisherman,' he said.

Wing Fat-hei prostrated himself on the floor.

'Tell him,' Douglas said.

'The communists who stole the black...' groaned Wing.

'Yes?' Sammy said, impatiently.

'I recognised one of them.'

'Yes?'

'I know him only as Dragon Fist.'

Sammy Chen folded his hands across his belly and looked sharply at Douglas. 'You are sure, fisherman?'

But Wing could not answer. He was sobbing and mucus dribbled out of his nose on to the polished marble floor. Sammy Chen nodded to Douglas who stepped forward and kicked the old man in the ribs.

'Kee Lung wants to know if you are sure?'

'Yes, Kee Lung, yes, yes. I know he did not think I would recognise him, but I have seen him in Aberdeen in his red car that sounds like a dragon. But what could I do. Who could I tell?'

Sammy Chen gave a long sigh. He had known from the beginning that whoever had stolen the opium had been from his own triad. Who else could have known the exact time and location of the handover?

He raised one finger to Douglas who dragged the old fisherman to the door and threw him into the foyer where two of his *sze kau* were waiting.

Sammy Chen pushed away his supper and brooded on this. 'Is he telling the truth?' he said to Douglas.

'It seems impossible. But why would he lie? He's terrified.'

Sammy Chen brooded. He studied this young triad with the limp. Sharkfin, they called him. He knew him by reputation from Dragon Fist himself. He was an unprepossessing creature, skinny, his face pock marked with the acne of his adolescence, and scarred from street fights. A soldier, an executioner perhaps. But not a planner. It was why Sammy was inclined to believe his story. But first it had to be thoroughly checked.

'You can go,' he said.

The young man looked disappointed, but he bowed and left

279

without another word. Sammy Chen picked up the telephone. In just a few minutes he had ascertained that a police launch had indeed gone missing the night of the *Fu Kwok*'s boarding, but the incident had been hushed up by the British authorities for political and security reasons. One of the missing crewmen was a Sergeant Tan Yam Keung, known as Louie Tan. His brother, Sergeant Tan Yam Kuan had been sponsored into the triad by Dragon Fist himself, and had even visited his apartment on several occasions.

The pieces of the jigsaw fell into place with abrupt and startling ease.

He made his decision. He went to the writing bureau that stood in one corner of the room, took out a pot of ink, an ancient lacquered pen and nib, and a piece of vermilion writing paper. He wrote quickly, and dried the ink with a blotter.

It was the order for Dragon Fist to be expelled from the Fei Lung triad. It was tantamount to a death warrant.

He had Douglas Ho brought back into the room, and handed him the warrant personally. He told him that on carrying out his orders he would personally sponsor his promotion to Red Pole.

62

Dragon Fist woke to the familiar ache in his bones. There were two girls sprawled in the bed; one had her thigh draped across him. He pushed her away, swung his legs off the bed and walked naked into the bathroom. There was a shower bag on the marble vanity; inside was a selection of syringes, some glassene packets and an adjustable strap. His fingers shook as he prepared the fix.

He heard a noise behind him, looked up into the mirror, saw a shadow in the bathroom doorway and the muzzle of a pistol. He spun around. But the intruder was quicker. The syringe was snatched out of his hands and the pistol shoved in his face.

He recognised the man behind the gun. Fishball Tak. There was another gunman waiting behind him, Jamie Wong. It didn't make sense ... his own people.

'What do you want?' he said.

They didn't answer. Fishball Tak propelled him out of the bathroom, towards the door. When they got outside he saw Freddy Yang floating face down in the pool, a brown stain spreading in the water around him.

Dragon Fist kicked out with his foot, took Jamie Wong in the heart, felled him, and then chopped down with his right hand, intending to knock the weapon from Fishball Tak's grip. But the drugs in his system had slowed him. Tak had anticipated the move and jumped back and away. He saw him aim the pistol low and fire. His leg buckled under him and he went down, breathless with pain.

Fishball Tak stood over him and pistol whipped him into unconsciousness.

They gagged him, tied his hands and carried him across the

foyer past two terrified tenants. They bundled him into the back of an ancient Austin. Dragon Fist came back to consciousness on the journey and immediately vomited with pain. The men in the car swore viciously and kicked him. He passed out again.

When he recovered he found himself on the deck of the *Fu Kwok*. His nephew was sitting in a deckchair on the poop, surrounded by half a dozen of his soldiers from the Walled City.

'Uncle, I'm glad you could come. We're going fishing. Did you bring some bait?'

Dragon Fist said nothing. If the gods willed it, he would survive. A man's fate was written on his forehead. It was useless to struggle.

They locked him in a stinking rope stowage, ankle deep in filthy water. He tried to reason what had happened but the pain would not allow him to think clearly. He could not move and he could not see, and his right leg was a searing agony. He slipped in and out of consciousness like a drowning man fighting to the surface for air, then losing the strength to stay afloat.

But as bad as the pain of the injury was his body's craving for heroin. He could think of nothing else. Even dying did not seem so terrible as being unable to soothe the hunger in his veins. He had once had an abcess on his tooth; this ache was the same, except it took over his whole body.

The air was oily and furnace hot, but he shivered and juddered with cold, his arms pinioned behind his back.

He felt the junk get under way, heard the throb of the motor, felt the vibration through the hull. He had vowed he would not show them his pain, but the movement of the boat took him beyond his endurance, and his demons pursued him to the limits of his sanity. He began to scream, and by nightfall he was babbling and incoherent.

Douglas was disgusted. He had respected his uncle. Now look at him. Sweating and shivering and screaming as if he had been tortured. He looked like one of the worst addicts in the street in Hak Nam. How could he let this happen to himself?

Douglas sat in a deckchair, a Beretta pistol resting in his lap, watching the sun sinking below the islands. Late-afternoon was a good time of the day for sharks, their feeding time. And just enough light to witness the spectacle.

'You've been sampling the profits,' he said.

Dragon Fist could not answer. He lay on the deck curled in on himself, shrieking and babbling. Several teeth were missing and saliva leaked from his chin. Blood from his knee had smeared across the wooden deck.

This was good. Douglas wanted his *sze kau* to see this.

He looked around at Wing by the tiller, grey with terror. It seemed to Douglas that the fisherman had aged ten years in the twenty-four hours of his captivity. What drug could be better than this sort of power?

'Where did Ho Chan-fu bury the opium he stole from you?' Douglas said to him.

The fisherman pointed to Joss House Island. It had been invisible that night, now it rose from the sea like a small, green whale.

'Where?'

'The beach. I saw lights on the northern end,' Wing said, repeating the words Douglas had coached him.

Douglas stood up and nodded. This theatre was for the benefit of his followers. 'You have earned the right to see your wife and children once more,' he said.

Wing smiled, uncertain.

Douglas nodded and three of his *sze kau* went below. They hefted a forty-four gallon drum up the companionway, and dragged it towards the stern.

Douglas grabbed Wing by the shirt and pulled him over to the gunwales to watch.

'Your family,' he said.

The three youths upturned the drum. What tumbled out into the sea was offal and meat, raw chunks, crudely chopped from the carcasses. Wing stared uncomprehending as the dismembered corpses of his family splashed into the ocean and drifted with the current.

His wife's head bobbed to the surface like a cork and he screamed. Douglas shot him in the back of the head and let his body fall into the water.

Dragon Fist was only half conscious of what was happening.

He writhed on the deck as if he had swallowed acid. How disappointing, Douglas thought. He will not be able to enjoy my show as much as I had hoped.

'Give him what he wants,' he said.

Two *sze kau* squatted down beside him. One of them tied a piece of rubber tubing around the upper part of his arm to distend the veins in his forearm. The other emptied the syringe into a vein. Dragon Fist moaned with relief and trembled and vomited.

By the time he had recovered the first shark had scented the blood of Wing's family and come to join the feast.

'Put a lifebelt on him,' Douglas said.

Dragon Fist did not understand what was happening, would have been unable to resist if he had. His eyes were glassy with opiate dreams, his face composed in the euphoria of the drug. Two triads forced the lifebelt over his head and shoulders then re-tied his hands behind his back. They dragged him up the steps to the poop deck. They attached a lifeline around his body, and the other end was secured to the stern.

Douglas took out the death warrant and held it up for them all to see. 'I shall not steal from my sworn brothers in the Hung family,' Douglas shouted. 'If I break this oath I shall die by a myriad of swords.' And he grabbed his uncle by the shoulders and threw him into the sea.

The sharks were slow to come. Dragon Fist floundered in the water for fully five minutes before one of the great fish summoned the courage to attack. But after that it was over very quickly, and Dragon Fist's screams were a memory on the wind.

Douglas turned and smiled at the young triads who were gathered around him in the stern. They would remember this, he knew. He had carved a legend for himself. They would say he had a supernatural affinity with the sharks. The name Sharkfin would become synonymous with terror.

He would return to the beach and find Sammy Chen's shipment. The credit it would earn him in the eyes of the 489 would be worth far more to him than the money. After all, what was a few million dollars when the fortune he dreamed of was so vast?

63

Saigon, August 1967

Saigon had changed, perhaps irretrievably, Baptiste decided. Instead of wide boulevards filled with bicycles, the streets were choked with convoys of olive drab trucks and jeeps spewing black diesel smoke. There were American and ARVN soldiers everywhere, their fingers nervously hovering over the triggers of their M-16s. Just kids, he thought, until he realised that he had not been much older when he came to Indochina with the French air force.

And there was the *bui doi*, the street kids, orphans and refugees, the scum tide of the war, beggars and pick-pockets and street thieves, roaming in their thousands. The older ones were called cowboys, they had Honda motorcycles and snatched bags and cameras as they rode past.

The tension in the city was palpable. Saigon was safer than it had been three or four years ago, when Viet Cong guerillas had blown up the My Canh floating restaurant and bombed the Brinks BOQ and the first US Embassy. But the sandbags and checkpoints and barbed wire all attested to a city still ostensibly under siege.

Gerry Gates and Colonel Tran van Li arrived together. The three men exchanged handshakes. A uniformed waiter brought them glasses of Thirty Three beer while they studied the menu.

Baptiste and Li watched each other warily. Baptiste had not forgotten Li, but for now business took precedence over pride.

'Good to see you back in Saigon,' Gates said to him. 'How's Vientiane?'

'It is just the same.'

'Haven't been back for a while. Anyway, I hear you're in business again.'

'Possibly.'

'Things have changed a lot in Viet Nam. Most of the old problems don't exist any more. I'm sure you and Mr Li here can come to some arrangement.'

'We always have before,' said Li, and his thin mouth split into a smile.

Baptiste wanted to dash his glass in his face. But instead he smiled also and returned his attention to the menu.

The noon rush was under way, as the stores and government offices disgorged their workers into the streets for the siesta. Pretty ebony-haired girls in flowing *ao dai* filled the boulevards, joining the crush of Renault taxis and siclos, rushing home to the suburbs. The Tu Do was a cacophony of horns and tinkling bicycle bells. One by one, the Chinese and Indian merchants brought down the steel shutters in front of their stores.

They made small talk as they ate, discussed the forthcoming elections. Colonel Nguyen Thieu and Air Marshal Cao Ky had allied on one ticket to try and beat off the threat of a civilian administration. The whole process seemed to amuse Gates.

'Democracy! What a crock of shit!' he chortled, and ordered another round of beers.

The afternoon rains began, but their table on the L-shaped colonnade was sheltered by a woven bamboo canopy. A police jeep raced past, its red lights flashing. The waiter appeared with a linen-draped trolley of French pastries.

'Let's talk about business,' Li said, finally.

Baptiste lit a cigarette. 'What's the deal?'

'There is no opium business any more in Saigon unless it comes through me,' Li said. 'These days the Air Force can bring the opium straight into Tan Son Nhut. We'll deliver it anywhere in Saigon, at a fixed price per kilo. After that, it's up to you.'

'And if I want to export?'

'The director of the Saigon Port Authority is Vice Premier Ky's brother-in-law. Again, I am sure we can come to some arrangement.'

Baptiste looked at Gates. 'Where does all this money go?'

Gates shrugged. 'Beats me.'

'It assists in maintaining the security of South Viet Nam,' Li said.

'Well, of course, if it is for a good cause. I would not like to think anyone was profiting by it personally. After all, *I* am supposed to be the gangster.'

'Well, let's not get too caught up in job demarcation,' Gates said. 'The reality is, we screwed up here. The do-gooders in Congress wept their tears over corruption and South Viet Nam being a police state, and forced us to get rid of Diem. Look what happened. The bad guys blew up our fucking embassy! That's why someone finally got some sense and backed Ky. The only thing that can guarantee security in this fucking place is a big surveillance network. Informers on every street. But that takes cash. So, okay, maybe you got to overlook a little graft, some stuff going missing at Tan Son Nhut, a little opium. Way I see it, we're just encouraging the local administration to access the private sector.'

'I have always been conscious of my civic responsibilities, you know that, Monsieur Gates.'

Gates drank his beer and watched Baptiste over the rim of his glass. 'Sure you are. Lucky, too.'

'Lucky?'

'Hell, you know. Rocky dying when he did.'

'It was a great tragedy. He was not an old man. His doctor said it was a heart attack.'

'Hell, I thought the old buzzard would live for ever.' Gates gave him a look that Baptiste could have interpreted a thousand ways. 'You just never know, do you?'

The rain had stopped. The streets were quiet now, only the hawkers with their watercolours and lacquer boxes remained, piteously chasing every Westerner they saw. Two newsboys were involved in a vicious knuckle and blood fight over territory.

'Yes, this life, she is strange. You can never know what is going to happen next.'

It was late-afternoon by the time Baptiste finished his business in the city. He drove home through the snarl of blue and yellow taxis, pedal cycles, motor scooters and army trucks, the exhaust fumes casting a grey and foul pall over the city.

Fate and ambition and anger had driven Baptiste Crocé back to Saigon.

Bonaventure had been right about General Rattakone. Less than a year after Baptiste had taken over the Bonaventure family business, the General had refused to order further *réquisitions militaires*. He had thought his Air Force could handle the opium traffic without private operators being involved, and he wanted to keep a larger share of the profits himself. Ironically, the war against the Pathet Lao escalated soon after, and the Lao Air Force was now almost totally occupied with bombing sorties over the Ho Chi Minh trail. Now it was the Vietnamese who ferried most of the mud into Saigon from Pakse and Savannakhet.

Baptiste was not surprised by what had happened. Opium was no longer a backyard business, as it had been in Bonaventure's day. The potential profits were too large to be ignored.

He had stayed on in Laos for two years, running the Amicu, occasionally organising a little gold and piaster smuggling out of Saigon. And waiting for his opportunity.

Now it had come and he had the Americans to thank for it. With the best of intentions they had once again inadvertently delivered his fortune into his hands.

Baptiste and Noelle had moved into the family villa on the old Rue Pasteur. It was large and expensive, having once belonged to a senior *fonctionnaire* of the old colonial administration. A long sweeping driveway led to an ornamental pond, shaded by plane trees, and a massive white porte cochère. Red and orange hibiscus sprawled up the pale blue stucco walls.

Noelle was upstairs in Lucien's bedroom. He was lying on his belly, asleep, Noelle stroking his hair. The back of the villa looked on to the roofs of the wash house, and Baptiste could hear the servants shouting at each other in their sing-song language as if they were yelling across a *paddi* field.

Noelle looked up as he entered, a frown on her face, as if she had been interrupted in the middle of a complex mathematical problem. She was always like this these days, vague and distant. Like a ghost, he thought. The ghost of someone he had loved.

'Is he sick?' he asked her.

'Just tired. A busy morning at school.'

He put his hand on her shoulders and kissed her cheek. She neither responded nor pulled away. As if she wasn't really there, like she had shed her skin and scuttled away somewhere to hide leaving just a husk behind.

'I brought you something,' he whispered.

He produced a velvet box. She opened it. Inside was a necklace, the Burmese rubies, cabochon-cut, rich like blood on the purple velvet. She did not even take it out of the box.

'Where did you get it?'

'A jeweller's on the Tu Do. Do you like it?'

'It's lovely. Thank you, Baptiste.' She gave him a wan smile and closed the box. She returned her attention to the sleeping boy.

Thank you Baptiste, he thought. Nearly five thousand American dollars. *Thank you, Baptiste*. That was it?

How was he ever going to win her back? How long would she make him burn at the altar of Jean-Marie Pepin? When it wasn't his fault!

It was she who had said to him: 'Do you want to chase clouds for ever?' All he had done was follow her ambitions. She had awakened this ache inside him, had started him on this road. Now they were going to have it all, and damn her, damn her.

She had become his most bitter obsession. All his life he had had any woman he wanted, but the one he could not possess was his own wife. In his more sanguine moments even he saw the irony of it.

He would not give her up, not ever. One day I will make her love me again, he promised himself.

Perhaps then I can let her go.

64

Dale navigated his 2CV through a press of cycles and scooters along the Tran Hung Dao Boulevard. Porters struggled with their tottering loads on their way to the markets. He heard the hooting of tugs and sampans on the river, and the stench of sewage and rotting water weed was overpowering.

As he drove further into Cholon the traffic jammed solid, horns blaring. He left the 2CV parked on the footpath and walked the rest of the way to the Trung Mai. He went inside. Flies buzzed on a sticky gold ringlet of flypaper on the frame of the little office door behind the reception. It was Sammy Chen himself who emerged from the back room, his chubby Buddha's face breaking into a vacuous grin. 'Mr Dale!' he said.

'Hello, Sammy.'

Sammy wore a suit jacket over a net singlet and a white *longyi*. He had a cheap watch with a chromium band on his wrist. As usual, there was absolutely nothing to betray the fact that he was one of the most prosperous businessmen in Saigon. A wise precaution with both the Viet Cong and the government collecting taxes in Cholon.

'This way, this way,' he said, and led Dale behind the desk into his office.

The rug was stained by tea and food, and the plaster was peeling off the dirty blue walls. On the desk were some account books and an abacus. A fan laboured in the corner, stirring the pages of a calendar that had been tacked to the wall above the desk, a plump girl in a Chinese opera costume grinning at them. In the other corner was a little spirit shrine with incense and offerings of fruit arranged around a plaster effigy of a Chinese god.

'Sit down. Please. You want whisky, Mr Dale?'

He nodded.

Sammy Chen opened a drawer and pulled out a bottle of Johnny Walker and filled two shot glasses.

'You wanted to see me, Sammy?'

'Maybe I have some information for you, okay?'

'What kind of information?'

'Perhaps is only a rumour.'

'Tell me anyway.'

'New VC cell here in Cholon, planning to throw grenade in the Café Verlain and then the Continental.'

'When?'

'Tomorrow. Lunchtime, when there is most people.'

'Do you have names?'

Sammy Chen tore a piece of paper from a pad in front of him, scribbled a name and address, folded the paper four times and handed it to Dale.

Dale put it in his pocket and drank some of his whisky. It was oily warm. 'Thanks, Sammy.'

Sammy Chen did not expect to be paid. Information of this kind was part of the tax the government expected from him in return for his opium franchise. It was a reasonable trade-off. These days the police even escorted his opium from Tan Son Nhut to his downtown *fumeurs*.

But Sammy had stipulated that he would only pass his information to the Americans, not Li's agents. Dale supposed he was looking to the future, when connections with American intelligence services might prove valuable. Sammy Chen had been negotiating the dark waters of Vietnamese politics for over ten years and he knew how it was done.

'Mr Dale, it doesn't mind I help you this way. But this is not how you can win this war, okay?'

Dale felt himself bridle at criticism from a Cholon gangster. 'Let us worry about that. The United States has never lost a war.'

'Perhaps that is what you do wrong, okay. Everything you do is trying not to lose. You bomb Hanoi, but you do not invade. You fight in Saigon, but not in Haiphong. Like fighting when all you do is try to block other fellow's punch. Soon you must

291

get tired and he will make you hurt, make you bleed.'

'I don't make the rules. Our government does.'

'Your government is stupid.' Sammy smiled in apology, flashing the gold tooth. 'Do not be angry, Mr Dale. Sammy Chen is a great friend of America. Without you, I never do such good business, never mind.'

'We have to weigh the lesser of two evils. Communism against a little opium.'

'I understand this. But does your government understand?'

'We're fighting a war, Sammy. The greatest war the world has ever seen. For freedom.'

'Freedom!' Sammy said, and chuckled and drank his whisky.

'And we're going to win.'

'I hope you win, Mr Dale. But first you need money. Like from opium.'

Dale found it repugnant to be sitting here with a man who traded in misery, having to endure his taunts. 'Sammy, one day, when this war is over, you and I may no longer be on the same side. Not if I have the choice.'

Sammy removed his spectacles and wiped them on the front of his jacket. 'I will tell you something about me, Mr Dale, okay? I have a cousin, live in Swatow. Once he has big business, hotel, also cotton factory, makes shirts, makes trouser, many. When communists come, he lose everything. When he try to run away, to Hong Kong, communists they shoot my cousin, his wife, his children. So I do not love communist, okay? Think I will always be your friend, whether you want or not.'

Dale finished his whisky and stood up. 'Stay in touch,' he said. He left, ice cold with rage. Where had his country gone wrong that now they had to trade with Chinese gangsters behind the government's back?

Noelle sat in the back of the Mercedes with Lucien, cocooned from the steamy heat and the rank smells of gasoline and sewage. Saigon was like a paved swamp; the hot, gamey winds never brought any relief. Even the plane trees seemed to sag in the noonday heat.

They took the same route every day to fetch Lucien from his

school, which took them past Truong Minh Gian street, now a mecca for American soldiers looking for drugs and girls. At night it was a twitching mass of people and cars and neon. Girlie bars had grown like cancers all over Saigon. There were more and more wounded on the street too, Noelle noticed, and the street children hunted in packs.

They were stalled on the corner of the Cong Li. She looked out of the window and without warning found herself looking into the face of Jonathan Dale.

He was hunched behind the wheel of a ridiculously small 2CV Citroën. Their eyes locked and she saw him lean forward and shout something out of his window which she could not hear. And then the traffic moved on.

She whipped around in her seat, saw him stop his car and leap out into the traffic. The snarl of bicycles and Hondas and Vespas and taxis and lorries exploded into a cacophony of horns. He ignored them and ran after the Mercedes, waving frantically.

She reached forward and tapped her driver, Khan, on the shoulder. 'Faster,' she said.

'But the traffic, madame. Cannot go faster,' Khan said helplessly.

Lucien sat up on the seat. '*Maman*, there's a man knocking on the window.'

'Ignore him.'

'It's an American. What does he want?'

Dale's face was pressed against the glass. 'Noelle! Noelle!'

'*Maman*, he knows your name!'

'Drive, Khan!'

A Vietnamese traffic policeman – White Mouse, the Americans called them – was in the middle of the intersection, on an ice cream cone pedestal. He raised a white gloved hand and waved them on. The Mercedes lurched forward.

'Hurry, Khan!'

Anxious and confused, he stepped on the gas pedal and the big car lurched forward, careering between a rumbling US Army truck, and an ancient rattling bus.

Noelle looked out of the rear window and saw Dale standing in the middle of the traffic, looking helplessly after her.

'Who was it, *Maman*?' Lucien shouted, thrilled and afraid. 'Who was that man?'

'Nobody,' Noelle said, her face white. 'Nobody at all. Now turn around and be quiet for your *maman*. You are giving me a headache.'

65

Lucien was becoming too heavy for pilot training, Baptiste decided. He collapsed, breathless, in a rattan chair on the verandah, and Lucien crawled back on to his mother's lap. Baptiste felt a pang of resentment. There was always a distance between them. This was not the kind of son he had wanted, and he blamed Noelle for that. She was turning the boy against him. The only time he ever came to him was for the aeroplane game.

'So Lucien,' he asked him, forcing a conversation. 'What did you learn at school today?'

'We had to learn our alphabet sounds. And we did numbers. And then we played chase with the girls.'

'Did you catch any?'

'I can't run fast enough,' Lucien mumbled.

'Well, did anything exciting happen today?'

'An American chased our car,' he blurted out, and felt his mother stiffen as he remembered that was supposed to be a secret. He hid his face in her blouse.

Baptiste looked up sharply at Noelle. 'An American?' he said.

'It was nothing,' she said, and waved her hand dismissively. 'Just some drunken Marine.'

Baptiste was silent a few moments, watching her face. She was so transparent. Did she really think he was such a fool? 'Dale,' he said.

'What?'

'Was it Dale?'

Noelle's hesitation confirmed it for him.

'Of course not.'

Baptiste got up and went outside. The screen door slammed behind him.

Lucien started to cry.

Noelle patted his head. 'It's all right, Luc,' she whispered. 'It wasn't your fault.'

66

Lucien was fascinated by his mother. She always smelled of flowers, and he loved to nuzzle her soft neck and enjoy the fragrance of her, loved the shimmering of the silk blouses that she wore, and the soft musky warmth of her breast. He could sit for ever and watch her comb out her long black hair.

Some day he wanted to save her.

He did not know what it was that gave him the idea that his mother had to be saved. Perhaps it was the sadness that seemed to follow her, cling to her like the perfume she wore, or the whispered and angry conversations he sometimes heard late at night behind the bedroom door, or the time he found her weeping silently under the simpoh tree. But he promised himself that one day when he grew up, he would make her happy again.

But for now it was enough that she allowed him to keep her secret.

The secret was for the times when his father was away. She would shut the door to the bedroom, go to the little locked drawer in the bureau and take out the long pipe and little spirit lamp she kept there. Then she would lie down on the bed, and take a little packet from a carved teak jewellery box. The box contained a funny-smelling black jelly. She would put some of the jelly on a hair pin and hold it over the spirit lamp and then put the jelly in the bowl of the pipe. After she smoked the pipe she always fell asleep.

He had never seen any other women smoke, especially pipes. In Vientiane, his father's friends sometimes came to the house with their wives, but he only ever saw the men smoke cigarettes. He imagined this was why his mother wanted him to keep it a secret.

While she did this he would play in the corner and the sweet-smelling smoke made him drowsy and sometimes he would fall asleep too.

But he knew he could never ever give up the secret. This sleepy, dreamy goddess was his, and he loved her with all the passion that a little boy can have for his mother. And in his innocence and his love he would have done anything for her.

He was still ashamed that he had told that other secret to his papa the day before he went away. He knew she had lied to his father about the big American who had banged on the window of their car. He knew because he had seen the American again, that very morning.

He had come to the house.

Dale drove along a boulevard of high walls and plane trees, the lavender and cream walls of the old French villas partly hidden by banana palms. He turned into a long driveway, stopped the car in front of the porte cochère. When he climbed out of the Citroën, his chest was tight with excitement. He had no idea what to expect. He did not care. He only knew he had to see her again.

An amah opened the door a fraction and peered out at him as if he were an ancient ancestor returned to haunt her. *'Que voulez-vous?'* she said.

He gave her his best smile. *'Madame Crocé, s'il vous plaît.'*

'Comment vous appelez-vous?'

'Dale. Jonathan Dale.'

The door shut again.

He looked up at the first floor, saw the movement of the chintz curtains at a window and a shadow quickly withdraw.

'Noelle!'

He waited, knocked again. The shadows grew longer, the twilight came quickly. No lights at any of the windows. Finally he gave up, got into the Citroën and drove away.

*   *   *

He drove into Cholon. It belonged to Saigon's night, a Chinese city of clashing cymbals and clicking mah-jong game tiles, of fan tan parlours and opium dens, of taxi girls and brothels and hotels like the Trung Mai, a caravanserai of illicit pleasures.

Sammy came down from his mah-jong to attend to him personally. He took a key from one of the pigeonholes above the desk. 'This way Mr Dale.'

Dale followed him up the creaking wooden stairs to the second floor. He opened a door and Dale went inside. Sammy grinned, handed Dale the key and left.

The room was shabby but clean. There was a stained washbasin with a cracked mirror and an ancient armoire in one corner, the single bed covered with a thin cotton pad. The shouts of the Chinese at their mah-jong filtered through the open window.

Dale lay down on the bed. A few moments later there was a discreet knock on the door.

'*Entrez*,' he said.

A tiny Chinese girl in a high-collared cheongsam slit to the thigh came in and without a word sat down beside him on the bed.

He reached up and stroked her cheek. She was young, no more than eighteen, he guessed. He suddenly felt like an old man.

'I'm lonely,' he said.

She undressed and laid her pale ivory body beside his on the bed.

Later, he lay in the darkness and stared out of the window at the rooftops of Cholon, and listened to the hubbubb of the night. It was past two o'clock and Cholon was still awake and gambling and shouting and eating and fornicating and doing business.

He felt desolate.

He thought about Michael and Jennifer in San Francisco. What would they be doing now? He tried to remember what time it was in California. Then he thought about Noelle sleeping just a few miles away, in the crook of her husband's arm, her son asleep in the next room. Everyone he cared about was separated from him, by distance, or by circumstances, while he, the warrior monk, fought his wars. It occurred to him, with a sudden stab of pain, that he had been fighting wars all his life and he wondered if he was ever going to win.

He was suddenly tired of the crusade. The Grail was as far away as it had ever been.

67

Bangkok, Thailand

The terrace of the Alliance Française was lit with paper
lanterns; music and subdued laughter drifted on the warm
evening. Some of the guests danced, others wandered on to
the balcony to watch the lights of the small boats moving
on the Chao Phrya.

Marcel Rivelini indicated, with a slight nod of the head to
the two young Thai girls who accompanied them, that it was
time for them to withdraw discreetly and powder their noses.

He had aged badly, thought Baptiste. The black hair had
thinned, there were slack pouches under his eyes, and red spider
lines of broken capillaries on his nose. The deadly combination
of the tropics and too much drink, Baptiste supposed. Rivelini
overcompensated with vanity. He wore too much jewellery, jade
rings, gold at his throat, a bracelet, a diamond-set Piaget on his
wrist. His suit was black silk.

Perhaps time had not been kind, but opium had been good
to Marcel Rivelini.

If he bore any ill-will towards the Bonaventure family in
general, and Baptiste in particular, he did not show it. Noelle
Bonaventure was, after all, just another woman; but business
was business.

'I suppose you've heard what is happening in Europe? The
Americans are putting pressure on the Turks.' He took a black
box of strong Russian cheroots from his jacket pocket and put
one in his mouth. He offered one to Baptiste. 'The Turkish
government have agreed to eradicate all poppy cultivation
on the Anatolian plateau in return for American economic

aid. My connections in Marseille are desperate to find an alternative source. Suddenly opium supplies from this part of the world have become very important.'

Baptiste nodded, but said nothing.

'You still have your connections in Laos?'

'How much do you need?'

'I am sure I can find buyers for whatever you can provide. But not opium, it's too bulky. In Marseille they want morphine bricks.'

Morphine. That's going to be a problem, thought Baptiste. But he understood the reasoning. The sheer bulk of raw opium made it far more difficult to smuggle through customs checks.

'You think you can do it?'

He nodded. 'I'll find a way.'

'You can get it out through the port?'

'I can arrange it.'

'Good.' Rivelini coughed again. It sounded as if he had a chest full of custard.

If this is what it does to you, perhaps I should give up, thought Baptiste. 'You're looking well,' he lied.

'I feel like shit. My doctor says I should go back to France. He wants me to give up these things, too.' He held up the cigarette. 'Fucking idiot.'

'You've been in Asia a long time.'

'I couldn't go back to France now. Too cold. Besides, I'd miss the women.'

On cue, the two girls returned. Baptiste realised he couldn't remember which one was his. Rivelini leaned forward and whispered. 'Naree puts chilli in her pussy. Incredible. Have you ever tried it?'

Baptiste admitted that he hadn't thought of it.

'By the way, how's Noelle?' For a moment he saw the ashes of an old fire flare in the other man's eyes.

'Beautiful,' he said, out of spite.

'You're a lucky bastard.' Rivelini pulled one of the girls towards him and squeezed her breast. She giggled, appalled, and squirmed away. All these years in Asia and Marcel still understands so little about these people, thought Baptiste.

His own girl was looking at him, obviously curious about his disinterest.

I suppose sex is like anything you can buy with money, he thought. When you are rich, your biggest enemy is boredom. The things that cannot be bought suddenly become important.

He had never expected it would be love.

Saigon

The old embassy, down by the river, had been bombed by the Viet Cong earlier that year. The new structure, recently completed, was encased in concrete to protect it from rocket and shell fire, and there were white pillboxes at each corner, manned day and night by US military police in green flak jackets and steel helmets. Marines with polished boots and gleaming belt buckles conducted elaborate security checks at the gates.

In the carpeted foyer a sculptured eagle, beak gaping and wings outspread, glowered down from a cluster of flags. She waited in line. When it was her turn, a young and meticulously polite clerk in a well-tailored uniform looked up and enquired whether he could assist her. His face betrayed neither surprise nor disapproval when she said the name. He spoke quietly into a telephone.

Reckless, she heard her father whisper. You never listened to me when I tried to warn you. Always so reckless. Now look what you're doing.

'Damn you,' she muttered.

But he was right. Beyond the grave, he was still right about her. Why was she here? What did she hope to gain from this?

For a moment she almost turned and ran back out of the building. But spite and desperation made her stay. She had to see him again. There was nothing else in her life.

Suddenly he was standing in front of her. He looked bewildered, relieved, disbelieving. 'Noelle?' he said.

Too late to run now.

Reckless! her father shouted. Will you never listen to me?

68

Vung Tau's peninsula jutted into the South China Sea eighty miles to the south-east of the capital. Its beaches were the closest to Saigon and so it had always been a favourite resort of the Saigonese. The French called it Cap Saint Jacques and had come here since the nineteenth century when they first colonised Indochina. The promontory was dotted with villas that had been built by their army officers and *fonctionnaires*.

They drove down early one morning in Dale's Citroën. It took longer than they anticipated, the road congested with army trucks and taxis and the inevitable bullock carts and bicycles.

It was an overcast, humid morning. Already their clothes were damp with sweat, and it was cramped and hot inside the little car, even with the windows open. Dale's legs were too large for the Citroën, and his knees rested against the metal dashboard.

She stole a glance at him as he drove. There were a few wings of grey in his hair now, but otherwise he was just the same. But his manner had changed. Finally Jonathan Dale had declassified his life.

'Susan and I separated about four years ago,' he was saying. 'Separated ... we were always separated. I've spent half of my life on the other side of the world. It was my fault, not hers.'

'You never get a divorce?'

'We talked about it.'

'But?'

He gave her a sad grin. 'She's one of the papal legion, like you. Doesn't believe in it.'

'And you?'

304

'I'm on God's side, sure. Just my God goes to a different church. Hell, mixed marriage. My old man said it would never work.'

In fact it was her father who had told him to consider carefully. Her old man had liked him, he supposed, looking back on it. Dale came from a good family, his father was a partner in a law firm, he had a college education, had served with valour in the Pacific.

But he wasn't a Catholic. As long as we have each other, it doesn't matter to us, Dale had told him. And he was right. As long as they had each other. It was only when their marriage fell apart that it had seemed important.

'What happened?' Noelle asked him. 'You no longer love each other because you're away from home for so long?'

'I guess at first my work was the reason we spent so long apart. But later, it was more the excuse.'

'Excuse?'

They had reached the outskirts of a village, and a water buffalo wandered into the middle of the road from one of the rice paddis. Dale slowed to go around it.

'You try and sort these things out in your mind ... but I guess I don't really understand it all. I know I loved her when we were first together. I mean, I think I did. It was just before I went to the Pacific. You feel things sharper then, thinking perhaps you won't be coming back.'

'The whole world make mistakes,' Noelle said, thinking of her own.

'We were just young, I guess.' He was silent for a long while, thinking it through in his head as he had done countless times before. 'She wrote to me every day when I was overseas. Christ I used to stare at her picture all the time, especially at night. I guess I made up a lot of stuff that wasn't there.'

'And then you are trapped.'

'We make our own traps. I made her into whatever it was I thought I wanted. We had kids. I had a career. Shit, it isn't a career, it's more than that. It's a destiny.'

My God, Noelle thought. *A destiny.*

'I tried not to notice.'

'Notice what?'

'When I came back ... the edge just wasn't there. Whatever it was I felt before I went. But what do you do? She'd waited for me. I had to marry her. For a time it didn't matter. We had babies. Wife, kids, a home. She was the American dream. What I was fighting for.'

They slowed again, trapped behind a convoy of slow-moving ARVN trucks, coughing black smoke.

'A few years later I was sent overseas. Indonesia, the Philippines. They came with me, but as the kids grew older it got harder. Then I got this.' He tapped his shoulder. 'Right outside the base where we were living. Michael and Jennifer were just a few yards away in the car. After that we decided it was too dangerous for them, for her. She took them back to the States. I guess that was the end of the story, the rest is just epilogue.'

Noelle touched his cheek. She did not feel sorry for him, realised only that like her he was trapped in a life he had thought he wanted: but also like her, he didn't have anyone else to blame.

'Sometimes I get angry,' he said. 'Not at her, just myself. Mostly, I feel sorry for Susan and the kids.'

'What is she like?'

'Susan? I don't know how to ... we had this fight once. I remember I called her a whore in the kitchen and a cook in bed. Shit, that must have hurt. It wasn't fair to her. She's not a bad cook.'

'What does she call you?'

'What?'

'You call her a bad thing. She calls you something back. That is the way, yes?'

'I guess.'

'So what does she call you?'

He didn't answer straight away. His face twisted into a kind of grimace. 'A warrior monk.'

Noelle laughed.

'It wasn't funny then, it's not funny now.'

'I'm sorry.'

There was a tense silence, and then he gave her a wry grin. 'Yeah, she was right, wasn't she?'

They drove out to the northern end of Back Beach, changed into their bathing costumes and leaped into the breakers that rolled in off the South China Sea. Afterwards they found a secluded hollow in the sand dunes and lay in the shade of the fir trees. He rolled towards her, content to stare at her, the sun glinting on the tiny, fine hairs on her forearms and thighs.

'You like what you see?' she said to him.

'Why didn't I meet you twenty years ago?'

'Because then I am only eight years old.'

He grinned. 'I guess that could have been a problem.' He ran his hand along her thigh, leaned forward to lick the salt from her shoulder and breast.

'No, you mustn't.'

'No one can see us,' he said. 'Right now there's only us in the whole world.'

Reckless, she heard her father groan.

'You're beautiful,' he whispered.

'That's my trouble.'

'What do you mean?'

'Dale, do you ever think God is watching you, through the clouds, counting up your sins? One by one. What happens when he runs out of fingers?'

'I don't imagine God like that.'

'How do you imagine God?'

'I don't know. Not as vindictive as that. Maybe I'd like to think that just now and then He'd be grateful.'

Her eyes widened. 'Now I see why you are not Catholic.'

'Whatever mistakes I may have made, I'm still on the side of the angels. He'd better remember that.' He stroked her back, brushing away the tiny grains of sand. He traced the curve of her spine with his finger, down to the cleft of her bottom. She shivered.

'I do not think He will like me doing this, Dale.'

'Tell me this is wrong,' he whispered.

'If it is right we would not have to run away to Vung Tau.'

'When it comes to me and you, I don't give a damn what's right and wrong any more.' He leaned across her, kissed her temple, her cheek, her neck. She tasted of salt. 'What changed your mind? Why did you come to the Embassy?'

'I am going to blow it up,' she murmured. 'I am really VC.'

'I'm serious.'

She hid her face in her arms. After a while, she said: 'Because for three years I can not forget you. Now I know how Susan feels.'

'I don't want you to forget me. Ever.'

He made her roll over on to her back. She let him explore her again. They made love slowly, in rhythm with the waves, withdraw with the sucking tide, in with the breaker, deeper with each fourth wave. And God watched from the clouds, counting her sins.

69

When Baptiste returned from Bangkok the old amah whispered to him what had been going on in his absence; three days in a row the madame had spent all her daylight hours gone from the house and Khan had to fetch Lucien from school alone. She thought the monsieur should know.

He thanked her, but decided to say nothing for the moment.

Instead he went to visit a former Sûreté detective who occasionally did certain surveillance and liaison work that he found too delicate to handle himself. Two weeks later he met the man in the Café Givral and received a full report. Noelle had become more circumspect on his return but that was all. She had met Dale four more times, each time in the morning while Baptiste was in the city on business and Lucien was at school. Twice they went to Dale's apartment on the Ngo Duc Ke, once to a hotel in Cholon, once they met in a park at the end of the Tu Do, near the waterfront.

He paid the retired detective handsomely for his efforts, took the three-page typed report home, and burned it.

He considered discussing the problem with Gerry Gates but immediately discarded this solution. His rage at this latest betrayal ran too deep. But there was also business to consider. After his conversation with Rivelini, an ill-considered response might put too much at risk.

No, what was it that Bonaventure had said to him once? *The problem requires a more Corsican solution.*

The cell was bare brick, and all the windows were painted black. A single light bulb hung from a flex in the ceiling. The only objects in the room were a rope and pulley, and a tub of soapy water.

A Vietnamese woman hung naked by her feet from the rope; her hands were tied behind her back and her head was suspended over the tub. Her wet hair hung like a mop and there were suds all over the floor and on the uniforms of the soldiers gathered around her.

One of them was holding her weight on the rope. Colonel Tran van Li nodded to him and he lowered her down so that her head disappeared into the bucket. For a moment her pale ivory body bucked and squirmed like a fish on a line. When it finally went still, the soldier pulled on the rope and lifted her out.

She blew soapy water from her mouth and nose, shaking her head like a wet dog. She gasped in a deep lungful of air. Colonel Li asked her a question and when she did not answer the soldier lowered the rope and dunked her again.

'I'm going outside,' Dale said.

'I thought you'd be interested in seeing this,' Gates said.

'Why would you think that?'

'It was your friend Sammy Chen who gave us this one. Remember that name and address he scribbled on a piece of paper? This is her.'

Colonel Li said something to the woman and she gasped out an answer. Dale heard the terror and desperation and shame in the woman's voice.

'Listen to her,' Gates said. 'She's babbling out names as fast as she can talk. I thought these VC were supposed to be tough.'

'She's a woman, Colonel. Hardly that even. A girl.'

'Don't get precious on me, Jack. She's the enemy. It doesn't matter what shape they come in.'

Li gave the order for the soldier to dunk her again. Dale went outside.

Gates followed him. He opened a packet of Lucky Strike and handed one to Dale.

'What's the matter?'

'Is this the way we make war, Gerry?'

'This isn't a game. The whole of Asia's resting on the outcome of this one.'

'So we torture little girls?'

'It's little girls like that who have been throwing grenades in restaurants and killing a dozen of our boys at a time.'

Gates lit their cigarettes. The smoke tasted bitter and acrid. Or perhaps that's just the bile, Dale thought. 'I just thought we were the good guys, Gerry.'

'Sure we are. Don't ever doubt it.'

'Well, sometimes I do.'

'Don't make me worry about you, Jack.'

The girl was screaming now. Dale heard the sound of a whip. Jesus Christ, this was like a nightmare.

Gates shook his head. 'Don't try and tell me you never knew what went on in here.'

'I still don't have to like it.'

'Sure you don't. You just have to like communism a whole lot less. No one ever said this was going to be easy. It's a war, the greatest war there ever was. Sometimes we have to make tough choices.'

Dale ground out his cigarette with his heel. 'I think I want to go back to the embassy.'

'Sure.'

Gates went back into the room. For a moment Dale was afforded a vision of the girl, her back striped with the pink welts made by the wire whip. One of the soldiers was throwing quick lime into the wounds.

If this was being on the side of the angels, he was glad he never had to work for the devil.

70

Their affair had settled into a rhythm. They could meet only in the mornings, so if she was able to get away from the villa, she would ring him at the embassy, whispering a few short words into the phone. Usually they went back to his apartment, where they immediately fell on to the bed, hungry for each other. Then they would sit and talk until either Noelle had to rush away to pick Lucien up from school, or Dale had to return to the embassy.

She asked him only once what he was doing in Viet Nam. 'Do you still advise on agriculture?'

'Classified,' he had said.

But when she asked about his children he had produced a family photograph, a more recent image than the one she had found in his bungalow in Vientiane. There was Susan, prettier and younger than Noelle had imagined; Michael, a tall, good-looking boy with chestnut brown hair like his mother; and a teenage girl with long bangs and braces on her teeth, self-consciously grinning at the camera.

'That's Jennifer,' he said. 'She's the bright one. We plan to send her to Berkeley. Michael's just Michael. A typical boy.'

'Do they miss you?'

'I guess.'

'How often do you see them?'

'This isn't for ever,' he said, avoiding the question, but begging another.

'No, it's not,' she said.

'Why do you stay here, Noelle?'

'What else can I do?'

'You could come back to America with me.'

'And be your Susan? I will see more of you here.'

'Then leave Baptiste and come and live here.'

'He would kill you.'

'I'll take my chances. Please think about it. I love you.'

He said it with a look of such sweet earnestness that she believed him. 'It doesn't make any difference,' she said.

He shook his head. 'I just don't understand why you stay with him.'

'It is so strange that a woman stays with a man because of a child? You never hear of this before?'

'I just don't want this to be all there is.'

'It's enough for now,' she had said. But she knew it wasn't true.

After they finished at the embassy, Gates and Dale went into a bar on the Tu Do called the Arizona and pulled up stools. It was dark and noisy, a juke box pulsing out a Beach Boys song. The bar was filled with off-duty soldiers, some of them openly smoking joints. Dale felt uneasy. This new trend of drug-taking among the young was something he had never been happy about. He had witnessed the burgeoning hippie culture on his trips back to San Francisco, and he feared for the future of the next generation, his children's generation. He already suspected Jenny had been involved in dope at school, but he had no proof. Michael? He wasn't sure about Michael.

They were pounced on by two twittering bar girls in tight blue jeans and sweaters. One of them had a long curly hairpiece and lipstick that could have been smeared on with a chisel. She was tottering on heels that must have been three inches high. She grabbed Dale's hand and placed it on her crotch.

'You bamilam,' she whispered. 'You number one, Joe.'

'My name's not Joe,' Dale said, and pulled her hand away impatiently. He tried not to get angry with her. Most of these girls still had mud on their feet from the *paddi* fields, country hillbillies come to Saigon to try and make a living for their parents who had probably lost their crops and perhaps even their homes to the war. Hard to see some of these poor creatures as sex objects, no matter how much make-up they wore, how tight their western jeans.

313

'What's wrong, Joe?' the girl said. 'You not like?'

'Nuts shot off,' Dale told her. 'Big mine. Kaboom! Nothing left, okay?'

The girl seemed doubtful. 'Number ten,' she spat at him. She said something to her friend and moved off.

The other girl sat on Gates' lap, and slipped an arm around his neck. She pulled down one side of her halter top to reveal a small, coffee-coloured breast and a dark button of nipple. 'I'm not in the mood either,' he said, and pushed her on the floor.

She got up and shrieked a stream of invective at him in the harsh peasant dialect of the countryside.

Gates ordered two beers. 'What's the matter, Jack? You look unhappy about something. The thing with Li still bothering you? Listen, she gave us the names of every one of her little comrades. We rounded them up this morning.'

'I'm a soldier, not a torturer.'

'Yeah, but soldiers don't win wars without knowing what the enemy's doing. A little gentle persuasion is all part of it.' Gates lit a Lucky Strike.

'It's not just that.'

'Okay, so what's really bugging you?'

'What's bugging me is we're losing the war, Gerry. I don't mean militarily, though I'm having my doubts there too. I mean, we're losing the big war.'

'What are you talking about, Jack?'

'Look around you. These are United States soldiers. Soldiers? They're kids. All they want to do is smoke dope. There's something going wrong.'

'It's just a little pot.'

'You're wrong, Gerry. Now it's just a little pot. But what's it going to be tomorrow?' He shook his head. 'I don't know, America's heading some place I don't want to go.' He finished his beer. 'I'm not good company tonight. I'm heading home.'

'You've been sitting behind a desk for too long. Maybe we should send you back upcountry to get your feet wet again.'

Dale thought about Noelle. 'No, I'm okay.'

*   *   *

314

As he left the bar he looked at Gates. The girl had come back. She was sitting on his lap giggling and his hand disappeared under what was already a very short leather skirt. Good old Gerry, Dale thought. He just loved wars. He would have been just as happy on the other side. If Hanoi had bars.

71

Noelle was shocked at the change in Marcel Rivelini. He looked dissolute, his hair was thin and his flesh hung in little pouches under his jaw and cheekbones. This was what my father had wanted me to marry, she thought. If I had not been so reckless.

They drank *les sundowners* on the verandah together while Rivelini dutifully reminisced about her father. The evening was hot and heavy, and the city smelled of rancid gasolene. Soft violet clouds silhouetted the plane trees against the sky.

Noelle excused herself to bathe Lucien and dress him for bed. Baptiste and Rivelini turned the conversation to the business that Rivelini had come to Saigon to discuss. And from Lucien's bedroom window, as she read him his bedtime story, Noelle heard every word.

'When can you make the first shipment?' asked Rivelini.

'Two weeks. One hundred kilos of morphine.'

'Good. A freighter, the *Cochin* will be docking in Saigon on the fifteenth. Her captain's name is Carbone – reliable, a Corsican. Have one of your people contact him to make the arrangements. Any problems, let me know.'

'There won't be any.'

'Try and buy up as much morphine as you can.'

'The *Cochin* is headed for Marseille?'

'No, Manila, then Panama.'

'Panama?'

'I have contacts there. A man called Ricord, he went there after the war.'

'A collaborator?' said Baptiste, amused.

'He was fighting the communists. The Resistance was riddled with them. Anyway, it is good for us. Latin America is an ideal shipment point for the United States.'

Baptiste was silent for a moment, thinking. 'So that's why you want me to find so much black.'

'America is a growing market, Baptiste. They are developing a taste for heroin. Remember the old days barnstorming sacks of opium around Laos? It was ridiculous. We were just playing cowboys. This is a proper business now. We have to be good managers, which means influencing the producers as well as getting our goods to market. Do you understand?'

'I think so,' said Baptiste.

'I'm sure you do.' Rivelini gave him a knowing grin. 'You always did have an eye to the future. I knew that from the very first time I saw you. Still, things have turned out for the best in the end, *hein*?'

Rivelini joined them for dinner. They ate to the usual accompaniment from the war zone ten miles to the north, a faint but persistent rattling of the windows, as the B-52s carpet bombed the jungle.

It sounded to Noelle like the oncoming rumbling of a thunderstorm, and underlined the foreboding she felt, a cold chill that gnawed at her all through supper and ruined her appetite. The word 'heroin' echoed over and over in her head. She had often wondered why her husband had decided they should leave Laos and come to live in Saigon.

Now she knew.

After Rivelini had gone, Baptiste adjourned to his study. Noelle followed him, shutting the door behind her. 'Why is Marcel in Saigon?' she asked him.

Baptiste went to the cabinet in the corner and took out a bottle of cognac. He poured three fingers into a crystal glass. 'Just business.'

'Just business,' she repeated.

'You wouldn't be interested,' he said and lounged behind the desk with the brandy.

'Try me.'

'Marcel is a business associate. I do not have to discuss everything I do with you, Noelle.'

'So he's a business associate now? Once he nearly broke your jaw.'

'That was a long time ago.'

'I have a right to know what you are doing. It is my father's business.'

'Not any more. He's dead.' He suddenly he lost patience. 'Look at you. Do you ever want for anything? Do you? Why do you treat me like this? What is it I have done that is so bad, huh?'

Well, I could answer that question for you, he thought. But once you murder one man, the second is not so hard, even when he's related by marriage.

'What have you done that is so wrong?' Noelle mused aloud. She made a great show of looking at her watch. 'It's late. I don't have time to go through the list if we're going to get any sleep tonight.'

'Stop carping at me! Where does this house come from, the fancy clothes you wear? Unless you're willing to starve, don't try and interfere with my business!'

'I really loved you once,' she whispered.

'And you will again.'

She shook her head. 'You've sold your soul.'

'Yes, but I got a good price.' He stood up and stamped past her out of the room.

72

They met in a waterfront park at the end of the Tu Do, near the Saigon River.

Noelle waited for him on a bench, watching a group of American sailors gathered around a bookstall flicking through copies of *Playboy*. A *bui doi* was trailing after them, trying to sell them little packets of number three heroin and marijuana.

She saw Dale striding towards her, his face creased with concern. He sat down beside her. 'Are you all right?'

'I must talk to you.'

'You could have come to the apartment.'

She shook her head. 'I want to talk, not to love.'

'What is it?'

'Day after day I pretend. Then today I wake up and I don't think I can pretend no more.' She looked up at him. 'I don't know what to do.'

'Is this about us?'

'No, it's about Baptiste.'

'Then it is about us.'

'Is it?' She looked around the park. Some street urchins in Brooklyn Dodgers caps were arguing among themselves, and a few feet away a cat cried as it nosed some discarded rubbish. So much misery everywhere, but she had never thought of herself as the cause of any of it before.

She took a deep breath. 'If I tell you Baptiste is exporting heroin to your country, what will you do?'

Dale did not answer her straight away. When he did his voice was slow and deliberate: 'You have proof of that, Noelle?'

'What proof do you want? I hear him talking to one of his business partners from Bangkok. I hear everything.'

She had thought he would be shocked by the news, but instead he appeared very calm. 'Where do they get this heroin from?' he asked her.

'No, not heroin. What they use to make it. What is it? Morphine. They want to make it into heroin and send it to America.'

He shook his head.

'What?' she said. 'What is it? Tell me.'

'I just wish there was something I could do about it.'

She stared at him, astonished. 'You already know this?'

'For the moment your husband and certain of his associates are under the protection of the Vietnamese government.'

'I am not talking about a few *fumeurs* in Cholon. He is exporting refined narcotics to your own country. Do you understand what I'm telling you?'

He looked away. 'Believe me, I don't like it any more than you do.'

'You will not do anything to stop this?'

'You're being naïve.'

Naïve.

Well, perhaps. Baptiste was right about her; she had been happy enough to enjoy the proceeds of the trade until now. First her father, now her husband. She hated what they were doing but as Baptiste liked to remind her, the food she ate, the clothes she wore, the luxurious villa she lived in, all were bought with opium. She had been living in a dream world, cocooned by dirty money. She always had.

'I must go,' she said.

'Wait. Can we just talk for a while?'

He reached for her hand but she pulled away. She needed time to think. The world had turned upside down. 'You always make it sound like you are guarding the Holy Grail, or I don't know what. You talk to me about freedom and saving Asia from communism. Maybe sometimes I think you are crazy, but still I am very proud. Now, I don't know. I think once you are such a good man. But you are just like my father, just like Baptiste. When you want, you can just pretend you are innocent.'

'Noelle . . .'

'Leave me alone. Just leave me alone.'

320

He would have run after her but knew it would not do any good. He would give her time to cool down. Then he could explain this to her. He watched her flag down a taxi and jump in. A moment later she was gone.

He did not think for one moment that he would never speak to her again.

73

Noelle would have needed a mountain of trunks to pack all the clothes Baptiste had bought her over the years. She left most of them in her wardrobes. When he left at eleven o'clock that morning she pulled out two suitcases and packed one for herself and one for Lucien. Khan had driven Baptiste into Saigon in the Mercedes so she went out on to Rue Pasteur and hailed a blue and yellow taxi. In the circumstances the suitcases were a luxury. All she really needed was in the crocodile skin bag she clutched to her lap; all her jewellery and two one way tickets on that afternoon's Air France flight to Paris.

They sped down the Cong Ly to Tan Son Nhut.

An embassy clerk handed Dale a phone message he had taken for him very early that morning; Noelle wanted to meet him at the Café Charles at eleven-thirty.

Since their meeting in the park he had thought about nothing else but her. For the first time in his life he was no longer convinced of his grasp of the truth. He thought he had always known the right way to examine any conflict, and now she had made him doubt his own integrity. He did not know what to do; all he knew was that he loved her and wanted her, and the thought of losing her was unbearable.

He had decided to talk over the problem of Baptiste's involvement in narcotics with Gates.

The Charles was on the Tu Do, two blocks from the Continental, between an Indian tailor's and a Chinese antique shop. There were a few bentwood tables and iron chairs on the pavement but customers rarely risked these any more, most taking their seats inside the café behind the wire mesh grille that offered some protection against VC grenades.

Dale was ten minutes early. He went inside, ordered a Tiger beer and waited. The streets were clogged with traffic, the café's radio battling to be heard over the din of the Hondas in the street. The clientele was mainly American soldiers, a few journalists. Dale detected the sickly sweet smell of marijuana.

He did not see Baptiste enter, but suddenly he was standing beside the table, a soft smile creasing the handsome olive face. The eyepatch made him remarkable in any crowd and some of the soldiers were staring at him openly. The black silk shirt was open at the collar and a thick rope of gold nestled among the matt of hair at his throat.

'You look surprised, Monsieur Dale. You were perhaps expecting someone else?'

So he knew. It was only a matter of time anyway. 'Sit down,' Dale said.

Baptiste accepted the offer.

'Beer?'

'Let's drink and be friends, yes?'

Dale nodded to the proprietor who hurried over with two more Tiger beers. Crocé lit a cigarette but did not offer the packet to Dale.

'Where is she?' he said.

'My wife? At home, I imagine. Where else might she be?'

'Let's not play games.'

'But I enjoy games. I am very good at them. In Vientiane I always play *vingt-et-un* with Noelle's father. He said I am a born gambler.'

A Vietnamese boy came into the café carrying a brown paper bag loaded with cigarettes and chewing gum, which he tried to hawk to the customers. The proprietor shouted at him angrily and the boy slouched away.

'You know I've been seeing her,' said Dale.

'In fact you have seen everything, yes?'

Dale was quickly tiring of this. 'What do you want?' he snapped.

Baptiste toyed with the Suntory ashtray. 'I did not come here to ask for anything. If I want anything, it is just to kill you.'

'Talk is cheap.'

'So is life in Saigon.'

'Let's get this straight. Are you threatening me?'

Baptiste shook his head, apparently amused. 'You think I am so crude? You misjudge me, Monsieur Dale.'

'Then why are you here?'

'I come here to say goodbye.' The waiter arrived with their beers. 'I do not drink beer,' Baptiste said and walked out, leaving his cigarette smoking in the ashtray.

Dale stared after him. What the hell was that about? He felt the tension draining out of his body. He had been waiting for Baptiste to throw a punch, pull out a knife, or a gun. He felt both relieved and cheated.

His disappointment was quickly replaced by alarm. What had happened to Noelle? And why goodbye? What was he planning?

Holy Christ.

The cigarette seller had left his paper bag in the corner.

He shouted a warning and leaped to his feet.

Noelle gripped Lucien's hand tightly as the taxi pulled in to the civilian departure terminal at Tan Son Nhut.

I'm finally doing it. I'm finally getting away.

She thrust a handful of piasters into the driver's hand. She didn't wait for change. She wouldn't need piasters where she was going.

She got out, pulling Lucien after her.

She searched the crowds inside the terminal: American servicemen, military police in their white helmets, smaller Vietnamese carrying their possessions in boxes tied with string, women in swirling *ao dai*. She half expected to see Baptiste already here, all swagger and mockery. Perhaps he had somehow anticipated her plans.

There was no sign of him.

He had said to her once that she could never get away from him; well, no one could be right all the time.

*   *   *

324

Gerry Gates was with Colonel Tran van Li on the terrace of the Continental when they heard the explosion of glass followed by a wave of heat. A plume of black smoke billowed from the shattered windows of the Charles, and debris rained down into the Tu Do. Gates knew the Charles was a favourite haunt of American servicemen and he immediately jumped to his feet and ran out of the hotel and down the street.

A shocked silence, broken only by the crackle of flames darting along the shattered concrete and corrugated iron. Then the moaning started. Bodies twitched in black pools. A woman sat on the ground nursing the remains of her baby on her lap.

A soldier started to scream, then another. Gates stumbled over the debris, pulling the wounded clear of burning rafters, his hands blistering on hot lintels, stopping only to brush burning sparks from his clothes.

He almost did not recognise Jonathan Dale. His face was blackened from the blast, his hair matted with blood, most of his clothes torn off his body by the force of the blast.

'Gerry...' he mumbled.

'Jesus H!' Gates said, and kicked away the wreckage from around him. Dale's right leg was a sodden mess of raw meat, two of his fingers were hanging by tendons. There was blood on his shirt but Gates couldn't find the wound. In the distance he heard the police sirens and the bells of the first ambulances.

The leg was bleeding badly. He fashioned a makeshift tourniquet from his belt and tied it around Dale's thigh. 'Hang tough, Jack. You'll be okay,' he lied.

'Noelle,' Dale said, and passed out.

The customs official carefully studied her passport, checked the photograph against her face. Then he calmly pushed it to one side and picked up the phone.

'Is there some problem?' she asked him.

He didn't answer her.

A few moments later another official joined him in the booth,

325

picked up her passport and told her, in French, that there was indeed a problem. Would she accompany him please?

He led her to a small interview room. It was painted a dirty green, and was quite bare except for a desk and two chairs. He told her to wait. As he went out, he locked the door.

Noelle pulled Lucien on to her lap and waited. She couldn't believe it. She felt the fight go out of her. She wanted to weep.

Almost an hour later the door was unlocked. An airport official ushered Baptiste into the room and shut the door behind him.

'Noelle. Going on holiday?'

He looked so smug. 'Can you buy everyone?' she asked him.

'Just about.' He sat down, smiled at Lucien and patted his head. 'Seriously, *ma chère*, where would you go?' He took her bag and pulled out the airline tickets. 'Paris? Who do you know in Paris?'

'I make friends easily.'

'How would you live?'

'I was going to become a prostitute. Try and improve my lot in life.'

His eyes flashed with anger for just a moment, and then he recovered. 'All right, I admit it. I'm hurt. I never thought you'd do this.'

'How did you know?'

'I'm ashamed to say that I have had someone following you. For quite a few weeks now.'

So he knew about Dale as well. 'You never tried to stop me before this?'

'You never tried to run away from me before this.' He tore up the tickets. 'My car is outside. Let's talk some more on the way home. It is stinking hot in here.'

He led his wife and son through the press of people and luggage, keeping a proprietary hand on her shoulder. The black Mercedes Benz was waiting in the forecourt. Khan opened the door. She climbed in the back with Lucien. Baptiste got in beside her.

'Don't feel too badly,' he said, as they drove back into Saigon. 'Even if you had got to Paris, I would have come after you. And little Lucien.' He chucked the boy under the chin. 'You can hide in a cave in the middle of Russia and I will find you. You're my wife. Nothing will change that.'

'It's like a curse,' she muttered, turning away and staring in dull pain out of the window.

'It doesn't have to be,' he said.

When they got back to the villa he sent Lucien to play in the garden, in the care of his amah, and ordered the rest of the servants out of the house.

The air of conceit and triumph evaporated. His face turned dark, like a thunderstorm passing over the sun. He took two steps towards her and slapped her face. 'Why are you doing this to me?'

She drew back her arm and slapped him back, as hard as she could. She would have hit him again but he caught her wrist. The outline of her hand showed livid against his cheek. 'I could break your neck,' he hissed at her.

'Then why don't you?'

'Because I love you. I have always loved you. It is just that you have never loved me.'

'I did once. I made myself stop. It was just a bad habit.'

'Why? Why? I have done everything for you! Phong Savan was for you!'

'Was it?'

'Yes. Yes! Okay, so there were women. Just whores, taxi girls, they meant nothing! I was young, I was stupid!'

'It's not just the women.'

'Jean-Marie.'

He looked desperate, like a cornered animal. Why am I so important to him? she wondered. Or is it just his monumental ego, wanting the one thing he cannot have?

He ran his fingers through his hair, his hands shaking. 'You are not to run away from me again.'

'You can't spend your whole life chasing after me, Baptiste. You'll never have time to do anything else.'

'Why are you doing this? Our life could be so good. Anything you want, I can give it to you. One day I will

327

be one of the richest men in Asia. You can ... you can be a queen.'

She shook her head. 'You disgust me.'

'You're such a fucking hypocrite! Your beloved papa, he was a gangster, smuggled opium all his life, you knew that, it was no secret. But you wept tears in buckets at his funeral, didn't you, huh? And he was a murderer too. He was the one who killed Jean-Marie! I tried to stop him but he did it, not me!' He jabbed viciously at the air, his finger hovering a few inches from her face like a dagger. 'But you! You are such a saint, such an angel, you accuse me. Everything bad that happens, it's Baptiste! Your straw man, the sacrifice to your conscience! You treat me like shit. And what is my sin? That I love you!'

'Have you finished?' she said.

'No, I have not finished,' he said, and grabbed her wrists and pinned her against the wall. He tried to kiss her and she bit down on his bottom lip. He drew away, blood welling from his mouth. He swore, then suddenly bent down, threw her over his shoulder and carried her to the bedroom.

She pummelled him with her fists, pulled up his shirt and sank her teeth into his back. She heard him gasp, but he did not release her. He kicked open the door to his bedroom and threw her on the bed. 'Now you're going to be my wife,' he said.

He rolled away from her. There were raised red welts on his back where she had bitten him, already turning an angry purple. His lip was swollen and she had drawn blood from his shoulder. Noelle stared at what she had done, appalled.

He got up, buckled his trousers, ripped off the shirt which she had shredded with her nails and teeth. He threw it on the floor. 'I will never do that again,' he said, his back to her. She sensed that he was somehow ashamed.

'If you do, I'll kill you.'

'Just understand this – I will never give up my son. You can stay, or you can go. But I will never give up my son.'

He walked out of the room, shutting the door gently behind him.

Noelle heard him leave the room. She remembered what the

Blind Bonze had told her: *'If you abandon your baby son, a new fate will be written. That is the only way.'* If that truly was the only way she would ever be free of him then she was trapped. How could she ever leave Luc?

329

74

San Francisco

Dale's memories of the bombing were vague; the boy with the paper bag of cigarettes, the look of horror on the proprietor's face when he understood what was about to happen, nothing more. A vague recollection of terrible pain, a montage of sounds and images, ambulance sirens, the smell of charred meat, Gates' voice telling him he was all right, surgeons asking him questions, their heads haloed by the bright lights of the operating theatre. Even the aftermath of the surgery, the roller-coaster of pain dulled by the gelatin warmth of the morphine, was now a distant memory. He knew it had somehow left a scar somewhere, deep in his brain, but he could not recall the contours of that pain. Its geography had mercifully vanished.

His final conversation with Baptiste had been erased. He could not even remember why he had gone to the Café Charles that day.

They shipped him back to the States. Because he was not officially a member of the military, they sent him to San Francisco General, and a private ward. A young man whose name he did not know, and who made no attempt to identify himself, came to visit him on the second day, and told him not to worry about the medical bills.

Through the window yachts tacked across a blue bay, the white caps swept before the wind – a world so far removed from the banana palms and the smell of durian and kerosene and steamy heat that it might not have been real. Only the pain was real.

The doctors told him he was lucky. Fragments from the bomb had lacerated an artery in his lower leg, but the surgeons at Cong Hoa had done a good job, and although he would still need further grafts, he would keep the leg. He had lost two fingers from his right hand above the first knuckle, and they had removed a damaged kidney. There were twenty-seven stitches in his scalp.

'Will I be able to ride a horse,' he asked them.

'Sure.'

'Great. Because I couldn't ever ride one before.'

They laughed dutifully. They had only heard that one a thousand times before. But if it helped him get better . . .

Michael had been his first visitor, but Dale had only just arrived from the airport and he was too drugged to talk much after the flight from Saigon. Next morning when he woke up Susan was there.

Her eyes were wet, and he felt both grateful and sorry. He wondered sometimes why she gave a damn. 'Well, look at you soldier,' she whispered.

'Let this be a lesson to you,' he said slowly, his tongue feeling twice its size, his lips numb, 'never smoke in a gas station.'

She squeezed his good hand. 'I prayed for you.'

Oh, no. Not God already. What did He have to do with this? 'Hey, thanks.'

'The doctors say you're going to be just fine.'

'Feel fit enough . . . for a couple of sets of tennis . . . already.' He was surprised what an effort it was to talk.

He drifted away into the soft buzz of morphine dreams. He dreamt Noelle was beside the bed, holding his hand. When he woke up Susan was still there. He smiled at her, and she said something to him, but the words seemed to come to him from a long way away.

When he woke up again Michael was there. The windows were black and he realised he must have been asleep all day. A lamp beside the bed threw soft shadows on his son's face. No, wait. The shadows were a fringe of stubble. Michael had started shaving. When did that happen?

'Dad?'

'Growing a beard?' he mumbled.

Michael shrugged, embarrassed. 'Hairs on my chest too, eighteen of them. One for every year.'

'Hey, me too. Two hundred and forty-eight. At least that's what it feels like.' He winced at a sudden, sharp pain in his leg.

'Want me to call the nurse?'

'A little pain never hurt anyone.'

Michael just stared, looking young and very pale.

'Hey, that was a joke.'

Michael went out to call the nurse who told him he was not due for more morphine for another three hours. 'It's addictive,' she said. Michael tried to argue with her, but she shook her head and stamped out.

'I'm okay,' said Dale.

Poor Michael, he thought. His all-star jock suddenly looked pale and fragile. Dale raised his good hand a few inches off the bed. 'Come here son.'

Michael took his hand, put his head on the bed and wept.

Susan and Michael were regular visitors, but Jennifer did not come and the subject of his daughter was pointedly ignored. Susan had mentioned in her letters that there were problems, that Jennifer had been neglecting her studies. Now he knew there was more to it than that.

'Where's Jennifer?'

Susan took a deep breath. 'John...'

'She knows I'm here?'

Susan had looked at Michael and there was an odd silence.

'She says she doesn't want to see you, Dad.'

Another kind of pain, something indefinable, guilt and betrayal together. 'Why?'

More shuffling silence.

'Michael?'

'She blames you, Dad.'

'What for?'

He laughed, a broken sound, without humour. 'For everything.'

Then it all came out, the problem with Jennifer. She had derailed her life. She had been to four lectures in the last six months, none at all in the last nine weeks. She had moved off the campus and the address Susan had was in Haight-Ashbury. With the damned hippies, thought Dale.

'I went to see her when she moved out there,' Susan said, 'tried to talk some sense into her. But now she won't even open the door. I pray for her all the time.'

'Great.'

'I went to see her yesterday, tried to persuade her to come.'

'And?'

Susan shook her head.

'Well, I'd better get mended,' Dale said. 'If Mohammed won't go to the mountain.' He forced a bitter smile.

Oh, Jesus, my own daughter. What's going on?

75

Two months later

The architecture was known as Stick and Stick. It was emblazoned with 'gingerbread', and featured every gewgaw of the carpenter's art; cartouches, spindles, festoons, arches and rosettes. The tall front door and its extended porch was flanked by columns, and there were squared bay windows and horseshoe arches everywhere. She was a grand, if gaudy, Victorian lady, considered an embarrassment in her middle age, but rescued in her dotage by psychedelia and the hippies. The front of the house was now an explosion of reds, blues and greens, all clumsily painted. The effect was startling, a Christmas cake of colour and design.

'Jesus,' Dale said aloud, and went inside.

He made his way painfully to the first-floor apartment, walking with the aid of a stick, his right hand still heavily bandaged. Out of spite and wounded pride he wore his old USAF major's uniform, even though he was supposed to be officially retired from military duty.

He knocked twice and waited.

He barely recognised the girl who opened the door. Her fair hair was lank and tied in a red bandana. She had on a suede fringed jacket and torn jeans, and wore beads – not pretty ones, not girl ones – big bright gaudy things that reached almost to her waist. And no bra, he noticed.

'Hello, Jenny,' he said, and offered an uncertain smile.

She smiled back, but he could tell it was an effort. 'Dad,' she said.

'I would have rung but your mom said you had no phone here.'

She shook her head. 'That's right.'

'So this is the new place.' A beat. 'Can I come in?'

There was music playing, too loud. It took a little while for Dale to realise that he recognised the tune. It was 'The Star Spangled Banner' played on an electric guitar. Christ Almighty. A man with a beard was asleep on a bean bag. His T-shirt said:

ALL THE TIME MORE OF US ARE BEING BORN
AND MORE OF THEM ARE DYING

He smelled sweat, and mould, and marijuana. There was no furniture except for a few bean bags and some Oriental rugs. There were posters on the wall: Che Guevara, the Grateful Dead, Jefferson Airplane. There was also a hand-pasted collage: the now-famous photograph of a Buddhist monk burning in a Saigon street; John Lennon peering through wire-rimmed glasses; Mick Jagger, Jimi Hendrix, Eldridge Cleaver, Bob Dylan; showers of peace symbols; a mushroom cloud; stacked Viet Cong dead.

In the corner was a small bronze Buddha and incense burning in an empty jam tin. It was almost an affront, a parody of his own life. What did these kids know about Viet Nam, about Buddha, about the bonzes who had committed their self-immolation in protest against Diem?

'Nice place,' he said. He had not meant it to sound so derisive but she picked it up straight away.

'Yeah, well I like it.'

He turned around and tried to force a smile. 'How have you been?' he said.

'OK. Good. Great.' A beat. 'I'm sorry I didn't come to the hospital.'

He waited for the excuse, but it didn't come.

'They said you were going to be okay. Are you?'

He held up his hand. 'Can't count up to ten any more.' It was supposed to be a joke, but she didn't smile.

'How's the war?'

A sore subject, he knew, and one best avoided. On his last leave they had had a heated argument about America's involvement in Vietnam and she had said things to him that he would rather forget. Perhaps when she grew up, she would understand a little better.

'Looks like it might be over for me. Got a cup of coffee?'

They went into the kitchen. There was a pile of dirty plates stacked in the sink, and a roach scurried out of sight. Jennifer filled a kettle and the pipes clanked and groaned. She put it on the burner.

'How much do you pay for this place?' he asked her.

'Ninety,' she said. 'Three ways.'

Three? he thought.

They made small talk while they waited for the kettle to boil. 'How's college?' he asked eventually. He tried to make the enquiry sound as casual as possible but immediately he could sense her tighten up.

'Okay.'

'No problems?'

'No problems,' she said.

Dale thought about it while she poured the hot water into two cracked china cups and dumped in two spoonfuls of instant. *No problems.*

He followed her back into the living room. She flopped onto a bean bag. 'Take a seat,' she grinned, but there was little humour in the smile. *Let's see you in one of these.*

Instead he leaned against the wall. The stitches in his side started to bite, and the bulky dressing bit into his ribs. A film of sweat erupted on his face.

'Does it hurt?' she said.

No, you hurt. Everything else is just physical pain. I can deal with that. 'It's getting better.'

'What happened.'

'You don't want to know.'

'Why? Is it classified?'

She was sharp, he remembered. She always was the one with the smart mouth. Hit first, repent later. Michael referred to her privately as Lash.

'I spoke to one of your tutors,' he said.

'Shit...'

'What's going on, Jenny?'

A shrug. 'I dropped out.'

'Dropped out.'

'Look, I'm twenty years old. You can't tell me how to live any more.'

No, but I can worry about you. That's okay, isn't it?'

'Oh, yeah, you're worried. You worry maybe once every six months. You come back here and do the big father act and then you get back to your dirty little war. So worry.'

The bearded man on the bean bag started to snore.

Dale nodded towards him. 'Anyone I should know about?' he said, still trying to keep the conversation light.

'Anyone you should know about?' she mocked him. 'I fucked him last night but I don't know his name. Chuck or something.'

He knew what she was doing. For a moment he wanted to slap her face, but he knew that would only make things worse, was probably what she wanted. Another crime to add to the indictment.

'Is he a good fuck?' he said. The words were like ashes in his mouth, but he knew the reaction she wanted from him, and he was determined not to let her win this particular game. Let's get through this, he thought. We'll get through it and then perhaps we can talk.

'What do you want, Dad?'

'I want to know why my daughter is wasting her life in this slum. I want to know why she got straight As all through school but now she's decided to drop out of Berkeley in her second year. I want to know what I ever did that was so bad that you want to treat me this way?'

She stared at him, open-mouthed. 'You want to know what you did that was so bad?'

'That was my question.'

'Three things. You were never there, you were never there, and you were never there.'

'I'm here now.'

'Too late buster.'

337

He wore that, and ploughed on. 'I'm still your father, Jennifer. I still love you.'

For a moment he thought he had broken through, but then she got up and went to the large tin ashtray on the floor under the radiator. She took out a long flat cigarette and lit it. Dale recognised the pungent smell immediately.

'I just thought of a fourth thing,' Jennifer said. 'You left Mom.'

'We separated. There's a difference. It was something we both agreed...'

'You broke her heart. Look at her now, for Crissakes. She's found the Lord. Jesus, you fucked her up!'

'I didn't mean to,' he said, and knew how lame it sounded. This was rough, far rougher than he had imagined. He remembered the dumpy tousle-haired two year old whose favourite game was to have him throw her in the air and then catch her. Was this what she had grown into?

She drew on the cigarette, the tip crackled and sparked. 'Hey, this is good Moroccan. Chuck says he brought it back from Marrakech. Want to try some?'

Dale snatched it out of her hand and tossed it out of the window. Jennifer shook her head. 'Well, you sure just made someone's day.'

'Stop this, Jennifer. Please.'

'Come on, Dad. Big boys don't cry.'

She flopped back on to the bean bag.

'Are you enjoying this?'

'How long are you home for this time?'

'I don't think I'll be going back.' He saw a flicker of hesitation, perhaps of hope. 'I want you to come home,' he said.

'I am home.'

'Here? This place?'

The bearded man opened his eyes. He saw Dale's uniform. Still stoned, Dale thought. 'Shit. Who are you, man?'

'Army. I'm looking for new conscripts.'

'Fuck,' the man said, and scrambled to his feet and ran out of the door.

Jennifer did not smile but he could tell she was amused. She stared at the open door, listening to his footsteps on the stairs. 'Very quick, Dad.'

338

Dale went to the window, opened it, leaned on the sill. The pain was bad. He took deep lungfuls of fresh air. 'What do you want, Jennifer?'

'I want you and Mom back together.'

'You're twenty years old! You're grown up! What does it matter to you now?'

'It's up to you. You want a good little daughter, I want a father at home. How's that?'

She was serious. Dale could almost see the world lurch out of focus. He had seen his life through a crazy mirror for the last twenty years, and now he had turned around to find it wasn't that way at all. Had he really hurt them all so badly?

'She'll never take me back.'

'She might.'

'If I did this ... you'd come home and go back to study?'

She nodded.

In that moment he knew he would forget Noelle, would abandon his crusade. He had fought twenty years to save the world and had ravaged his own with neglect; he had thought his children had worshipped him from afar, and they had hated his guts; he had thought Susan had wanted the separation too, and he had torn out her heart; he had thought what he did really mattered but somewhere he had lost belief.

'Okay,' he said to Jennifer. 'Let's try it your way.'

76

Saigon, August 1969

Baptiste turned off the Hong Thap Tu into Cao Thang Street. Sammy Chen's villa was hidden away behind a high wall and tall fishtail palms. Baptiste had met Sammy many times since Bonaventure's death, usually in a back room at the Trung Mai. He guessed that the invitation to Sammy's house meant that this was not just routine business.

Sammy was waiting for him on a patio that had been shielded with breeze blocks. He greeted Baptiste effusively and offered him a glass of Chivas Regal whisky, but restricted himself to green Chinese tea.

'Double luck,' Sammy said, and raised his tea cup.

They observed the usual pleasantries, and then the conversation turned inevitably to the war. There were reports that Ho Chi Minh was ill, and they discussed his likely successor if he died, and what effect it might have on the stalled Paris peace talks. It was already apparent that the talks were a farce, another holding action by the North Vietnamese. It was also clear that the Americans were losing their war of attrition where it mattered most: in their own cities and universities.

Finally Sammy mopped at his face with a handkerchief and said: 'So, Kwo-chao, we talk business now, yes?' He could never manage Crocé and pronounced it Kwo-chao. 'You need more number four.' It was a statement, not a question.

'Are you selling?'

'All the number four you want.'

It was an astonishing declaration. Baptiste just stared at him.

Sammy took off one of his shoes and started to pick at the toe nails of his right foot. Baptiste was not sure if he was impressed or disgusted. Did the man have so much self-confidence that he didn't give a damn what other people thought of him? Or was it that he was from peasant stock and had made all his money before he ever learned better?

'I can buy here in Cholon?' Baptiste asked finally.

'In Vientiane. You talk about transport with General Rattakone and Colonel Li, okay?'

'You have people making number four in Laos?'

'I buy opium and protection direct from Rattakone. I get good cook from Hong Kong, can make China White, ninety-nine per cent pure. It is like franchise, okay. Like hamburger joint!' He giggled, and his spectacles flashed in the sun.

Baptiste drained his glass. Sammy poured him another one. 'We might be interested,' he said.

Sammy slapped his knee. 'No, you need! America they stop Turkey growing poppy, now try to stop Mexican too. Where else you get cheap number four now?'

Sammy was right and his timing could not have been better. Or perhaps, thought Baptiste, like any good businessman, he had simply anticipated the opportunity. The Turkish eradication program was indeed hitting their customers hard in the United States. Now the government was applying the blowtorch in Mexico as well.

Now the supplier has become the buyer, Baptiste thought. How the world turns. 'I could have some very big orders for the next opium harvest. We could be talking about initial orders of one thousand kilos of number four.'

At current prices Sammy could look forward to a cash advance of almost two million dollars, but he did not even pause for breath. 'Perhaps next year I will make this order more bigger.'

'How?'

'There is beaucoup Americans in Saigon now. Just like Hong Kong. Want good time, want girl, want whisky, want drugs.'

'Like soldiers everywhere.'

'Yes, like soldiers everywhere,' Sammy agreed. 'Only here not really soldier. Just short-time soldier. Twelve month in Viet

341

Nam. Then, if they not die, go home to America. *Beaucoup* short-time soldier.'

Baptiste fanned himself with his fedora. The breath of the city was as hot and fetid as a jackal and it reeked of decay and diesel. 'And?' he said.

'Not just soldier, Kwo-chao. For every man who fight in jungle, America has ten more who is clerk, or engineer, or cook. Very bored. Captive market.' Sammy shook his head. 'Big market, Kwo-chao. More bigger than *les pauvres* who come to the *fumeurs*.'

'You're going to use Saigon as a test market,' said Baptiste, and the realisation took his breath away.

'Imagine if all this soldier get taste for China White in Saigon, okay? Take appetite back to America, okay? User always become seller. Will make a big new market in America.'

'That's an interesting idea, Sammy.'

'No my idea, Kwo-chao. Idea come from biggest drug trafficker in history – Britain.' His eyes twinkled and he rocked happily in his chair. For a moment Baptiste had the bizarre impression of a fat, happy Buddha. '*Great* Britain. In China, before the British come, opium is banned, okay? Is against Confucius code. But Britain has beaucoup opium from India. Must sell somewhere. In China they buy tea, buy silk, have nothing to trade. So they import, never mind law, never mind opium war, make their own market. Soon is China has trade deficit. So. *With opium must make own market.* All big hongs in Hong Kong, Butterfield Swire, Jardine Matheson, all get fat on opium, all same. Now we get fat, okay?'

'But instead of having to invade another country, this time the invaders have come to you.' Baptiste had to admire the man. He certainly understood business economics.

'Yes, Kwo-chao. They come to us!' He raised his glass in a toast. 'Double happiness and double prosperity!'

A dream of enormous wealth is something that most men toy with, a harem fantasy of riches realised only in their dreams. Suddenly Baptiste felt the mirage form itself into something he could almost smell and touch. He touched Sammy's teacup with his glass. '*Salut*,' he answered.

77

The street pulsed with gaudy neon signs: Melody Bar, Blue Diamond, Dolce Vita. They hurried past pizza bars and hamburger joints filled with American servicemen. A Pat Boone song thumped from the doors of a nightclub.

A small boy followed them down the street, tugging at Rivelini's jacket. 'Mister, you want boom-boom my sister, mister?'

'Watch out I don't boom-boom you,' he growled, disentangling himself.

'Yes, mister, how much?' the boy called after him.

They found their way to Le Cigale, a nightclub run by fellow Corsicans. They took a table in the corner and Baptiste ordered two Martell brandies. A hauntingly beautiful Vietnamese with hair down almost to her waist was singing old Légionnaires anthems with the anguish of a Piaf.

Baptiste studied the other man. Rivelini's face looked grey, and the lines in his forehead and cheeks could have been carved with a chisel. 'You're looking well, Marcel.'

'I feel like shit.' Rivelini fished in his pockets for his cheroots. As soon as he lit one, he broke into a coughing fit which did not subside for almost a minute. When it was finished, he inhaled deeply. 'That's better,' he groaned.

'You should cut down,' Baptiste told him.

'What for? Coughing is good exercise.'

Baptiste shrugged. The brandies arrived. '*Salut*,' he said. '*Salut*.'

'So how have you been? You look like you've lost weight.'

'I could afford to. I'd put on a few pounds. We can't all drink from the fountain of youth, like you.'

343

'Clean living and a clear conscience.'

Rivelini grunted with derision. 'How's Noelle?' he asked, and thé familiar look of envy and prurient curiosity came to his face.

'She's well, Marcel. She told me to pass on her best wishes.'

'You are full of shit, Baptiste. She could never stand the sight of me.'

Well, true. 'She counts you as one of her closest friends.'

'You're a liar, you always were.' He drank his Martell. 'Remember that night in the Constellation.'

'I was drunk.'

'An understatement. Yet she loved you from the moment she set eyes on you. It was written all over her face. I knew I'd lost her even before she hit me with that bottle.'

'She didn't hit you with anything, she just pushed you, that's all. You fell over the chair.'

'She hit me with a bottle! I needed six stitches in my head. Lucky for you, or I would have killed you with my bare hands. I was so crazy I never heard her come up behind me. How would you remember, the state you were in!'

Baptiste decided to allow him this small victory. Poor Marcel. It seemed the memory of that night still burned so fiercely in him, he had been forced to reconstruct it in his mind and style his defeat in a more romantic light.

'You're right. I hardly remember a thing.'

Rivelini grunted, downed his brandy and called for two more.

'Something has come up, Marcel.'

On stage Miss Yen Hung was wailing a song about Algiers. Baptiste wondered at the irony. A Vietnamese girl who had never seen a desert singing in French about North Africa. Another of life's strange cocktails. Like two Frenchmen sitting in a Saigon bar planning to smuggle Laotian opiates to America.

'I hope it's good news, Baptiste. They're screaming at me in Marseille. This Turkish ban is biting hard.'

'Perhaps we can help them. Number four heroin, ninety-nine per cent pure.'

'From where?'

344

'Laos.'

'Laos? They can supply us in bulk?'

'Rattakone has come to an arrangement with a chiu chao syndicate here in Saigon. They are giving him experienced Hong Kong chemists to take over the morphine refineries at Ban Houie Sai. They buy his opium direct, and Army protection. It's like a franchise. His words.'

Rivelini exploded into another fit of coughing. When he had finished he lit another cheroot. 'You're saying they want to restructure the whole business?'

'That's not all of it. The chiu chao are also talking about flooding the Saigon market with cheap heroin. Creating a new generation of addicts in the United States.'

'We have enough trouble meeting demand right now!'

'Not for long, Marcel. They've promised me as much number four as we want.' He lowered his voice, like a lover. 'Just one ton will bring the syndicate twenty-five million dollars. How rich do you want to be?'

Rivelini was silent for a long time. 'I think it's time we talked to a few people,' he said finally.

The crystal wall sconces threw a soft yellow light over the room. Baptiste sat by the French windows, *en smoking*, a week-old copy of *Le Figaro* open on his lap. Noelle went to stand by the windows, watching the last of the sunset turn to rust. Shadows crept across the lawn. Two fat putty-grey lizards chased each other along a verandah post. Lust or murder? she wondered. The two were inescapable.

The distant rumble of artillery set the Limoges china rattling in its glass cabinet. From much closer came the short staccato bark of a light machine gun. 'Listen to that. Every day the war gets closer. Why do we stay in Saigon?'

'Business,' said Baptiste.

'Can't you do your business in Bangkok? Like Rivelini and the others?'

'Saigon is no more dangerous than Vientiane.'

'I worry for Lucien.'

'We're not Americans. We've nothing to be afraid of.'

Noelle saw a shadow move across the lawn, and for a

moment her heart leaped, imagining a Viet Cong. But it was just old Chi Hai, their amah, with a packet of Lucky Strike and an airline miniature of Johnny Walker for the spirit shrine under the simpoh tree.

Baptiste threw the newspaper on the floor and came to stand behind her. His fingers stroked her hair, and she felt his hot breath on the nape of her neck, and shivered, an involuntary ripple of pleasure. 'Don't,' she whispered.

How had life led her here? All she had ever wanted was romance and adventure; she had thrown her arms around the first handsome stranger who had fitted the role. But instead of a white charger, there was a red Packard, and instead of her white knight there was a man with a heart as black as the insides of a bear.

If she ran he would pursue her. If she stayed he would corrupt their son with his greed. Her life with him had become a chronicle of quiet desperation.

And then there was Dale. She had heard nothing more since the VC bomb in the Café Charles had nearly claimed his life. What did she expect? A letter perhaps, a phone call? Something to let her know he was all right. Instead it was as if he had never existed.

I have cried the last of my tears for that man. For any man.

Perhaps it was just as well. He had been corrupted too, as her husband had been. She remembered her last conversation with him. Yes, in many ways he was just like Baptiste, the reverse side of the same counterfeit coin.

'You are so beautiful,' he whispered.

He traced the contours of her back with his fingers and the nape of her neck with his lips. She tried to shrug him away but his fingers dug into the flesh of her shoulders and held her.

'I hate you,' she murmured.

'Not tonight. You can hate me tomorrow.'

'I hate you always.'

He was iron hard, pressing against her, between the swell of her buttocks. She was aware of the male smell of him, sandalwood aftershave, tobacco, the cognac he had enjoyed after dinner. He unfastened the ties of her dress and slipped the sleeves from her shoulders. She put up her hands to stop him but he grasped her wrists and drew them away, holding them tight to her sides. 'I love you, Noelle. You're the only woman I've ever wanted.'

She wanted to draw away from him, but she felt herself surrender. Her body was about to betray her again. He put his arm around her waist, holding her hands to her sides, and with his free hand slipped open the buttons of her dress down to her belly. Her nipples were tight brown buds.

She could not see his face, but knew he was smiling and could have torn at his eyes. 'You say no, but your body says yes.'

'Get away from me!' she hissed, and struggled with him, but he held her tight and his free hand cupped her breast, and gently rolled the nipple between his thumb and finger, and she heard herself moan. Her back arched, and she offered him her throat. She gasped as his teeth bruised the soft flesh.

His hands pulled the hem of her skirt to her waist and rolled the black tissue of her pants over her hips. They dropped to her feet. 'Not here,' she said, thinking of the servants, the hundred pairs of eyes that might be watching them from the darkness.

But he would not stop. His hands were under her arms, lifting her, she felt the heat of him between her legs and then he was inside her, so suddenly that she gasped aloud. They fell to their knees, their bodies locked in shadows and yellow light.

His fingers rubbed over her nipples in time with the hammering rhythm of their lovemaking. She felt the blood pounding in her veins, the din of the night insects rose in crescendo. It ended suddenly and unexpectedly, they both trembled together, their bodies shaken like puppets, and lay on the floor, breathless.

After a while she felt his weight lift off her back, and he withdrew. He got up and left the room, without a word.

She tried to stand up, but her knees were too weak. She leaned back against the jamb of the door, her knees drawn up to her chest. Her breath sawed in her chest and beads of sweat inched down her spine, her temples, and her throat. She felt the stickiness of his semen on her thighs.

She stared at the night, hating herself and hating him for the times like tonight when she was so lonely she would sleep with the devil rather than sleep alone.

347

78

Tiburon, San Francisco Bay

The mimosa was in heavy bloom, a tall cedar threw its shadow across the redwood deck. The air was spiced with sea-salt and the tang of charcoal and roasting meats from lunchtime barbecues on other decks and patios all around the bay.

Dale brought a bowl of salad out of the kitchen and put it on the table. He was dressed in fawn slacks, topsiders, and a pale blue open-necked shirt. Susan had wanted him to wear his Bermudas but he had declined. If he was going to play the weekend executive, he would at least do it with some dignity.

'You don't think it's going to be too hot out here?' she asked him.

Dale shrugged. Perhaps, perhaps not. In his experience San Francisco was the only place in the world where you could experience all four seasons in one day. 'They say it may snow later.'

Susan stared at him. 'Really?'

'No, I'm kidding.'

'We could set up the table inside.'

'No, hell, leave it here, it doesn't matter.'

She folded her arms and joined him at the rail. The yard dropped away under the deck, ending in a tangle of bramble and torn rock at the edge of the bay. A panorama of San Francisco was laid out in front of them, the Golden Gate and the mountains of Marin to the west, to the south the forests of Angel Island and the skyline of the city. The harbour was a riot of colour, yachts and catamarans weaving a tapestry of bright canvas and gleaming fibreglass hulls on the choppy bay.

348

I could have gone back, Dale reminded himself. The Company wanted me back. Gates had called long distance half a dozen times. But instead he had come home to Tiburon, to an Air Force pension and a salary package with benefits, and his father's law firm in the financial district.

Five days a week he put on a three-piece suit and took a commuter ferry to an office overlooking the Oakland Bay bridge, to advise harried men with sharp suits about corporate law. On weekends he sailed and played golf. He was no longer defending the American dream he had once deified; he was living it.

And he found it utterly empty.

He spent his days as a penitent, a decent man trying to do the decent thing. Jennifer came over every weekend, twenty-two now and in her final year. She had kept her part of the bargain, had moved back on campus, resumed tutorials and lectures, put her life back on the rails. She was majoring in political science, had worked as a volunteer for the Democratic party in the '68 elections. Dale's father had offered her a job at his law firm when she graduated, but she had told him, and Dale was there when she said it, that she was not interested in working for fascists.

He thought the old man was going to arrest.

She still wasn't sure what she would do. Perhaps get a job in welfare, or in the mayor's office. In that ambition he had understood her for the first time. He realised she was a lot like him. She wanted to change the world, only she was going to start a little closer to home.

His pocket liberal, he called her.

His life finally took on the outward appearance of normality, and he told himself his was the only moral choice. He stayed because of his promise to Jennifer, but he stayed also because something in him had died. He no longer believed.

'I wonder what this one's like?' Susan was saying.

'Sorry?'

'Jennifer's new boyfriend. I wonder what he's like?'

'Probably a 3-B like all the others,' Dale muttered. A 3-B. Their private code: beard, beads and a bandana.

'Don't forget. Be nice.'

'Hey, I'm always nice.' Lie. He felt as mean as a caged bear.

He looked down at his wife. The sun was in her face, and it high-lighted the small lines around her mouth and eyes. She looked for a moment childlike and fragile. 'I'm sorry,' he murmured.

'What for?'

'For every damned thing.' Regret wasn't the same as love, but he meant it just the same.

She put her arm through his and touched her forehead to his shoulder. He heard the tinny growl of Jennifer's Volkswagen bumping into the drive, the quick blast from the klaxon.

'Jennifer,' he said with relief, and pulled himself free.

Jennifer tottered in on black platform shoes with huge silver buckles. She wore bell-bottomed blue jeans, and a gauzy white blouse with frilled sleeves and collar. The material was so thin it was almost transparent, but Dale was relieved to see that she was at least wearing a bra. Out of deference to him, possibly.

The boyfriend's name was Scott, and he wasn't a 3-B. He wore a button down Oxford; it was hanging outside his jeans, okay, but he had ironed it. His hair straggled over the collar, but at least not past his shoulders, unlike the others. There were shoes on his feet – sand-shoes, anyway – and the jeans had been washed. Not recently, perhaps, but this year.

In fact he was an extraordinarily good-looking boy, with deep blue eyes and the face of a choirboy. Too baby-faced to grow a beard, he proclaimed his identity on the T-shirt he wore under the Oxford. Dale's first positive impressions were hastily revised as he read the message:

JOIN THE ARMY
TRAVEL TO STRANGE AND EXOTIC LANDS
MEET NEW AND INTERESTING PEOPLE
AND BLOW THE SHIT OUT OF THEM

Susan was watching him, her face a mask of apprehension. *'Guess who's coming to dinner,'* he mouthed at her.

Dale fetched drinks, and they sat on the deck and made small talk. Susan put Scott under the spotlight. In answer to her questions, Scott told them he was studying twentieth-century

American literature, and wanted to write novels one day. He might go into journalism when he graduated. He came from a small town in Arizona and had worked his own way through college. His father was a lineman.

Dale grudgingly conceded that Scott was handling his interrogation well. Perhaps we should put him under a little more pressure, he thought. Slide some slivers of bamboo under his fingernails.

Jennifer decided to rescue him. She suddenly turned to Dale and said: 'How's Michael?'

'In the Philippines, last I heard.'

'What's he doing there?'

'Snake School.'

'What's that?'

'Jungle survival training. Before he goes on to Vietnam.'

There was a sudden chill in the air.

'Conscripted?' Scott asked.

'He volunteered for the Air Force,' Jennifer said, in the same tone she might have used to admit that her brother was a serial killer.

'We're very proud of him,' Dale countered. 'He graduated from the Air Force Academy last year. He's been training as an FAC with the Air Commandos.'

'What's an FAC?' Scott asked.

'Forward Air Controller. They co-ordinate air support. He wanted to be a fighter pilot, but he didn't make it. FAC's the next best thing. So he tells me, anyway.' He didn't add, out of deference to Susan, that Michael would be flying slow, low-flying aircraft in open combat, and that the FACs had among the highest casualty rates in Viet Nam.

'My brother Mike's a hero,' Jennifer added tartly.

'I tried to talk him out of being a hero before he left,' Dale said. Yes, and I'll lie awake worrying about him for the next three hundred and sixty-four days. I was supposed to be here making up for the lost years. Instead I'm losing him to another war.

Scott turned casually to Dale. 'I understand you were in Vietnam.'

'That's right,' he said.

351

Scott gave him a small sympathetic smile as if he had just suffered a bereavement. Dale wanted to throw him out then but he kept his peace. 'Family tradition?' Scott said, giving Susan a winning smile.

'It's a masculine thing,' Jennifer said.

'What did you do over there?' Scott asked Dale.

'It was classified.'

'Oh, right.' A smirk at Susan.

Dale felt the old anger welling up again. Why do I have to apologise for my life?

'No regrets?' Scott asked.

Dale felt himself tense. 'What kind of regrets, son?'

'Look, I don't want to offend anyone here, I understand from Jennifer that you have a very military family, but I think I have to let you know right now that I am philosophically and intellectually opposed to what this country is doing in Viet Nam. I consider anyone who goes willingly to this war is morally, if not legally, guilty of war crimes.'

A long silence. Susan found something of particular interest out on the bay. A tacking duel perhaps. Jennifer just stared, like a spectator at a bullfight, waiting for Dale's reaction.

It wasn't what Scott had said, Dale decided later, it was his tone and his expression. The young man was too smug in his opinions, too assured of his own intellectual superiority. He has never faced a moral dilemma in his whole life, Dale decided, and thinks he understands the difference between right and wrong. It was suddenly overwhelmed by the desire to remove him from the moral high ground, by physical force if necessary.

'Well, now you've brought it out into the open, Scott, I must admit I do have one regret.'

'Oh?' He raised one eyebrow in an inquisitor's arch.

Dale leaned forward, lowering his voice in the manner of contrition. 'I don't think I should have tortured those women and children.'

Scott wasn't sure. Dale saw a moment's hesitation and was gratified by it.

'Daddy...' Jennifer's voice was low and menacing.

Dale threw up his hands. 'Okay, okay, so it was only one little girl. I shouldn't have brought it up. It's just the smell of all these barbecues, I guess.' He nudged Scott's arm. 'When the meat's cooked, I'll grab the pliers from the kitchen and show you this really neat trick.'

'Come and help me in the kitchen, please, Scott,' Susan said. She grabbed his arm and practically jolted him to his feet. She led him off the deck, leaving Dale alone with his daughter.

He took a long swallow of his whisky and soda. 'Seems like a nice young boy.'

'Jesus Christ!'

'I wouldn't go that far. He might, though.'

'You always manage to fucking embarrass me.'

'Please don't say "fuck", Jennifer. I'm a traditionalist, you know how it upsets me.'

'That was unforgivable.'

'Being rude to your host, you mean? No, not unforgivable. He's just young, that's all.'

'I meant you.'

'Oh, I was only kidding, you know that.'

'It isn't funny, talking about women and children being tortured. It's actually happening, for God's sake.'

'Well, sure, I know that. I've been there. But how do you know?'

'I can read.'

'So can most people. It doesn't mean they've learned to analyse.' Dale was astonished to find himself defending the war. How had she managed to do that? He didn't believe in it any more either. Sure it wasn't funny that women and children were being tortured. But you had to know Tran van Li to really understand how unfunny it was.

'I don't know how Mom stands you,' she said.

'I don't know either. But it was your idea.'

She gave him a pitying look.

'Is this what you really wanted?' he asked her. 'Or are you punishing me?'

'You want to leave us again and go back to your war?'

'Well, as it stands, I wouldn't be leaving you kids any more. You can't stand to be with me anyway, and me and Mike sort of crossed in the post. So it's really only Susan. Does she know you're fighting her battles for her?'

'Is that what you believe?'

'If you want the real truth, I don't know what I believe any more. You and Scott make me feel very old.'

'Maybe you are. That's why there's a revolution going on.'

'Well, I've seen plenty of revolutions. Real ones. But my daughter wasn't in any of them. I guess that's really what I care about.'

'Isn't it a bit late to start caring now?'

'Yes, it is. You're right. It is too late. But I'd give anything to be able to go back to when you were still young enough not to hate me.'

'Yeah, well, you can't,' she said.

God damn, but she can be mean, Dale decided. He was suddenly very tired of this. 'Look, Jen, I don't give a damn what you think about me. I'll reap what I've sown, same as every man. But I figure you're too old to be doing this. You're twenty-two. Time to get on with your own life and stop trying to change me, and stop wallowing in the past. You can't make me responsible for the rest of your life.'

'You don't know what it was like! I might as well have been an orphan!'

'I thought I was doing the right thing at the time.'

'No, you didn't. I don't think you even thought about it. You love your country, Dad, no doubt. You just don't like the people in it.'

Susan and Scott came back on to the deck and the conversation ended. Dale cooked the steaks and then Susan made increasingly desperate efforts to keep the conversation going while they ate them with coleslaw and potato salad. When they had finished Susan said she had bought pastries from the Sweden House but Jennifer said she could not fit in another thing – even though she had only pecked at the salad – and Scott claimed a backlog of study.

After they left Dale and Susan sat on the deck, staring at the debris of the meal, finishing the Stag's Leap cabernet he had bought for the occasion.

'Well, that seemed to go well,' Dale said.

Susan said nothing. She got up and went inside with an armful of plates. He heard her crying in the kitchen.

79

Dale lay in bed, fighting the pain in his leg. The old wound was his personal weathervane. It had healed well and left him with a limp that hardly anyone noticed, but when the weather turned cold it began to ache like a rotten tooth. It would be cold tomorrow. On cue, a sudden rush of wind rattled the window pane behind the curtains.

There was Talwin in his drawer, but he resisted all pain killers unless it got so bad that he started to sweat. In the hospital he had found himself becoming addicted to the morphine and it had frightened him. The fuzzy gelatin dreams of the opiates still induced in him something like nostalgia.

So he lay with his hands behind his back, apparently just staring at the ceiling, but concentrating on the pain, forcing it back.

Susan came out of the bathroom in a nightgown of blue silk. She had kept her figure over the years and he was aware that she was still attractive, while remaining personally unaffected by her. This feeling of detachment frightened him; he supposed it had to do with being in love with another woman.

Or did he just dream that? Even before he had left the hospital, it was as if Noelle had never happened. When he went back to Susan, he went back to his old life. It was like slipping into an old cardigan he had found at the bottom of a drawer. Their marriage took on an almost surreal quality, both of them avoiding the past, as if the last twenty years had been a bad dream. They had become two people without a history.

But the fragile truce held.

He still wondered why she had taken him back so readily. Perhaps it was to justify a lifetime of waiting; or perhaps she really loved him. Really loved him! It was an uncomfortable thought and it made him wince.

'What were you talking about with Jennifer?' Susan asked him as she got into bed.

'We weren't talking. We were sparring.'

'Well, you were being provocative. It's your own fault.'

'I never denied it, did I?'

'Still. That Scott ... son of a bitch deserved it.'

Dale smiled. Susan rarely swore. In her mouth the words sounded quaint rather than offensive.

She insinuated herself in the crook of his arm and toyed with the hairs of his chest. 'Was any of it true?'

'Any of what true?'

A stilted silence. 'Is there anything you regret?'

The question caught him by surprise. She never asked him anything about that other life. He knew that if he said 'No' that would be the end of it. Susan would be satisfied and the question would never be raised again.

So he said: 'Perhaps.'

'You do regret things.'

'Yeah.'

'You want to tell me?'

He turned to look at her. She was chewing on her bottom lip, the same expression he had seen once when she tried to light the barbecue with kerosene, wary, frightened, waiting for the explosion. There were many answers he could have given her. He chose what he thought was the soft option.

'Jennifer,' he said.

'She's the reason you wanted us back together.'

He looked away again. 'It was part of the reason.'

'Are you sorry?'

'Of course not.'

'You're not a very good liar.'

'Never claimed to be. I was a good soldier, a passable spook. Everything else, I get Cs.'

'Jenny's angry at you right now but she'll come round in time. She's young, she thinks she knows everything.'

'What if she's right, Susan? What if the last twenty years was all a mistake?'

356

'You did what you thought was right.'

'And what do you think?'

Her fingers went beneath the sheet, and she smiled. 'I think he still wants me, even if you aren't sure.'

That's the trouble with being a man, Dale thought. What's between your legs betrays you every time. There's never a chance of being noble, or loyal. Sex and love are always getting mixed up. Women never make that mistake.

So he wanted to make love to his wife. Why did he feel as if he was cheating?

He wished he loved Susan. She deserved his love, and his passion, but in the end, like tonight, all he could give her was his imitation of it.

80

Saigon, February 1970

Tet, the Chinese New Year, had come and gone. The sprigs of plum tree blossom that had decorated the house were losing their blooms. The riot of flowers that had appeared in the gardens and in the markets, the chrysanthemums, Buddha flowers, rooster combs, mandariniers and dahlias, had withered and died.

'It's too hot in Saigon at this time of the year,' Baptiste told Noelle. 'I've rented a villa in Vung Tau for a few days.'

She nodded her approval. The heat had been intense and she was sleeping badly. 'When do we leave?'

'I've told Khan to be ready to take you first thing tomorrow morning.'

'And you?'

'I have business to attend to here. You take Lucien. Khan will take care of you.'

Ah, he was planning something. She should have expected this. Nothing he did could ever be taken at face value. 'What are you going to do, Baptiste? Have you got a woman somewhere? Is that why you want me out of the way?'

'Don't be ridiculous. I am reformed.'

'Men like you don't reform, Baptiste. They just learn subtlety.'

He lit a cigarette and grinned at her. 'You think sending my wife and my son to Vung Tau, so I can entertain a mistress in my house is subtle?'

'For you.'

He liked that. 'I'm sorry, but this time I shall disappoint you.'

'Disappoint is not the word I would have chosen.'

'I will be good, I promise.'

'What are you up to?'

'As you insist on prying, I am inviting some associates here this weekend for a conference.'

'Which associates?'

'No one you know. They are from America.'

She shook her head. 'Crooks.'

'Not to put too fine a point on it, *chérie*, it is how some people characterise us.'

'You, Baptiste, not me.'

'It is guilt by association, I think.'

'What are you doing, Baptiste? What is it this time?'

He put his arms around her waist. 'It is very boring.'

She pushed him away. 'Don't patronise me!'

'It's just business. Do you really want to know, *chérie*? If you don't know, you can at least protest your innocence when the police come to knock down our door one night.'

'It's drugs, isn't it?'

He lowered his voice, conspirationally. 'The Vietnamese want me to smuggle fish sauce into the United States. They are going to put it in the hamburgers and break the will of the Americans.'

'Is it heroin?'

His smile fell away, and he fixed her with a cool stare. 'Don't try and get in my way, Noelle. I love you with my life, but you will not interfere with my business. Okay?'

'When will it ever be enough, Baptiste? How much do you need before it's enough?'

He seemed bewildered by the question, as if he had always thought she understood. 'I just like to play the game.'

'What game?'

'I don't know what it's called. But when you die, the one with the most money, wins.'

She thought it was another of his jokes, but he did not smile. He kissed her gently on the cheek. 'Enjoy Vung Tau,' he said and left the room, calling for Khan to get the car ready to take him into Saigon.

* * *

In the dining room of the Crocé villa there was a long table of polished Burmese teak. The men who gathered around it one evening three days later were not the kind of men Baptiste Crocé was accustomed to doing business with. They were not chiu chao triads or Yunnanese traders or Lao warlords; they were Italian Americans in very expensive suits. There were three of them: Santo – 'Sonny' – Trinca was from San Francisco, an unremarkable man, his skin so pale he looked like an insect that had spent its whole life under a rock. His suit appeared to be two sizes too large for him and he wore the pained expression of a man who has just stepped in a puddle of vomit. He was at work on his gums with a toothpick.

By contrast his son Aldo was big-boned, with the easy assurance of someone who has had everything they ever wanted. He looked around the room with a bullying smile that seemed to pity everyone who was not lucky enough to be born a Trinca.

On the other side of the table was Giovanni Bonetti from Miami, known as Johnnie Knee from a time in his troubled youth when he had nailed a man's legs to a wooden pier. Bonetti was a big man who had gone to fat, although the impeccably tailored pearl grey Dior suit was designed to camouflage the extra pounds. Strands of black hair were pushed across a speckled brown pate like guitar strings. There was a Rolex Oyster Perpetual on his wrist and thick gold rings on his fingers. He had the gravelly voice of a parade ground sergeant and the forced bonhomie of a restaurateur.

The other guests were Jean-Luc Vellard, a *paceri* from Marseille, and his godson, Rivelini.

Other men stood around the tables or sat on the verandahs flicking through newspapers and magazines; either paid-up muscle or brain, decided Baptiste. It was not hard to distinguish one from the other.

The bells of the Basilica called the faithful to six o'clock prayers. It was that time of the day when the city's energy was at its lowest ebb, wilted from the heat and dust and pollution of the day, before the frenetic sexual hum of the night.

Baptiste presented his terms and conditions, including price per kilo and transportation costs. When he had finished there was a long silence.

360

Bonetti was the first to speak. He cradled his drink – the finest VSOP cognac, and he had adulterated it with ice and soda water, Baptiste noted – in one huge paw, while his *consigliere* reached over his chair and lit his Havana. Sweat poured in little rivers down his face. 'You can guarantee us supply?' he said.

'Within two months of your order,' Crocé answered.

'Price?'

'Twenty-five a kilo. Half on order, half on delivery.'

Bonetti grunted, poker-faced.

Now it was Trinca's turn. He tapped the table with a gnarled forefinger. 'What about this trouble with the communists?'

'The war in Laos works for us and against us. The American bombing, and communist gains, have driven many of the Meo – the tribespeople who grow the opium – out of the growing areas. But the villages that remain have lost most of their men to Vang Pao's mercenary army. Growing opium has always been women's work, so now it is the only crop that many villages can grow. And whatever happens, if there's opium we will find a way to get it out. Besides, it is the only export they have.'

Bonetti interrupted. 'Opium is one thing. Heroin is something else. I don't want no shit. It's like the dope those Mexicans have been trying to bring in. A lot of my customers won't take that crap.'

'This is top quality product, Mr Bonetti. We have tested in the market here in Saigon. On Americans.'

Trinca had extracted a piece of the chicken he had eaten for lunch from a molar and studied it carefully before swallowing it, and getting back to work. There was a gurgling sound and he suddenly leaned forward and winced in pain. 'Jesus Christ, my guts are on fire. I hate this fucking country.'

'Asia has a way of punishing sensitive stomachs,' Rivelini said.

Trinca was not sure if Rivelini was mocking him. He gave him the benefit of the doubt. 'All I done since I been here is shit and sweat. I don't know how people live in this dump.' Another cramp squeezed his bowels and he groaned again. 'I can't wait to get out of this fucking place.'

'Is there anything I can get you, Monsieur Trinca?' Baptiste asked him.

'I'm okay,' Trinca said, and relaxed as the cramp left him. Sweat ran down his cheeks. 'We were talking about product. You say you can arrange transportation?'

Vellard spoke for the first time. He was a tall, stooped man with fine grey hair, a slide rule parting and a distinguished appearance. In the street Baptiste might have mistaken him for the curator of an art gallery. 'If I may?'

Baptiste nodded.

'As you know, until now we have brought the black to Marseille, refined it there, and then used couriers and freighters to deliver it to the United States. Now we will be able to bring refined heroin into Panama via the Philippines. Panama's narcotics regulations are liberal, and many of the customs and police are already in our pocket.'

'How come?' asked Aldo. His father gave him a look of patient forbearance.

Vellard assumed the expression of a teacher having to remind a teenager of his alphabet. 'After the war certain of our country-men were accused of collaborating with the Nazis. Some of them found it convenient to take early retirement in Latin America.' Vellard again addressed the rest of the table. 'From Panama our people will arrange delivery to any city of the United States.'

'What protection you got?' Bonetti wanted to know.

'The Vietnamese government guarantees security,' Baptiste answered. 'They must. They cannot survive without their share of these incomes.'

'But you're handling this?' Sonny Trinca asked him. 'I don't do business with no gooks or chinks.'

Baptiste had spent so long in Asia he sometimes forgot the prejudices of the other side of the world. '*Bien sûr*. You will be buying direct from us.'

'Sounds good to me. Let's get down to details. I want to fly back to the States in the morning.' He flicked the toothpick on to the floor, and stood up quickly. 'Jesus, I got to take another dump.'

And he fled the room.

81

A few days after she returned from Vung Tau, Noelle took a 'phone call at home from her father's former accountant, Paul Delavane. The conversation was a short one. They arranged to meet the next day at ten o'clock in the Continental.

The last days of Rome, Noelle thought sourly as they drove through the morning traffic on the Tu Do. The city of wide boulevards and bicycles of her memory was gone. The tamarind trees were dying from the pollution, the cafés were being replaced by girlie bars with names like Nevada and New York and Arizona.

She saw a child, no more than eight years old, selling packets of *ma thuy*, heroin, to a group of American soldiers. Nearby a black soldier sat in a doorway under a neon palm tree, crying and shivering in spite of the heat.

Suddenly in these last few months heroin was everywhere, on the streets of Saigon, not hidden away in the *fumeurs* of Cholon. Schoolgirls sold it from roadside stands on the road to Long Binh, or stuffed vials in the pockets of Marines as they walked down the street. She had begun to wonder how much of this new trend was the work of her husband.

The 'Ode to Billy Joe' was playing from speakers mounted on the corner columns of the Continental terrace. An old man in khaki shorts and a pith helmet was leaning over the stone fence, trying to sell a wooden flute to an Australian journalist.

Delavane was sitting at a table near the street. He was a large man, with a grey waxed moustache and a bushy beard, a few sparse strands of hair plastered across his head. A jade-handled cane rested against the arm of his chair.

He rose to greet her, and kissed her hand with elaborate charm.

Delavane was an old friend of her father's, and had handled all of his business affairs for thirty years. Like Bonaventure, he was a member of the *Union Corse*.

'You look enchanting,' he told her.

'Thank you, Paul,' Noelle answered. Delavane liked to think himself a rogue and a womaniser. She thought he was insufferable but felt it imprudent to tell him so, especially as she was here to ask a favour.

He signalled the waiter to bring two *cafés au lait*.

'Baptiste knows nothing of our meeting?' she asked him.

Delavane toyed with his moustaches. 'Of course not. At least, not from me. But I am curious. Why the secrecy?'

'I think you can guess.'

'You are going to leave him?'

'Not exactly. I just wish to go my own way financially.'

He nodded his understanding. 'Well, that should not be too difficult.'

'Not for you perhaps. That is why I asked you to meet me.'

Delavane took a pair of half moon spectacles from his breast pocket and placed them on his nose. Then he took out a small black leather notebook, licked his index finger with a flourish, and flicked through the pages until he found what he was looking for. He glanced at her over the rim of his spectacles. 'I jotted down a few figures to jog my memory.' He returned his attention to the notebook. 'Your father left you a handsome estate. Nine hundred and eight-seven thousand francs, at my latest estimate, in cash, bonds and gold bullion, held in the Banque de l'Indochine in Bangkok, the Hong Kong and Shanghai Bank in Hong Kong, and the Banque Nationale de Paris in Marseille. You also possess the deeds to the villa here in Saigon.' He looked up again. 'As a citizen of France, you are also entitled to a share of your husband's assets.'

'I have no idea what my husband now earns, or what he owns. All he inherited from my father was three aeroplanes, which he promptly sold a year after his death when Rattakone closed down his opium business.'

'Well, legally, it would be rather difficult to recover anything, anyway. He is now beyond the reach of a French court.'

364

'I want nothing from my husband. It's Lucien I am worried about. His future. That is why I want you to set up a trust fund for him and administer it for me.'

'I would be delighted.'

'Half a million francs. I want it invested beyond my husband's reach. Until Luc is twenty-one.'

'How soon?'

'Can you do it before you leave Saigon this time?'

'For you, Noelle, of course.' He put his hand on hers and it stayed there. His lips spread into an unctuous smile.

For God's sake, Noelle thought. He actually thinks he might get me on the rebound.

She removed her hand. 'Thank you so much, Paul.'

They made desultory conversation, she finished her coffee and left. She should have done this a long time ago, she realised. It was the only way. Baptiste had made her life a hell. He was not going to destroy her son as well.

That night after dinner she discussed with Baptiste what she had seen that day in Saigon.

'There were soldiers using heroin in the street.'

He sat in a Louis Quinze armchair, a brandy balloon of Martell on the console table beside him. 'Americans.'

'It frightens me, Baptiste.'

He looked up from his newspaper. 'Why should it frighten you?'

'Before there was opium, then this *ma thuy* they smoke. But now you can see them injecting. I saw one of them right there on the Tu Do, doing *that*. It's evil.'

Baptiste sounded bored. 'It's what the Americans want. The Chinese like to smoke, the Americans like to stick needles in themselves.'

'Is this you, Baptiste?'

'What?'

'Is this you? Is this your business now?'

He took a moment to answer, and she knew he was considering his reply. 'No. If you must know, it's the Chinese.'

'Would you tell me if it was you?'

'Of course not.'

'Thank you,' she said. 'You are nothing if not candid.'

He threw his newspaper on the floor and stood up, angry now. 'Let me tell you something. Before you criticise me, remember this: every big fortune ever made has been amassed on other people's misery. Opium, for instance. When the British forced their way into China, opium was almost half of their colonial revenue. Half! The canals and the railways and the great stone buildings they built during their Queen Victoria's reign, almost half of them built with dope. Think of it! And *la belle France*. By World War Two opium was a quarter of all our revenue from Indochina. We imported it from India and sold it to the Chinese to sell to the Vietnamese! This is nothing new, these drugs you see on the street, they are not some great new evil. This is just business. That's all. Business.'

'Thank you for the history lesson.'

'Perhaps your papa should have given you a proper education in real life.'

'He left that to you.'

'A thankless task, *chérie*.'

'Tell me, Baptiste, is this what you want for Lucien? You want him to peddle drugs and build a great new empire for himself?'

'Lucien is my son. When he is old enough I will let him make up his own mind what he will do with his life.'

'Will you, Baptiste? Will you?'

She walked out.

When she reached the sanctuary of her bedroom, she locked the door and threw herself on the bed. Oh, Papa, what a life you dragged me into! You made me pay a big price for my one million francs.

The next day she was not there to pick Lucien up from school. He had noticed her absences more and more frequently.

Your maman is tired.

Your maman has a migraine.

Your maman is feeling the heat.

Khan held open the door of the Mercedes and he climbed into the back. They drove home in silence.

The villa was dark and quiet. Chi Hai told him that his

maman indeed had another headache and had gone up to her bedroom to sleep. He was to go into the garden and play.

Khan and Chi Hai withdrew to the servants' quarters. When there were out of sight Lucien climbed the simpoh tree in the back garden, up to one of the tallest branches. The shutters to his mother's bedroom were partly open and he saw her moving inside the darkened room. She wore just a white silk slip.

As he watched she took out the little camphor box that contained her opium pipe and the little gauze packet of opium, and lit the spirit lamp on the table beside the bed. Then she lay down, disappearing from view, but occasionally he could see the little puffs of opium smoke drift upwards towards the window.

She thought he didn't know. She thought it was just her secret. She thought her headaches and her mysterious women's problems and illusive sicknesses that she complained of hid from him what she was really doing.

But Lucien knew.

He knew what she was doing was a very bad thing and he also knew that somehow it was all his father's fault.

82

They were in a little air-conditioned restaurant across the street from the Continental and the old opera house which now served as the Vietnamese lower house. It was called the Givral and was a favourite of Baptiste's; they baked their own croissants fresh every morning, and he often came here for a late breakfast and *café au lait*. It was where he had told Delavane to meet him.

'You had a meeting with my wife two days ago,' he said.

'It was a confidential discussion.'

'She's trying to hide her money from me.'

'She is making adequate provisions for the future.'

'What kind of provisions?'

'Baptiste, please, you know I cannot tell you that.'

Baptiste smiled. He was an imposing man, thought Delavane. The eyepatch could appear either menacing or debonair, depending on his mood. He still had a mane of thick blue-black hair at an age when many men found theirs thinning or turning grey. He exuded a scent of sandalwood and tobacco, but never seemed to sweat, never appeared uncomfortable even at this time of year. It was unnatural.

Now he fixed Delavane with a powder white smile full of humour and bonhomie. 'I'll strangle you, you little shit,' he said.

'Baptiste?'

'Monsieur, to you. No, I can do better than strangle you. One of my friends is Colonel Tran van Li. I believe it would not be too difficult to persuade him to hold you on suspicion of communist sympathies. You don't want that to happen, believe me. His favourite trick is to hold a Zippo lighter under a man's testicles. He uses one lighter in particular. It has an American flag on it, with the WHAMO symbol. Winning Hearts and Minds. It's his idea of a joke.'

Delavane broke into a sweat. 'You wouldn't dare!'

'Don't gamble on what I would or wouldn't dare to do. You have no idea. This is Saigon, and there's a war on. You've lived in Asia all your life, like me. You know anything is possible.'

Delavane started to get up. Baptiste clamped a hand on his wrist and stopped him. 'I'm not a nice man. Never was. I admit I was once just an easygoing fellow, but that was a long time ago. I'm in this business too deep. I'd cut out your liver and eat it if I had to.'

'If Rivelini hears about this...'

'Your friend Marcel won't give a shit. He wouldn't lift a finger against Colonel Li, he'd rather gouge his own eyes out. There are people in Marseille who need Colonel Li more than they need Marcel Rivelini now.'

Delavane found he was trembling violently. Now he could not stand up if he had wanted to. 'What do you want?'

'In my pocket I have two million piasters. A lot of money to carry around at one time. Perhaps I should give it to you for safekeeping.'

'In return for what?'

'First tell me what Noelle wants from you. Then I'll tell you.'

'Rocco trusted me!'

'Rocco's dead.'

'I promised him I would take care of Noelle's affairs.'

'That was very honourable. Why don't you tell that to Colonel Li when he's lighting his cigarette off your blazing genitals. You've gone pale. Do you want another drink?'

'I won't let you take all her money!'

'I don't want her money. I don't need it. I just need to maintain some control over my family's life, which is only right and proper for a man in my position. Don't you agree?' He reached into his pocket and took out an envelope. 'Inside here is a banker's cheque drawn on the Banque de l'Indochine payable to the account of Monsieur Paul Delavane. Two million piasters is a lot of money. Here, take it.' When

Delavane did not move, Baptiste tucked it into the accountant's breast pocket. 'Now then, tell me what Noelle wanted and then we'll discuss some compromise that will accommodate your conscience and my needs. You don't look like the sort of man who could endure a long conversation with Colonel Li.'

The next day, when Khan came to pick him up from school, Lucien saw his father in the back of the Mercedes. At first he thought something must have happened to his mother, and felt the cold settling of fear in his stomach. He got into the car and waited for the blow to fall.

Instead Baptiste smiled down at him and asked him if he had had a good day at school.

As they drove, Lucien sat rigid. Khan did not drive home the usual way. They headed out of the city, away from the wide boulevards and grand stone buildings into the Oriental quarter. Vertical signs in Chinese script crowded up the walls of the shophouses, and occasionally he caught glimpses of the port, the greasy waters of the Arroyo Chinois, wooden houses suspended on stilts over glistening black mud. This was Cholon, he knew, a part of the city he had never been before. He was filled with excitement and dread.

'Where are we going?' he asked.

'There's something I want to show you, Lucien. Something you have to understand.'

Khan turned off the main thoroughfare, leaving the tangle of taxis and siclos and motor cycles behind. They were in a quiet street of shophouses and arcades. It was past noon and it was deserted. Lucien saw oil drums filled with rubbish, piles of fruit peelings and human excrement, a dog nosing at a pile of ordure.

Khan stopped the car outside an ancient house with a dilapidated wooden balcony and a door with cracked green paint. The door opened on to a dark flight of stairs. A Chinese youth sat outside on an orange box, in a pair of voluminous blue shorts and a dirty white singlet.

Baptiste took Lucien's hand and got out of the car. The youth jumped to his feet and bowed his head in their direction.

Baptiste ignored him, and led Lucien inside.

At the top of the stairs was a locked and barred iron door. Baptiste rapped impatiently. A shutter opened and after a moment Lucien heard the sound of bolts being drawn back. They went inside.

Because of the darkness it was the stench that struck him first; the sweet treacle-smell of the opium mixed with the overlaying taint of unwashed bodies. As his eyes grew accustomed to the gloom he realised the room was full of living skeletons, stacked on narrow wooden benches, some asleep, others awake but with eyes that were glassy and unfocused. It was utterly silent, except for the occasional gurgling sound of an addict drawing on his pipe.

'Have you ever seen *un fumeur* before?' Crocé asked him.

I have seen *Maman*, thought Lucien. But that was never like this. And besides, I cannot tell you about that. It is our secret.

He shook his head.

'These people drink smoke,' whispered Baptiste. 'They need it, like you and I need air. If they go a day without it, they get sick. You see, Lucien, some people are strong, and some people are weak. That is the way the world is divided. Not into countries, like they teach you in school, but into the weak and the strong. There are the ones who need smoke, and the ones who give it. If you need something you are weak, and you will be weak for ever. But if you are a giver, you are strong, and you can have anything you want. Anything. Do you understand?'

Lucien nodded. He thought about his mother. He had never before thought of her as weak.

'Never forget you are one of the strong ones,' his father went on. 'That is your heritage. Everything else they teach you, about God, about society, about laws, none of that matters. You live and you die, that's all you need to know about God. And if you are strong it doesn't matter about society, or about laws. You can make your own rules, and everyone will love you for it. Do you understand?'

Lucien nodded. But he did not understand. He only knew these people had on their faces the look of suffering, the same

371

look he saw on his mother. They were trapped, as she was, and his father was somehow glad of it. He did not think he could ever be like his father; he was his mother's son. But he feared that he would never be free of his father's pernicious influence, not until the day he died.

83

They ate their dinner at the great carved teak table where Santo Trinca and Giovanni Bonetti had sat a week before. Chi Hai had prepared grilled fish with coriander, followed by coconut ice cream. They ate in silence. Afterwards their *boyesse* cleared away the plates, and brought a bottle of Martell reserve to the table. Baptiste poured two fingers into a cut crystal balloon and lit a Russian cheroot, a recent affectation.

'I spoke to Delavane today,' Noelle said.

'Did you?'

'Is that all you have to say?' Her eyes glittered in the dull yellow light of the wall sconces.

'Yes.' He drew on his cheroot, watched the smoke spiral towards the ceiling. The cicadas beat in rhythm in the gardens. What did she suspect? Surely Delavane had not hinted anything of their conversation to her?

'He said you tried to persuade him to give you power of attorney over my affairs.'

The little bastard. He had more balls than Baptiste had given him credit for. He would have to call Colonel Li tonight and have him teach the little shit a lesson.

'How did you intend to arrange that?' she asked him.

No further need to be coy. 'I thought a man of Monsieur Delavane's experience must be able to find a way to set the papers in front of you among a mass of others. I did not think you took much interest in documents.'

'And so you wanted to defraud me of my inheritance.'

'I merely wanted to protect you and Lucien from your recklessness.'

'You are a thief and a liar.'

373

He sipped his brandy. He loved her best when she was like this. She had been too pliant of late. He preferred it when she had the fire in her belly. It fed his own appetites.

Noelle traced the rim of her own glass with one long pearly fingernail. 'What did you discuss last week with your visitors?'

'Just business, I told you.'

'You murder your best friend, you try to steal from your wife and son, you keep whores, you deal in death and misery. Is there anything else I should know about you?'

He grinned. 'It doesn't seem much, I admit. I am sure you must be overlooking something.'

Noelle looked down at her hands, at the band of gold on the third finger of her left hand. She slid it off and tossed it down the table. 'We're done, Baptiste.'

'I told you before, Noelle. We are not finished until I say it's finished.'

'And how will you keep me?'

He laughed, genuinely amused at this little tantrum. 'You know you can't get away from me.'

She stood up and walked slowly towards him, snake-hipped, a seductive smile on her lips. She picked up the bottle of cognac that stood at his elbow and poured the contents over his head.

He gasped and jumped to his feet, furious. 'You little bitch!' he shouted, and then his jaw fell open and he stared at her in utter horror. She had grabbed his gold Bronzini lighter from the table and now held the flame inches from his face.

'It would be so easy,' she said.

'Noelle!'

'You would burn like a crêpe, with a blue flame. I should like to watch your head burn, Baptiste. See it fry.'

'Don't.' He started to back away, and he looked for the door. She jerked the flame closer.

'Noelle!'

'One more move and I'll torch you, I swear it!'

Now she stood between him and the door. He thought of making a grab for the lighter but the flame was too close. He might knock her arm towards him.

Her face was a demon's, and she no longer looked beautiful. Her lips were twisted into a snarl of disgust.

'Put it down!' he begged her.

'I always tried to tell you smoking was bad for your health.'

'For the love of God!'

'God? God doesn't love you, Baptiste. In fact I am sure he has a special corner of hell reserved for you. But if I touch you with this flame, do you think he will still be able to recognise you at the gates?'

'Please!' He was horrified to hear his own voice was as shrill as a girl's.

'In a few seconds you would burn like pork. Do you remember the monks who used to pour petrol over themselves to protest against Diem? Their skin turned black. But then some women like black men, Baptiste. What do you think?'

He kept his eyes fixed on the small blue flame. He took a deep breath and blew. The flame extinguished and he snatched for the lighter. But Noelle was too quick for him. She snatched her hand away, relit it, and pushed it back in his face. He cried out and took a step back, falling over his chair and landing on his back on the floor. She crouched over him.

'Next time you burn, I swear it!'

'Putain! Tu es fou!'

The brandy had run down his forehead and into his eyes, blinding him. He could smell the reek of it in his hair, on his shirt. He was hypnotised by the tiny blue flame as it danced in front of his eyes.

And then it was extinguished and Noelle took a step back.

He felt the breath go out of him. He did not try to stand, his legs were trembling too violently for that.

'I want you to understand,' she was saying, 'that I cannot tolerate living with you any more. I think for a long time a part of me still went on loving you, and that made me weak. But now I am leaving, and I am taking Lucien. You can stop me this time, if you want. But if you do, I will kill you. Or you can kill me first. That is your choice. But just accept that if you try and get in my way, one of us is going to die. I don't care which one.'

She left the room.

Nom de Dieu de bordel de merde.

She means it, thought Baptiste. She really hates me this much. Despite everything I have done for her, she hates me to her bones. I really think she would kill me. One morning I'll wake up with my throat cut. The realisation left him numb.

And yet, I could never harm her, not even to keep Lucien.

Women. After everything I have done for her. This time I really will have to let her go.

84

Northern Laos, January 1970

The hills were ablaze with red and white poppies, brilliant against the sombre purple backdrop of the mountains. Already the petals were dropping, and every evening, as the day began to cool, Li May went into the field with her family to help with the harvest.

She worked diligently, using a special three-bladed knife to scour the green seed pod, the thick white sap oozing out of the cuts. The white sap would congeal in the cold night air, turning the colour of molasses, and they would all rise at first light to scrape off the new opium before it spoiled in the sun.

The mist around the mountains was tinted with the violet of twilight when Li May, her mother, and her three elder sisters headed back to the village. The smoke of cooking fires hung above the trees and thatched roofs, and the village dogs began their barking.

Li May ran ahead, laughing. When she reached the outskirts of the village she heard a familiar thunder, saw a silver jet plane roar down the valley towards them. Like all the villagers she was accustomed to the planes; the scream of the sleek fighter bombers that patrolled the mountains and the rotor hum of the helicopters that brought them their rice each week were as familiar as the grunts of the pigs under their house, or the squawking of the chickens. Even when the jet began its strafing run, Li May did not realise the danger.

Neither did her family.

The hammer of the T-28's machine guns shocked her into stillness. The red earth exploded into the air, passed her

377

in a stinging cloud, cracked down the mountain towards her mother and sisters. Li May opened her mouth to shout a warning but it was already too late. She watched them fall, saw the silver bird continue down the valley, the dipping sun glinting on its wings.

And then it was gone, out of sight beyond the curve of the valley. The roar of its engines faded to a distant hum.

Li May did not cry, or run; she barely understood what had happened. Her mother and sisters lay in the middle of the path, like a pile of bloody rags. Her mother convulsed, a bloody foam on her lips, and lay still. Her sister's insides had spilled in the dirt, and she knelt down and tried to scoop them up for her and put them back. Someone dragged her away. She looked up at the shocked and frightened faces of the villagers.

It was silent now. Even the dogs had stopped barking.

85

Two months later

'Cleared in hot. Hit my smoke.'

A Thunderchief rolled out of the clouds towards the white plume of phosphorous, firing its cannons. The answering roar of the North Vietnamese 37-millimetre guns was deafening.

'We go home now!' Smiley shouted from the back seat of the Bird Dog.

Then Michael heard another sound, almost inaudible beneath the barrage of the guns; the pap-pap-pap of 12.7-millimetre machine guns. He saw the green tracers arc across the sky towards him. A shell smashed a hole between the accessory case and the engine block.

'We gunna die!' Smiley wailed from the back seat.

Michael called up Cricket, the daytime airborne command post. 'This is Raven six-three. I've taken a hit on Route 4, east of Xieng Khouang. I'm heading for Alternate but I don't think I'm going to make it. The engine doesn't sound good. Try and get a fix on me.'

Burning oil left a tail of black smoke. More oil spewed over the windscreen and flames licked out of the casing. They were losing altitude.

'Cricket, this is Raven six-three. I have a fire, I'm shutting the engine down now. Hope you have a tracking beam on me – looks like I'm going in.'

He fired off the rest of his Willy Pete rockets to buy a little more height, and tried to maintain an easy spiral as he searched for somewhere to land.

'We gunna die!' Smiley moaned.

Maybe, Michael thought, surprised at how calm he felt.

With the engine shut down they were alone with the eerie silence, the sound of the air battle left behind. Razor-back ridges jutted through the clouds, the green shadows of the mountains loomed around them as they fell deeper into the valley. There were scars on the mountain slopes, some hill tribe family's opium patch.

Nowhere to land. The mountains would just swallow them up.

Smiley began to sob a prayer to his ancestors.

There!

Through a swirling bank of gauze Michael saw the *paddi*, emerald green in the fold of the valley, almost on the edge of the plain. He rolled out of the spiral, just a thousand feet AGL, and glided towards it.

The *paddi* was dissected by mud dikes about every two hundred yards. He knew he would have to clear the first dike as low as he could; but on the last fifty feet of the approach he realised he wasn't going to make it. Fighting the nose against a stall he felt the undercarriage slam into the dike and the Cessna bucked like a frightened horse and the tail sheared off. The plane skidded across the *paddi* on its belly.

The Cessna bounced and lurched. The world went black as oil gushed across the windshield. A jarring impact and all the breath went out of his body.

Silence.

For almost a minute, he did not move, shocked not only by the physical buffeting his body had taken but by the miracle of simply being alive.

It was Smiley who shook him from the torpor. He felt arms go around his neck and a wet kiss on his cheek. 'You numbah one!' Smiley shouted.

Michael fumbled with his shoulder harness and scrambled out of the cockpit, cursing himself for the wasted time. During their descent they had been spewing black smoke, an easy trail to follow from the ground. They had to get clear of the Bird Dog and out of the open.

'Smiley, hurry!'

'You numbah one, Mai Koo! We not die more! You numbah one!'

'Hurry!'

They opened fire from the tree line, four hundred metres to their left. Michael recognised the uniforms of North Vietnamese regulars. He hauled Smiley out of the cockpit and tried to drag him away from the wreck, but he was too shocked to move.

'Haul ass, Smiley!'

Smiley stared at the soldiers running towards them from the treeline. The smile fell away. 'We gunna die,' he said.

He was only a small man. Michael grabbed him and threw him easily over his shoulder in a fireman's lift and started to run.

Michael took stock. The map, the revolver, the survival kit, the radio, the food and the water were still in the Bird Dog. They were surrounded by enemy troops, and the Air Force Jolly Green Giants would not land without having first secured proper radio contact. And pretty soon it would be dark.

But it isn't all bad news, he thought. I still have my Swiss Army Knife in my belt.

He started to laugh, silently, on and on until his ribs ached. Hysteria, he thought, and it was as if he was watching himself from a distance. Smiley was staring at him as if he had gone insane. Which, in a way, he had.

'Why you funny, Mai Koo? We fucked,' Smiley whispered.

A Skyraider roared down the valley, banked over the wreckage of the Cessna. Michael heard the North Vietnamese open fire from the ground, the Skyraider pilot looked for altitude, then made the wrong guess and continued his patrol on the other side of the valley.

'It's going to be one of those days,' Michael whispered to Smiley.

They had run blind into the jungle for several minutes, away from their pursuers. They were now on a forested ridge overlooking the *paddi* field. He could hear the Vietnamese calling to each other as they searched the undergrowth. Michael was aware of a ripe odour very close. Smiley had soiled himself.

'This way,' he whispered. He led the way up the ridge,

through stands of elephant grass and bamboo ten metres high. The grasses sliced their skin like razors, but Michael would not slow the pace. Already a twilight gloom was falling over the jungle.

When they reached the crest of the ridge, he slashed down a long pole of bamboo with his knife and pulled off his olive green fatigue trousers. Smiley's eyes widened in shock. The *falang* had definitely gone crazy.

Michael peeled off the red silk boxer shorts he wore underneath his flying trousers. 'Christmas present from an old girlfriend,' he said to Smiley. 'We'll make a signal flag.'

'Never happen,' he said.

'The Skyraider will see us.'

'Never happen.'

'I'll get you out of this.'

'Never happen.'

'I promise.'

'We gunna die.'

He put his trousers back on – if the bad guys got him, he sure as hell didn't mean to die bare-assed – and hoisted the makeshift flag above his head. The Skyraider was still droning up and down the valley. He just hoped the Vietnamese were not watching from the *paddi*.

The bamboo pole was heavy and Michael and Smiley took turns with it, resting their aching arms between shifts with the flag. Smiley soon gave up. 'Never happen, Mai Koo. We die. We go to ancestor. We see Buddha. We come back, another life, try again.'

Michael heard the Skyraider turn and head for home. His arm and shoulder muscles started to cramp, but he kept waving. Twice the Vietnamese fired their assault rifles at shadows in the undergrowth. They were getting closer.

Almost sunset. Do we keep running?

Then he heard it, the unmistakeable *whump-whump-whump* of a helicopter. Smiley, sitting with his head in his hands, looked up, eyes wide with excitement.

It was getting closer.

'They're coming right at us. They've seen us.'

Smiley jumped to his feet, yelling and waving his arms.

'Shut up!' Michael hissed. He heard the Vietnamese shout a warning, then they were crashing towards them through the long grass.

It came at them suddenly, flattening the elephant grass with the pressure of the rotors, an Air America Huey. It whirled and descended, hovering a few feet away from the ground.

Michael pushed Smiley towards it, then grabbed him by the seat of the pants and shoved him in through the door. A Hmong loader dragged them in, and they collapsed on to the cabin floor. Smiley threw his arms around Michael's neck. 'You not numbah one, Mai Koo, you Buddha!'

The crew chief turned around and grinned at him. 'Nice underwear, son,' he said, and they took off. Michael heard the staccato chatter of automatic weapons fire.

The other loader, an American, leaned over him. 'You peed your pants, son,' he said. Michael looked down. He had too.

The chopper pilot's name was Neil Esterhazy; he had CRAZY ESTERHAZY stencilled on his helmet. He was out of Vientiane. His T-shirt said: 'Fly the Friendly Skies of Laos', and had a stencil of a T-28 diving with all guns blazing.

'You're a lucky son of a bitch,' he said. 'I was making a delivery for the customer on the J when I heard you call in. Damned if I would have seen you if it wasn't for those crazy shorts.'

'Thought I'd be spending the night in the jungle,' Michael said, feigning bravado.

'Don't want to do that, man. Facilities are fucken terrible.'

Michael patted the canvas sacks he was leaning against. It wasn't rice. One of the bags was split and a pungent black jelly-like substance was oozing out. 'What's this shit?'

Esterhazy gave him a pitying look. 'Not been in Laos long, have you, son?'

'A few weeks. What the hell is it?'

Esterhazy grinned and shook his head. 'Believe me, son, you don't want to know.'

383

86

Michael went back to the hootch. There were two AA pilots sitting in a corner of the bar, and they nodded as he walked in. 'How was your day, Raven?'

'Got a little tense,' Michael heard himself say. He went to the bar and poured himself a large White Horse. He felt ice calm now, and the twilight colours were vivid as neon. Dusk was rush hour at Long Tieng, as the Cessna 0-1 'Bird Dogs', the Air America Hueys and Sikorskis, and Royal Lao T-28 fighter bombers, all scrambled to land before nightfall. Down on the ramp hard-faced Americans in jungle fatigues led exhausted Hmong troops out of the helicopters; and Royal Lao pilots paralysed with cramps were lifted from their cockpits by groundcrews.

There was a sense of unreality to it all. Instead of lying dead in the cockpit of his plane, or on the jungle floor, his body bloody and riddled with bullets, he was in the hootch drinking whisky. Tonight he would probably get a little drunk with his fellow Ravens, and the story would gain in the re-telling. And, at the same time, it would diminish.

There would be laughter and backslaps and it would be forgotten. Tomorrow he would get up and climb in another Bird Dog and do it all over again.

He felt someone watching him. He turned around. It was a little girl, a Hmong. Some people called them Meo, the derisory name the Chinese gave them. But Smiley had told him it was like calling a black American a 'nigger' so Michael avoided it. They were hill people, numerous in the mountains of the

384

Golden Triangle, and the war that was raging in the north of Laos was decimating them.

They were a handsome people, and this little girl was no exception. She was no more than eight or nine years old, and she squatted on the floor, staring at him, her hands folded gracefully in her lap like gloves. She had huge dark eyes and an expression as solemn as a priest's.

'Hello,' he said.

'She don't talk,' one of the chopper pilots said, without looking up from the letter he was writing.

'What's wrong with her?'

The man shrugged his shoulders. 'She just don't talk. Guess she don't understand nothing either.'

'What's her name?'

'May or somethin',' his companion said.

Michael guessed she was one of the orphans who lived at Long Tieng. The Hmong warlord, Vang Pao, had his headquarters on another part of the base. When one of his soldiers died in battle he assumed responsibility for the man's wife and children. But the war had raged for so long that in some parts of Laos there were few Hmong males left alive between the ages of sixteen and forty-five and so the number of orphans at the base had grown alarmingly. The USAID school was just down the road from the hootch and sometimes the children stopped by on their way to try and coax small change and chewing gum from the Ravens in the bar.

Michael fetched a Coke from the bar and handed it to her. She took a sip from the bottle and gravely handed it back to him. As if she was taking Communion.

He studied her more closely. She had a fine, coffee brown skin and exquisitely carved features, framed by bangs of midnight black hair. The hazel brown eyes were as big as a doll's.

He squatted down to her level. 'May or somethin',' he said, grinning. 'That your name?' He tapped his chest. 'My name's Michael.'

She just stared at him.

'Michael,' he repeated, more slowly.

'Might as well make faces at yourself in the mirror for all the good that's gonna do,' one of the chopper pilots said.

He tried again: 'Michael.'

'Wasting your time, man.'

Little Ly May turned and ran outside. Michael shrugged, turned away, and concentrated on getting drunk.

87

He was up before dawn, his head clear, his body tingling
with adrenalin. The alcohol had not touched him. He might
have been drinking water all night.

The shower was a fifty-gallon barrel with an immersion
heater in it. They told him that in winter ice formed on the
surface overnight and the first man up had to break it to get
the heater started before he could shower. Something else to
look forward to.

He had been in Laos only two weeks. Before that he had
spent almost six months in Vietnam flying Rustics, but his
frustration with both the suffocating 'Rules of Engagement' –
the so-called Romeos – and the army bureaucrats who policed
them, the remfs – rear echelon motherfuckers – had quickly
disillusioned him with the war.

In his first month he realised what he was up against. One
morning he had been flying low over a montagnard village in
the Central Highlands. He saw Vietnamese regulars dragging
villagers out of their huts and shooting them. His OV-10 was
armed with two thousand rounds of strafe so he asked for
permission to fire. He was told to stand by.

Fifteen minutes later, with most of the villagers now slaugh-
tered in front of his eyes, permission was refused.

Then a week later he was threatened with court martial for
refusing to drop napalm on a thatched village. He had seen
children in a rice *paddi* not twenty yards away.

He and his fellow FACs soon came to hate the remfs more
than the Viet Cong. A pilot from his squadron volunteered for
the secret Steve Canyon program, and wrote to Michael from
Laos telling him that although the work was probably more

dangerous even than Viet Nam, it was a chance to get away from the military and the bullshit.

He signed on.

Which was why he now found himself in Laos, a country he knew nothing about, at a place called Long Tieng, a village he had never heard of. It was in a bowl-shaped valley, a tiny Hmong village that had now become one of the biggest military installations in South East Asia. It was also a complete secret to the outside world. Shangri-la with barbed wire, someone had described it.

The air-conditioned comforts of similar US military bases were absent at Long Tieng. The pilots lived in thatched houses in the village, which was no more than a tangle of dirt streets and hastily installed power cables. Their houses were raised on stilts to keep out wild animals and save them from the floods in the monsoon. In winter temperatures often fell below freezing at night. They had open latrines and did their own cooking.

But here at least they were fighting a war without regulations. A righteous war, Michael decided. The Pathet Lao had become minor players; it was ostensibly a fight between North Vietnamese regulars and the Hmong. But the clandestine nature of what they were doing in Laos still disturbed him. If they were the good guys, why was it such a closely guarded secret?

He shaved and went to the hootch to make himself coffee. He sat and stared at the map of Laos on the wall, as he did every morning, trying to absorb every contour and every landmark, knowing that such knowledge might one day save his life. A cool and dirty-coloured dawn broke over the mountains. He heard Floyd and Mama, the pet Himalayan black bears, stirring in their cage next to the bar.

He suddenly realised he was not alone.

'Ly May,' he said.

He had no idea how long she had been there. She was squatting inside the doorway, her eyes huge and unblinking like some silent night animal's. Her black smock and skirt blended with the shadows.

'What are you doing here?' he said. He crossed the room and squatted down beside her. 'You scared the hell out of me.

I felt a pair of eyes staring at me, I thought one of the bears had got loose.'

No response.

Michael patted his chest. 'Michael,' he said slowly. 'Michael.'

He searched in his shirt pocket and found a stick of gum. He gave it to her. She held it tight in her fist and stared back at him. Michael performed a little pantomime that she should eat it. She chewed it three times and swallowed.

'You're supposed to make it last, kid.' He took off his Giants baseball cap and put it on her head. Ly May did not move.

'Giants,' he said, and mimed a batter. 'Greatest baseball team in the world. Well no, that's not true. They never even won a World Series. I used to go watch them all the time when I was a kid. That's where I got an appetite for lost causes. Like this one.'

The little girl watched him with an intensity that suggested he was the most fascinating and bizarre creature she had ever seen. He felt like a monkey in a zoo.

'I guess you don't understand a word I'm saying. Wouldn't make any difference if you could talk, would it?' He tapped himself on the chest once more. 'Michael. Mi-chael.' He pulled the cap further over her eyes. 'Keep the sun off. Damn, if you aren't the prettiest little kid. Where's your mom and dad? Dead, I guess. I wonder if you got any brothers or sisters. It's a damned shame, Ly May. What's happening to you people, I mean. First time I felt like I was on the right side of the war was when I came up here, you know that? And I volunteered. Thought I'd be holding back the red army. Soon found out that was a whole crock of shit. Whoa, sorry. Forget I said that word even though you don't know what it means. Shit is a bad word. Anyway, what was I saying? Viet Nam. You know Viet Nam? In Viet Nam, next to nobody wants us, and we tell the whole world what we're doing. Up here, we're doing something right and we want to keep it a secret. But then I guess it was us that got you into this shit – whoa, that bad word again – so that's why we don't want anyone to know. That make sense to you?'

'Who you talking to, Mike?'

Michael looked up. It was Chad Burke, the Head Raven. He

was dressed, as usual, in a checked shirt and denim jeans.

'The little kid here.'

'Hell, Mike, she don't understand a word. She don't talk either. Hasn't said a word to anyone since she got here.'

'How come?'

'Father died fighting for Vang Pao. Couple of months ago the rest of her family were mowed down right in front of her. Some fighter jock made a strafing run right through the village.'

'Jesus.'

'Must have been one of those boys from Udorn. Fast FAC maybe. Those mothers don't give a shit.' Chad clapped his hands. 'You go home now, Ly May.' He shooed her out. 'Poor little kid. What can you do? Place is full of them. Come on, let's get some breakfast.'

Bedraggled groups of Hmong soldiers, barefoot and wearing black pyjamas, waited on the edge of the runway for Air America choppers to airlift them back to the jungle. Some of them were as young as eight or nine years old, dwarfed by their own Armalites. Their brothers and sisters, too young even for Vang Pao's army, hefted Willy Pete rockets and pumped gasoline on the runway.

Michael made his way from the maintenance shack on to the ramp, Smiley beside him. Smiley was his Backseater, one of a squad of Laos trained by Vang Pao to help the Ravens differentiate between friendly and enemy targets. Smiley had earned his nickname for his committed and unwavering pessimism.

'Weather no good,' he announced when he saw Michael that morning. 'Cannot fly.'

'It's not so bad, Smiley.'

'Very bad. Cannot. We die.'

'Hey, I'm Buddha, remember?'

'No, even Buddha not fly in this. Never happen.'

It was true the weather was bad, but then, the weather was always bad in Laos. All the Ravens joked there were only three flying conditions in Laos; foggy, cloudy and lousy. It was still burn-off season, the time of year when the tribesmen set fire to the forests to clear new opium fields, and a smoky-blue haze fell like a shroud over the whole of northern Laos. Sometimes a cloud bank of smoke rose two miles into the air above the fields.

Today the cloud ceiling was down to fifteen hundred feet. It wasn't going to be easy, but Chad told them the bad guys were on the move and they had to fly.

'Mai Koo!'

Michael stopped and turned. It was Ly May.

'Jesus. The kid talks.'

She ran across the ramp, held something out to him in her fist. He took it. It was a tiny jade Buddha on a leather thong.

'What is this, Smiley?'

Ly May spoke rapidly to Smiley. 'It is lucky Buddha,' he translated. 'She says you have bad *phi*, bad spirit that follow you. Buddha will protect you now.'

Michael smiled at her and she suddenly, disarmingly, grinned back. 'Tell her thanks for me, Smiley. Hey, and ask her how she got this?'

There was another rapid-fire exchange.

'She sells hat you give her,' Smiley said. 'Says is very urgent you have Buddha. We go home now?'

'Hell, no. We've got some flying to do.'

'If you have bad *phi*, we die for sure. Must give Buddha time to chase *phi* away.'

'Get in the plane Smiley.'

'We die, Mai Koo.'

But he clambered into the cockpit.

Michael bent down to Ly May. He slipped the Buddha over his neck and held out his hand. Ly May stared back at him, non-plussed. He picked up her hand and shook it. 'Thanks, little Ly May. You come to the hootch tonight and I'll buy you Coca-Cola, okay?'

He stood up and strode across the ramp to his airplane.

There were no other Bird Dogs in service so Chad had given Michael command of a Cessna 0-17. There was no back seat. Instead Smiley sat directly beside him in the cockpit. As he clambered in, the little Hmong was rocking back and forward, pale and sweating. 'We die today.'

'For Christ's sake, Smiley!'

391

'We go home now. More better.'

'This is the last goddamned time I'm flying with you. You're getting on my nerves.'

The haze had settled over the valley, reducing visibility to less than half a mile. Michael took off blind into the clouds, counted to fifteen, then turned the nose of the Cessna hard left to miss the nine thousand-foot mountain directly in front that the Ravens knew as the Vertical Speed Brake. There was an opening in the surrounding mountains shaped like a saddle, and he knew that if he performed the manoeuvre correctly he was lined up for the saddle and the PDJ.

If not...

The curtain of white parted for a moment and Michael could make out the plain directly in front. He slapped Smiley on the thigh. 'It's going be okay,' he said. 'Trust me. Buddha's on my side!'

Smiley rolled his eyes and resumed his glum meditation on the Fates.

Michael followed Route 5 and the edge of the plain towards the west, looking for targets. There were rumours that enemy troops had circled behind the Vang Pao line that ringed the southern edge of the J.

The milk bottle haze obscured everything. Occasionally peaks and ridges jutted through the gauze, slashed to razor backs by wind and rain, and once, Michael made out a mountainside scarred by the slash and burn of the Hmong. Once verdant with hardwood, the slopes were now covered in poppies, or lay fallow under savannah grass.

They had been in the air less than ten minutes. The shell fire came from nowhere.

The legend of the Golden BB was part of Raven folklore: stories of pilots who had flown at a hundred feet through storms of anti-aircraft fire and come out unscathed, to cruise the next day over open country at five thousand feet and be shot through the chest by a single rifle round.

It sounded like firecrackers exploding. A series of holes appeared in the floor of the Cessna. Smiley screamed and clutched at his leg. Blood spurted over the interior of the windshield. Michael thought the blood was his and looked down at his own body, searching for a wound.

Instinct took over and he put the Cessna into a steep climb, turning away from the gun that had targeted them. Smiley was thrashing and screaming in the seat beside him. Michael thought: Perhaps he was right, perhaps the bad *phi* did follow us into the plane.

He levelled out at six thousand feet and banked one eighty, on a heading back to Long Tieng. Smiley's left leg was in tatters, blood pumping from the wound. He realised the little Hmong was going to bleed to death long before they arrived back at Long Tieng.

He kept the plane steady with his feet on the rudders, then ripped off his belt and fashioned a tourniquet around his thigh to stop the bleeding. Smiley flailed with his arms and the Cessna bucked and swooped as Michael fought to keep control. Smiley's eyes rolled back in his head, and he passed out.

The bleeding had stopped now, but Michael had no idea if Smiley was alive or dead. Blood slopped on the floor under his seat like bilge.

'We go home now,' he said to Smiley, who lay slumped and bloody in the seat beside him.

He helped the ground crew lift Smiley out of the plane and into a waiting ambulance, then walked back to the hootch and poured himself a shot of White Horse. Then he realised he didn't need it and left it on the bar. He caught a glimpse of himself in a mirror, his face and shirt spattered with a spray of blood. 'I don't know about the bad guys, but you sure terrify me,' he said to his reflection and walked out, laughing.

Chad was waiting for him on the ramp. 'I think you should take the rest of the day off,' he said.

'I'm okay.'

Chad shook his head. 'That's twice in two days. Better take a break.'

'I feel fine.'

'Go back to your hootch. Rest up. No one's going to fly with you today anyway. The Hmong all say you've got bad *phi*. Go on.'

Michael shrugged and walked away.

The next morning he felt in a buoyant mood as he walked across the ramp. Smiley had been flown down to Vientiane where surgeons had operated on his leg. He was going to live.

He reached the cockpit of the O-17 and froze. His muscles turned to iron. He began to shake, and he had to sit down, right there on the apron.

I should be dead.

He remembered the chatter of small arms fire he had heard when Esterhazy had rescued him two days ago; the NVA had been that close. And yesterday the bullets had passed through the cabin, either side of his feet, and he hadn't been hit.

He looked down at his hands and could feel Smiley's blood over them. He felt sick when he thought about it.

One of the groundcrew helped him to his feet. He weaved over to the operation shack, threw his gear in the locker and went back to the hootch. Chad found him there half an hour later, sitting on the floor, still staring at his hands. He put his arm around his shoulder. 'Delayed shock, son,' he said. 'I guess we better send you down to Udorn to rest up for a few days.'

88

Udorn, Thailand

After the privations of Long Tieng, Udorn was an air-conditioned heaven. Still shaken from what had happened, Michael refused an invitation from some of the AA pilots to accompany them into town to visit one of the bath houses. When he finally made it to the Air America bar, he ran into Esterhazy.

Esterhazy was a grizzled bear of a man, a former Marine pilot, with flying credits in Korea, the Middle East and the Alaskan oil fields. He had been crop dusting in Ohio when Air America found him. They had given him an offer he could not refuse; a thousand dollars a week and a box to come home in.

He was in his forties, with a salt and pepper moustache, skin tanned as weathered tobacco, his body as lean as a runner's. He had slightly mismatched eyes that gave him the lunatic look that had doubtless earned him his nickname. Like most Air America pilots he wore more gold jewellery than an Arab princess; two thick chunky rings, a gold Rolex, a gold identity bracelet with the initials NE, more ropes of gold around his neck. The pilots said it was to buy their own ransom if they got into trouble, but Michael had decided it was pure vanity.

Esterhazy grinned when he saw him. 'I know you! You're the guy with the red boxer shorts!'

Michael greeted him as loudly and shouted for a bottle of whisky for the bravest and best chopper pilot in the whole of the South East Asian theatre – and shit on those Jolly Green Giants! – and the two of them proceeded to get drunk.

*　　*　　*

'Tell me,' Michael said, after their fifth White Horse, 'what was that stuff in the sacks that day?'

Esterhazy lowered his voice theatrically. 'That, son, was opium.'

'You're kidding.'

'May the good Lord strike me down if I tell you untrue, brother. What they want to put in the back of my machine is none of my business. I just get paid by the hour.'

'Opium?'

'Look, the war has screwed things up for the people here, you know? I guess they don't have no other way of getting piggy to market.'

'But what happens to this stuff?'

Esterhazy shrugged his shoulders. 'I don't get paid to ask questions, man. They call. I haul.'

'But our own planes? Flying dope?'

Esterhazy poured two more whiskies. 'How do you think they pay for this war?'

'We're peddling drugs now?'

He frowned. 'Not us, man. The Generals. I hear Vang Pao even has his own heroin factory right up there at Alternate.'

'Bullshit.'

'Hey, it's the American way. Free enterprise pays for everything.' Esterhazy playfully tousled Michael's hair. 'No harm in being young. You'll learn.'

Later, when they were both very drunk, they reprised the story of the rescue for the rest of the bar. Michael took off his trousers, tied them to a bar stool and waved them over his head, while standing on a table which was meant to represent the ridge. Esterhazy climbed on the bar, and swooped down to try and grab them. But he missed the table by two yards, landed heavily and hit his head on a chair on the way down. Groaning, he passed out dead drunk on the floor.

Long Tieng

Ly May herself was not sure why she liked the American so

much. Like all *falangs*, he was pretty ugly, a clumsy and hairy giant with pale skin and huge feet; but there was something in his face that was very kind, and like all the Americans, he held a grotesque fascination for her.

She was also terrified and intrigued by the great silver machines the Americans climbed into every day. It was one of these terrible birds that had ripped her family to pieces. They belonged to the Americans, so it must have been an American who had killed her family. But why? Did they think her mother and her sisters were Pathet Lao?

The American, Mai Koo, was the first person since her family had died really to take an interest in her. At the orphanage they fed her, and gave her clothes; but they did that for all the children. She was grateful, but it was not special, and it did not take away her loneliness.

But Mai Koo had knelt down and smiled at her, and given her Coca-Cola, and the disgusting food the Americans all ate that was like eating poppy sap, and he had even given her a present, which had won her a lot of face with the other children.

She had thought she had found a new friend and protector, but then he had gone away again, and she did not see him any more. She had experienced this before. She guessed that Mai Koo had gone to the war, and that was why he had not come back. When people went to the war they very seldom came back. That was what had happened to her father and her brothers.

But then, one day, as she was heading back to the orphanage from the USAID school, she saw him again. She pushed her way through the legs of the Americans in the Coca-Cola place and tugged on his trousers to make sure he was real, and not a *phi* who was trying to trick her. He had looked down and grinned at her and said something in his strange language that she did not understand. Then he put his hands under her shoulders and hoisted her up on to the bar. 'Ly May! Want a Coca-Cola?'

She knew that word and nodded her head. He went behind the bar and came back with a bottle with the cold, dark, tingly liquid inside. He gave it to her to drink, and then started talking in his loud voice to the other Americans. She held on to his shirt with her fingers to make sure he did not go away again. She had been lonely for a long time. In the absence of her father she figured that this one would do just as well.

From that day Ly May refused to let him out of her sight, and whenever he was not flying she followed him around, a second shadow. She became a regular at the Raven hootch, she was there every morning when Michael got up, and was waiting for him at dusk when he walked from the ramp. She would have nothing to do with anyone else. She taught him to flick one of the little painted wooden tops the Hmong children loved, and in return he taught her how to blow bubble gum. The first time he ever saw her really laugh was when the gum popped and splattered over her nose.

At night she climbed on his lap while he sat at the bar with the other Ravens and later she fell asleep, curled up next to his stool. The other Ravens became fond of her too and she became an unofficial mascot.

Sometimes Michael would touch the jade Buddha at his throat and think about the morning she had presented it to him on the ramp, a few minutes before the stray 14.5-millimetre had taken Smiley's leg. He wasn't superstitious but he wondered if perhaps the bullets were meant for him...

If it was his bad *phi* that had almost claimed him on those two days in March, the little Buddha had since done its job. He flew his ten- and twelve-hour combat days without taking any more bad hits, although every evening when he returned he found new bullet holes in the fuselage and wing that had to be hastily repaired with typhoon tape.

Somehow Michael felt the presence of Ly May had changed his luck.

He tried to teach her a little English. She learned to say 'Coke' and 'Right on' and 'Mer-Ka' for America. One day one of the pilots taught her to say 'Sum-bich' when he wasn't there, and when he found out he was furious.

Some evenings he went up to the orphanage with a bag of Juicy Fruit and candy, and taught the children to play baseball in the street outside, using a rattan ball and a stolen MP baton.

One evening she hit a home run and he scooped her up on his shoulders and carried her round the bar.

But a month later it all came to an end. The Pathet Lao and North Vietnamese managed to infiltrate the Vang Pao line and attacked Sam Thong.

89

The haze and smoke of the burning season had hidden their movements. But on 17 April the communists attacked Sam Thong from the north, pounding the base with mortars. Forty thousand Hmong refugees took to the hills; the Americans abandoned the airstrip, took their wounded and flew south to Vientiane. Sam Thong was just twenty kilometres from Long Tieng, and the communists swiftly moved on to Skyline Ridge, to lay siege.

Michael woke to the sound of a mortar shell crashing down in the street. The impact jarred him out of his bed and on to the floor. He ran outside. Pigs were squealing, running from one side of the street to the other, a Hmong woman was chasing a naked toddler.

He saw Ly May running towards the hootch from the direction of the orphanage. 'Mai Koo! Mai Koooooo!'

He heard the sound of another mortar shell, knew what was going to happen. 'Get down! Ly May! GET DOWN!'

The shell slammed into a tin shack fifty yards away. Michael felt a blast of heat and suddenly found himself lying on his back. He raised his head, looked down at his body, astonished to find himself uninjured. He rolled over, shook his head, his ears still ringing from the concussion. His balance was gone, and it took him three attempts to get upright.

The shack had disappeared. Twisted sheets of tin and splintered timber littered the street. A pig lay on its back, its entrails smeared through the dirt. The Hmong woman and the toddler were a bundle of bloodied rags.

'Ly May?'

He found her crawling in circles on her hands and knees

beside an overturned jeep. Her face was covered in blood. 'Mai Koo?' she whimpered.

He scooped her up in his arms and stumbled through the wreckage of the street towards the hospital.

Michael and the rest of the Ravens climbed into their 0-1s and spent all that day co-ordinating the strikes against the mortar positions in the surrounding hills. From the air Michael could see long lines of Hmong on the road heading south. At the airstrip itself Air America Dakotas were still taking off every two minutes, ferrying out Hmong refugees, most of them small children and women with pathetic bundles of possessions on their backs. Outside the CIA compound men in sport-shirts were throwing bundles of paper into flaming gas drums.

As he touched down at the base later that afternoon Chad ran across the apron to meet him. 'I want you out of here, Mike. Once it's refuelled, take your Bird Dog down to Vientiane.'

'That bad?'

'It doesn't look good. I'm getting everyone out.'

'Let me just check in at the hospital. Ly May got hurt this morning.'

'Fifteen minutes. But then you haul ass out of here.'

The hospital was empty, most of the patients had already been ferried south. Ly May was alone, lying on her back in one of the wards. There were thick pads over both her eyes and a raw stitched seam on her head, just below the hairline.

Michael felt sick to his stomach.

He put his lips close to her ear. 'Ly May,' he whispered.

'Mai Koo?'

'I'm here.'

She groped for his hand, gripped it with surprising strength. 'Sum-bich,' she said.

His eyes felt hot. 'Yeah,' he said. 'A real sum-bitch.'

He wiped his face on the sleeve of his shirt. Jesus. 'Let me find the doctor,' he said.

She wouldn't release his hand. 'Mai Koo go Mer-Ka?'

'No,' he said. 'Mai Koo get Coca-Cola for Ly May.'

She accepted that. But as he crept from the room she whimpered: 'Mai Koo?'

'I'm coming back,' he said.

He found the doctor, a young Air Force surgeon by the name of Fairchild, in the casualty room. A body lay on one of the tables, an American in civilian clothes. There was a black jellied hole in the middle of the face.

'Don't even know his name,' a familiar voice said. 'I told him to duck. He turned around and said "Why?"'

Esterhazy was sitting on the other table, while Fairchild sutured a gaping wound in his shoulder.

'What happened?'

'Mortar round just as we were taking off. Thought I was about to check out. What are you doing in here? You bring me some grapes?'

Michael turned to Fairchild. 'There's a little Hmong kid out there.'

'One of your strays?' Fairchild asked him.

'Sort of.'

Fairchild shook his head. 'I've done the best I could. She took shrapnel in both eyes. She needs a good opthalmic surgeon.'

'What are you going to do with her?'

Fairchild finished stitching Esterhazy's shoulder. 'I've given her some morphine for the pain. I'm sending her down to Vientiane as soon as I can.'

'They've got eye surgeons in Vientiane?'

'I doubt it.'

'So what's going to happen to her?'

Fairchild dressed the wound and was going to put the arm in a sling but Esterhazy waved it away. Fairchild shrugged, flicked off his rubber gloves and dropped them into a kidney dish. 'Mike, I'd like to help every little kid in Laos, but I can't. It's not my fault.'

'You mean she's going to be blind?'

'I don't know.' Fairchild was not indifferent just exhausted.

'What's going on?' Esterhazy said.

'You got eye doctors in Udorn?' Michael asked him.

'Shit, we each got our own personal brain surgeon.' When he saw the look on Michael's face, the grin fell away. 'I don't know, it's got to be better than Vientiane. Hell, I can try for you. No skin off my butt.'

'You can fly her down?'

'The horse I rode in on had to be shot. It's in little pieces all over the runway. They're flying me back on some fucken useless thing with wings. But I'll take care of this kid for you, son. Neil Esterhazy, Angel of Mercy.'

'I owe you one.'

'You owe me two. Fact is, I own your ass, Dale.'

Ly May heard him come back into the room. He tried to imagine what it must be like for her, frightened, in pain, unable to see, aircraft droning overhead, shell fire, foreign voices. Knowing all her own people had fled.

'Mai Koo?'

'They're taking you to Udorn,' he whispered to her.

'Mai Koo!' He heard the pleading in her voice. She groped the air with her hand, reaching for him. Michael was frightened that if she caught him, she would never let him go. He couldn't stay with her, it was impossible. He had done everything he could.

'You'll be okay.'

'Mai Koo!'

'I'm not leaving you. I'll come and find you in Udorn. But I can't stay.' He knew she didn't understand what he was telling her.

'Mai Koo!'

He rushed out of the hospital. As the door slammed behind him he heard Ly May's voice.

'SUM-BITCH!'

A world of darkness, and pain, and men talking in the strange language she still did not understand. When she had heard Mai Koo's voice again she felt a little better, because she knew he would protect her. But then he went away again, and she had screamed his name over and over, but he did not return, and she knew he had abandoned her too.

Like her father, like her mother, like her brothers and sisters, everyone she loved only went away. Now she was alone in the night, and there was no one to help her, and nothing she could do.

Except hold on to life, for what it was worth.

*　　*　　*

That night the Ravens found whatever billets they could in Vientiane. Michael got the last room in the Settha Palace Hotel, and immediately collapsed on the bed in a black, dreamless sleep. At four o'clock his watch alarm woke him. He got a ride back to the airport, refuelled his Bird Dog himself, and was back in the air with the rest of the Ravens at dawn.

During the night North Vietnamese sappers had tried to infiltrate the perimeter at Long Tieng, but there had been no direct assault. When Michael arrived over the base, the surrounding mountains were still partially obscured by the drifting smoke of burn-off. Visibility on the ground was down to less than one mile. Michael spiralled down, looking for glory holes, breaks in the overcast where he could rendezvous with his air and lead them down. He spent the whole day finding targets and co-ordinating wave after wave of T-28s and Phantoms against the North Vietnamese positions. His memories of the day were a blurred montage of shouts and smoke, terror and rage, exhaustion and sudden, pumping adrenalin.

By the time he got back to Wattay, with dusk settling like dust over the Mekong, it was as much as he could do to lift himself out of the cockpit.

90

The two bell boys were asleep with their heads on the counter. Michael went behind the desk and looked for his key. It was gone.

He nudged one of the boys awake. 'Where's my room key?'

The young Lao shrugged his shoulders and settled his head back on his arms.

Michael picked up his flight bag and went up to his room. The door was half open. His canvas holdall was in the corridor, so crudely packed that the sleeve of one of his shirts protruded through the zipper.

He went in. A camera, notebooks, and a Pan Am flight bag were thrown across the bed. There was a pair of jeans over the room's only chair, and women's underwear draped over the overhead fan, which was revolving slowly. A home made dryer, Michael thought, with grudging admiration for the as yet faceless interloper.

The bathroom door opened. The woman who appeared was soaking wet, and wearing only a T-shirt that reached barely to mid-thigh. Her black hair hung over her face like a wet dog. She was holding a towel.

She stared at him. 'Who the fuck are you?' she said. Michael recognised a Brooklyn accent.

Shit, Michael thought. A New Yorker. Get ready for a fight. 'More to the point, who the fuck are you? This is my room.'

'You got a key, bud?'

Michael didn't answer.

'No, you don't got the key, do ya? You don't got the key, 'cos I got the key. So it's my room. Beat it.'

He didn't move.

'What are ya, a rapist or somethin'? 'Cos if you are, I better
warn you I got four brothers in my family, and they was all
in gangs. You want to try something with me, you better get
a spare set of balls stashed away some place.'

'When I left here this morning, this was my room. I haven't
checked out. So how did you get it?'

She came towards him, still drying her hair, as if they were
an old married couple having a routine fight. 'You been in Asia
long?'

'Seven months.'

'Shit, a slow learner. Let me give you a tip, bud. If you
got a room in the only hotel in town, you don't wanta give
the key to reception. Know why? 'Cos they think you ain't
never coming back. And even if they think maybe you might
come back, some cute little *falang* bats her eyes at them and
offers to pay a few bucks more for the same room, and they
give her the key. Now you got that, or you want me to
run it by you again but slower?'

'This is my room,' he said.

The girl threw the towel on the bed. 'So, you wanna fight
me for it? Ten bucks says you walk out of here singing like
Frankie Valli.'

She put her hands on her hips, one knee bent and out front
and looked at him like his sister used to when she had just taken
the last candy from the box. The T-shirt clung to her body and
her nipples were dark bruises against the white cotton. Her
smile let him know she knew what he was thinking.

Michael went out. The door slammed behind him.

'You are too acerbic, monsieur,' the manager, Mr Maurice,
told him later. 'You must be more malleable. We have other
nice rooms. No bath, no fan, perhaps mosquito net has little
holes, but nice room.'

Michael picked up his holdall and jumped in one of the *siclos*
waiting outside.

Chad settled him in on the floor of his bungalow and told
him they would find a place for him next day, or maybe the
day after. Definitely by next week.

All the Ravens were tired, too tired. Seven of them poured

into an ancient Renault taxi designed for four people and rode into town.

The Air America watering hole in Vientiane was the Purple Porpoise, run by a genial Australian called Monty Banks. Monty gave away as many drinks as he sold and affected a refined upper-class accent that became a little erratic after too many of his own large pink gins. He played host to most of Vientiane's diplomats, pilots and spooks. The reason for this was simple: Monty's bar was strictly off limits to journalists.

When they got there, a large group of Air America pilots had already taken up residence in one corner of the bar. Two of them were wearing Stetsons, another had a T-shirt which said: SHOT AT AND MISSED ... SHIT AT AND HIT. There were bottles of White Horse everywhere, and several of them were smoking marijuana.

The Ravens joined them. They were the same breed as Esterhazy, Michael found out, hotshot rotor heads, most of them former Marine pilots. One of them, a ginger-bearded and freckled Southerner called Okee, had two half bottles of White Horse strapped to the front of his shirt, like grenades. Two long straws led from the bottles to his mouth. His friend, a Texan who introduced himself as Ratface, had a small wooden box around his neck on a leather thong. Michael asked him what was in it.

'My toe,' Ratface said, deadpan.

'What?'

'Toe got shot off last year, just after the monsoon. So I cremated it and the ashes are in the box.'

Ratface felt the need to prove the point. He opened the box and held it out to Michael. Okee leaned forward and blew, and a little cloud of ash spilled on to the table.

Ratface rounded on him, furious. Okee grinned and settled back to suck on the straws. 'You needed to cut your toe nails,' he said.

Chad thought the incident at the Bungalow vastly entertaining, and regaled the AA pilots with the story of Michael's misfortunes.

'I give you a toast to Mike Dale,' he finished, raising his glass. 'Shot at, fucked with and homeless!'

407

Suddenly the bar fell silent. Every head turned towards the door. Someone swore under their breath.

She was wearing blue jeans and a white blouse, and her hair hung in a mass of black curls to her shoulders. There was a leather bag over one shoulder. It looked heavy. Michael remembered the notepads and camera he had seen on her bed.

His bed.

'That bitch,' he said.

She had balls, he gave her that. She ignored the stares, went up to Monty at the bar and ordered a beer. He stared through her, as if she wasn't there.

'Is that her?' Ratface said.

'You know her?'

'Reporter,' Ratface said. He might as well have said: 'The devil.'

'Planet Earth calling barkeep. I said, gimme a beer.'

'I'm terribly sorry, young lady,' Monty said, still sober enough to retain his accent, 'but you are not welcome in this establishment. I must kindly ask you to leave.'

'What did you say?'

'He said, we don't serve no reporters in this bar,' Okee told her.

'I ain't no reporter, bud. I'm a journalist. Want me to spell that for ya?'

'I know how it's spelt,' Okee said. 'S-H-I-T.'

There was a long silence.

'A time warp,' the girl said. 'I coulda sworn this was the twentieth century. I better check my diary.'

'Get your smartarse mouth out of this bar,' Ratface said.

Michael got up and went over. 'Remember me?' he said.

'What's up, bud? Did I forget to pack your toothbrush?'

Michael lowered his voice. 'You been in Laos very long?'

She did not look quite so sure of herself now, Michael noticed with pleasure. He leaned closer.

'Let me give you some advice now. We don't like reporters in this bar. Or journalists. Or New Yorkers. So feel free to fuck off. Now you got that, or you want me to run it by you again only slower?'

She stared back at him, and for a moment, just a moment,

408

he saw her lip quiver. Christ, she's going to cry, he thought, suddenly appalled. I thought she was tough.

She hitched the bag further up her shoulder and walked out.

The rest of the pilots cheered but Michael went back to the table and instead of savouring the sweetness of the victory, felt sour and suddenly depressed. Well, he had extracted a measure of revenge, but it just left him feeling petty and diminished.

He got a little drunk and went home early, thinking about Ly May.

91

Five days after the assault began heavy rain cleared away much of the smoke haze and improved visibility, turning the tide of the battle. Wave after wave of Phantom strikes now found their target, hitting the communist supply lines from the Plain of Jars. When Michael landed at Wattay that afternoon, he knew Long Tieng would be saved.

He got a Peugeot taxi back from the airstrip. The sun was setting behind the Mekong, turning the plain into ochre colours. The taxi driver was a dreamy, smiling Lao, with the disconcerting habit of turning around in the driver's seat to talk to Michael in the back. He said he wanted to practise his English.

'Watch the road!' Michael shouted.

The driver obeyed, but a moment later he twisted around again. 'In America, every people has TV, yes?'

'Yeah, please watch the road.'

'Yes, yes.' He turned around again. 'In America, every people has box where you put the cold? What is word?'

'Refrigerator. Fuck, look out!'

There was a buffalo cart directly in front of them. He swerved around it one-handed, and did not see the *siclo* coming from Vientiane. The other driver bleated his horn ineffectually and drove off the road into a ditch.

'Stop the car,' Michael said.

'Why?'

'Stop the car!'

He ran back to the scene of the accident. The *siclo's* front wheel was mangled and the driver was sitting in the ditch with blood dripping from his head. He smiled and waved his hand at Michael.

His passenger was not as sanguine.

'Which motherfucker did that?' she said.

'Oh, it's you,' Michael said.

'You driving that machine, bud?'

'No, ma'am,' Michael said. 'If I had been I would have backed up over you, and made sure of the kill.'

Michael's taxi driver had made the mistake of returning to see what all the fuss was about. He stood on the side of the road, grinning.

The girl went up and swatted him behind the ear. 'You nearly killed me!' she shouted.

The little Lao backed away, still grinning.

She swatted at him again, and he ducked. A bullock cart rolled by and the farmer on the running board stared at the scene, astonished.

Michael moved in to break it up. 'Hey, now that's not going to do any good, is it?'

'He damn nearly killed me!' she shouted again.

A police car stopped at the edge of the road and two Lao police got out. The Lao taxi driver shouted at them excitedly and one of the policemen took out his notebook and pointed to the girl.

'Now what's going on?' she said to Michael.

'You're the old Asian hand, you tell me.'

The other policeman unclipped his holster and came towards her, one hand hovering over the revolver.

'Jesus Christ,' she said.

'Looks like a night in the dungeons,' Michael said. 'If they torture you, I want to come and watch.'

'You gotta help me,' she said.

It was an astonishing declaration, but Michael found, to his own surprise, that he agreed with her. He reached into his pockets and took out a handful of American dollars. He waved them at the two police then pointed to the girl and touched his temple with his forefinger. 'It's okay, she's crazy,' he said. 'Crazy American! Woman! Time of the month. Got her period. Really cranky.'

The pantomime made them smile and they nodded their heads in understanding. He gave them each five United States dollars and they nodded and put the notebook away and the policeman with the revolver reclipped his holster.

Michael bowed his head slightly, putting his hands together in a *wai* of thanks, then grabbed the girl by the arm and led her back to the taxi. 'I'll give you a lift,' he said.

'It's not my fucking period,' she hissed at him.

'Christ, what are you like when it is?'

The driver shook his head when Michael indicated he wanted him to take the girl with them into Vientiane. Another five dollars in US currency persuaded him.

They drove the whole way in silence. The girl looked steadfastly out of the window. She was biting her lip and he could see she was replaying every move in her mind and regretting it.

At the Bungalow she got out. Michael got out with her. He paid the taxi driver the agreed fare and handed him another tip.

'How much do I owe you?' she said.

Michael shrugged.

She reached into her bag, took out a leather wallet and removed a handful of Laotian currency, everything she had. She crushed it into his shirt pocket. 'I'm not going to owe you for anything, bud.'

'Name's Mike.'

Her face softened. 'Amy Duke,' she said. 'Friends call me Dukes.'

'I imagine they would.'

'Why did you do that?'

'Do what?'

'Help me. I sure as hell wouldn't a helped you.'

'I don't know. Maybe I admire your guts. Maybe I think you're all bluff. And maybe you remind me a bit of my big sister.'

'Well, I appreciate it. I guess I lost it a little back there.'

'Yeah, well. We all lose it sometimes.'

'I ain't giving you your room back.'

'I never thought you would.'

'It's a dog eat dog world, Mike,' she said, recovering a little of her poise. 'You gotta remember that.'

'Sure, I'll remember that. So tell me, what were you doing heading out of town this time of night?'

'I had an interview with one of Rattakone's honchos. He's got a big villa out that way. Screw it, I ain't in the mood now. Woulda just been another snow job anyway.'

She shook her black curls from her face and looked up at him. He could not decipher the expression on her face. He was afforded a glimpse of the black lace edge of her bra between the buttons of her khaki shirt and the contradiction intrigued him.

'So tell me, Mike, what's going on up north?'

'I don't know, Miss Duke. I don't read the papers.'

She put her hands on her hips. 'Hey, pal, the airport's thick with unmarked airplanes and choppers. Some of them have got rockets. There's been C-123s flying in and out every day for nearly a week. You don't gotta be a Harvard grad to work out there's some big shit going on somewhere.'

'Do you write like you talk?'

'Look, pal, I write like I have to, I talk like I want to. Okay? So don't give me any crap. Now tell me about this war.'

'I can't tell you anything about the war, Miss Duke. You know that.'

'Why? What are you guys hiding out there?'

'Oh, you know, gas chambers, couple of missile silos· with nuclear warheads. Howard Hughes. The usual.'

'You know, you talk to the embassy, they say you guys are doing armed reconnaissance. What the fuck does that mean?'

'It's reconnaissance. Only we're armed.'

'I been talking to some of these refugees.'

'Yeah? They understand the accent? I don't.'

'I know a little French.'

'Yeah? How do you go with the grammar?'

She ignored him. 'Funny, some of these people they say they had to get out of their villages not because of the Pathet Lao, but because they was bombed out. By Americans.'

Michael remembered Ly May and her family, strafed in their own village. 'They're Lao airplanes, Miss Duke.'

'Why did you look like that?'

'Like what?'

'Just then, when I talked about the Meo getting bombed out of their villages. You got this look on your face.'

413

'It disturbs me. It's not something I like to hear. And they're Hmong. They don't like being called Meo.'

· She crossed her arms, deepening the valley between the edges of black lace. Deliberate? Michael wondered. 'You're not like the others, are you?' she said, softly.

'I just fly airplanes. I don't go in for psychology.'

'You go in for stories about American B-52s bombing the Plain of Jars?'

'I've got to be going, Miss Duke.'

'You frightened of a woman, Mike?'

He laughed, not taking that bait. 'Bet your ass.'

As he walked away, he heard her call out: 'You sure you're on the right side?'

92

The communist siege of Long Tieng lasted eleven days. By the end of the month, Vang Pao's army had driven the communists off Skyline Ridge and out of Sam Thong. That night, the combat weary Ravens and the rotor jocks of Air America met in the Purple Porpoise to celebrate.

In the argot of the Ravens crews, they were all a little tense. But Michael had now stopped thinking about his own mortality. Whenever he felt the empty feeling of dread in the pit of his stomach, he drowned it with White Horse.

He was in a huddle with four of his fellow Ravens when he heard Okee shout from the end of the bar: 'Hey, Ratface, d'you hear what happened to Crazy Esterhazy?'

'Fucked the Queen?'

'No, man, bought the farm. Golden BB, I heard. Shit out of luck.'

Michael twisted around. 'Esterhazy? Neil Esterhazy? When?'

'Don't know, man. Just heard it, that's all.' He grabbed his drinks from Monty and turned away. 'Some crazy bastard, that one,' he said, Esterhazy's only eulogy.

Michael stared at Okee's back. Esterhazy. He felt sick. The AA man had seemed indestructible. If they could get Esterhazy . . .

But there was another reason for this feeling of dread. Esterhazy had been his link with Ly May.

He heard her voice ringing through the hospital corridor at Alternate. '*Sum-bich!*'

The cold scum of guilt settled in his stomach. For Christ's sake, he thought, I didn't abandon her. I tried to help her. She's not my responsibility. I did the best I could.

He looked around the bar at the AA jocks, mercenaries, pirates and believers, at his own buddies, quixotic adventurers, happy with their lost cause. What the hell are we doing here? he wondered. If we're going to help these people, then let's do it. If we're not, then let's get out of their country and spare them any more misery.

We're saving the world from communism, his father had always told him. Did that make it okay to run dope in Air America helicopters? Did the United States government know that Vang Pao was said to have a heroin factory just a mile from where he was standing? If what they were doing was right, why were they keeping it a secret from people like Amy Duke?

Two Ravens had disappeared in their O-1 during the Long Tieng siege, the wreckage had never been found. In the end, would their deaths make a scrap of difference? Would any of their sacrifices count for anything?

He put his drink on the bar and walked out.

Chad found him in the White Rose. The bar was in a side street off the main street, sign-posted with a wagon wheel. The atmosphere was heavy with cigarette smoke. Groups of men sat around in little booths or on wicker chairs, mostly crew-cut men in wide-checked shirts. CAS, Chad decided. The rest of the customers were Air America pilots. The older fixed wing guys were at one end of the bar, loud and drunk, the younger ones in another corner, smoking a joint.

A Saigonese dance band played on a makeshift stage. 'Op, op and awaaaiiii, in my bootifoo baloo...'

Some Lao girls danced topless on one of the tables, enthusiastically but without rhythm.

Michael was sitting alone, drunk.

'I thought I'd find you here,' Chad said.

He pulled up a chair and lit a Lucky Strike. A girl in a tight red mini-skirt perched on the next table and opened her legs. She was not wearing underwear. She took the cigarette from Chad's mouth and placed it between the lips of her vagina and managed to produce a smoke ring.

'What do you think of this stuff?' Chad asked him.

416

'If I were you, I'd give up smoking,' Michael answered. 'That particular cigarette anyway.'

'You know the saying. Where there's smoke, there's fire.'

'A lot of other things too.'

The girl saw she had not attracted their interest so she threw the cigarette on the floor and moved on to look for a better prospect. Michael wondered if this was where May would be in a few more years. But then, he reminded himself, even that fate would be denied her. She was blind. Probably have to take up begging.

He indicated the bottle of White Horse on the table. 'Drink?'

Chad shook his head. 'You look like you've had enough for both of us.'

'I'll be okay to fly tomorrow. I don't get hangovers.'

'You left Monty's pretty fast, I hear. Even left your drink on the bar.'

'Hey, I can trust those guys.'

'What is it, Mike? If you're getting burned out, I can send you down to the Panhandle for a while. They got a country club in Pakse. Two hours flying a day, targets nominated by the enemy.'

'I'm fine. I can do my job, Chad.'

'Is it that kid?'

'Maybe. Can you get me down to Udorn again?'

'Is that where they took her?'

Michael nodded.

'There's plenty of orphans in Laos. You can't save them all.'

'I don't want to save them all. Just this one.'

Chad lit another cigarette. 'There's another O-1 has to get picked up. You can fly down tomorrow afternoon. Get an Air America flight from Alternate.'

'Thanks, Chad.'

'Take it easy. It's just another war. Okay?'

Chad left early. Michael stayed another hour, then decided to walk back home. After a while he got lost and found himself outside the huge US Embassy compound. A few blocks further on he passed the Russian and North Vietnamese

Embassies, and the Pathet Lao Legation. It all seemed surreal. They were the enemy, for Christ's sake. Finally realising he had taken a wrong street, he headed back towards the centre of the town, found himself staring at the Pratuxai, the Lao's *Monument Aux Morts*, built in the style of the Arc de Triomphe with cement donated by the United States for the Wattay runway. Michael remembered that Okee had told him they had rechristened it the Vertical Runway and that it was now a tradition for visiting American pilots to try and run up it when they were drunk.

'Anything those guys can do, a Raven can do twice as good,' Michael said aloud, and after a running start he took two giant strides up the sides of the monument and landed with spine-jarring impact in the dirt. He lay groaning on his back, staring up at a black sky.

'I thought you got to be smart to fly an airplane,' a woman's voice said.

'Miss Duke?'

'What else you do for fun? Slam your fingers in doors?'

Her face swam in and out of vision. He tried to get up, couldn't. 'I guess I drank a little too much.'

'Hey, look at me. I'm shocked and amazed. You want a lift or you wanta fly home?'

Michael rolled over, dragged himself to his knees. There was a *siclo* a few yards away, the driver staring at him as if he had just fallen from the moon. Amy helped him to his feet and dragged him on to the cracked leatherette.

'The Bungalow,' she said.

For the first time in his life, Michael woke with a hangover. A yellow border of light stained the sky. Christ, he should be in his Bird Dog. He sat up, too fast, and a wave of nausea left a patina of oily sweat over his forehead. He tried to remember where he was.

Amy Duke lay beside him in the bed. The sheet was pulled down to her waist, and she was asleep with her arms stretched above her head, sleek and langorous as a cat. In the shadowed half-light her nipples, he noticed, were tight buds of pink, the aureoles the colour of a bruise. Her lips were slightly parted, in the shape of a heart, the black curls spread across the pillow. His groin was as hard as a rock.

Sleeping with the enemy.

He quickly pushed back the mosquito netting and jumped out of bed, fumbling for his clothes. He found them on a chair in the corner, neatly folded.

'Love 'em and leave 'em, right?'

Christ, she was awake. 'I have to get out to the airfield.'

She sat up, belatedly pulling the sheet up to her chin. 'Can I come along?'

'I'm dropping a nuclear bomb on the Yunnanese. Nothing your readers would be interested in.'

'How's your head?'

Michael pulled on his trousers and shirt. 'I must have been very drunk.'

'You gotta be drunk to sleep with me, you mean?'

'Miss Duke...'

'Hey, I think, in the circumstances, Amy is okay.'

'Amy. I can't afford to be seen with you...'

'It's okay, no one saw us. It was dark and I pulled the shade.'

'You know what I mean.'

'If it's a boy, what should I call him? Ya know, in case I don't get to see you again.'

Michael stopped at the door. He didn't know what to say to her. How the hell had something like this happened? 'I'm not the kind of guy who makes a habit of this, Miss ... Amy.'

'So this stuff about us getting married, it was all crap, right?'

He stared at her.

Amy laughed. 'Oh, brother, I wish you could see your face. Mikey, wise up.'

'What?'

'Hey, it's okay. Listen to me. It didn't happen. Nothing happened. You was drunk. By the time I got you back here, you couldn't have raised your little finger, never mind anything else!'

He could have strangled her. 'We just slept?'

'*I* slept. *You* was unconscious.'

419

'I'll see you around.'

'Hey, Mike.'

'What?'

'Real shame. You got great landing gear.'

He went out, slamming the door.

Bitch.

Udorn, Thailand

No one at Udorn knew what had happened to Ly May.

One of the doctors had heard about a little girl who had been brought in on an Air America flight and had been treated briefly at the base hospital. He did not know where she was now. The doctor who had handled the case had been rotated back to the States. There was a rumour the patient had been transferred to a military hospital in Saigon, though that would have been highly irregular. But you know what those AA jocks are like...

Michael wanted to weep with frustration. The only one who knew the whole story was Neil Esterhazy and he was dead. Had he arranged to have her flown to Saigon for specialist treatment? There were flights out of here to Pakse and Saigon every day. But which hospital? He got the name and address of the doctor who had been rotated back home and scribbled a quick letter. But he knew it would be weeks before he got a reply, if at all.

What would happen to Ly May in Saigon? How would a little blind kid who did not know the language, did not have a friend in the world, survive? All her life she would think he had abandoned her. She would end up a beggar on the street.

He had to find her. If he was going to sleep at nights, he had to find her.

But how?

He headed for the O Club in a black depression.

There were three of them, combat pilots in their flight suits, sitting on top of the bar. It was a rule in the officers' club at Udorn that an ordinary officer – navigator, trash hauler, maintenance man – stood at the bar. Fighter pilots sat on it. They were the élite of the élite, and even at recreation they set themselves apart from the rest.

Michael vaulted up beside them. One of the pilots, a young man his own age with crew-cut blond hair, eyed him suspiciously. 'Who are you, buddy?'

'Name's Mike Dale. I'm a Raven.'

Immediately the ice was broken. The young pilot grinned. 'No shit. Name's Hal. Hal Brenner.' He held out his hand. 'This is Frank and JD. We're on fast FACs.'

Michael had heard of the fast FACs. The war had escalated so rapidly that there were not enough Ravens at Long Tieng to cope with the demand for air strikes. So the Air Force had come up with the idea of using FACs out of Udorn, using high speed jets.

Michael and the other Ravens felt they were worse than a waste of time; they were a liability.

'This guy's one of us,' Hal said to his two colleagues. 'What are you drinking, Mike?'

All Michael could think about was Ly May, and he was in no mood for condescension, no matter how well intentioned. 'I'm not one of you,' he said.

'What's that, Mike?' Hal said, still grinning.

'We fly at a hundred feet at sixty knots and get the shit shot out of us. You swinging dicks fly at ten thousand feet, the bad guys couldn't hit you with a moon rocket. How the fuck can you know what's happening on the ground? We reckon you kill as many friendlies as you do enemy.'

It was a deadly insult. The three pilots fell silent. Hal was still grinning but there was a menace in his eyes. 'What friendlies, Mike?'

'Hmong soldiers.'

'They're all slopes to me, man. What the fuck difference does it make?'

Michael was too astonished to respond immediately. 'They're the reason we're fighting the war,' he said finally.

'Gook's a gook,' the one called JD said. 'Hell, few times I save some strafe so I can shoot up a village on the way home.

421

Way I figure it, got to be some commies down there. I play the odds.'

Michael thought about Ly May. Perhaps it was this guy who did it, he thought. Or one just like him. It didn't really matter. They were all the same.

It happened so fast no one in the bar that night remembered seeing the Raven actually move. One minute he was sitting on the bar chewing the fat with these three jocks, the next minute he was running as fast as he could for the wall. Only now he was holding one of the jocks by the seams of his flight suit. When the guy hit the wall, they all swore you could hear his teeth rattle. Then the Raven hit him so fast you couldn't count the punches. Maybe a dozen in five seconds. The guy went down like a bag of shit, out of it before he hit the floor. Then his two buddies jumped on the Raven and if a colonel hadn't showed and broken it up, someone could have got killed.

93

The door was open. Amy Duke was on the balcony, her back towards him, hunched over a typewriter. There were green mosquito coils dotted around the room. The bed had not been made, and underwear was draped over the mosquito netting. There was a battery-operated cassette player on the bedside table. He recognised Mick Jagger's voice. 'Sympathy for the Devil'.

'Please allow me to introduce myself ...'

He wondered if she had heard him enter. 'Amy?' he said.

'Mister Vertical Take-off.' She kept typing.

'I came to apologise.'

'Well, I'll be dipped in shit!'

'I didn't thank you.'

'What for, fly boy?'

'For picking me off the street.'

'Hey, you could have got a lot more for your money, bud. Too late now. If you're sniffing around for seconds, forget it. Not in this canteen.'

He sat down on the bed.

'You figure on staying, do ya?'

'What are you writing?'

'Well, it ain't gonna win me the Pulitzer, I'll tell you that. It's just the crap the embassy feeds me but if I dress it up real good it gets to sound almost believable. They're real regular guys over there, you know? We got no secrets, they reckon. Any place you want to go, just ask the guys over at Air America. You can imagine, right? One lap of Wattay airfield maximum, and if they don't try and push you out the loading door, you got lucky.' She finally looked over her shoulder and then whistled in mock admiration. 'Look at you. Not just one black eye, you gotta have two.'

'You should have seen the other guy,' Michael said, and smiled. He felt his lip crack.

'Well, you two-fisted, hard drinkin', son of a gun,' she drawled in an imitation of a southern belle.

She turned completely around, straddling the chair, her arms resting on the back. The arms of the T-shirt were broad and again he glimpsed the black lace. A vision of her lying on her back on the bed, her arms flung over her head, came back to him, unbidden. You're a fox, Amy Duke, he thought. The body of a disco dancer and the manner of a drill sergeant. Why am I here even talking to you? You're trouble.

'What can I do for you, Mike?'

He shrugged.

'You want to know what you missed out on, don't ya? Typical of a guy. You get the scent once and you just can't get off the trail.'

'This was partly your idea.'

She sat up, feigning outrage. 'You calling me a whore?'

'One, I think you like me, same as I think I like you, don't ask me why. Two, as a writer you should know whore is only one syllable, not two.'

'Pardon me for living.'

'One thing I have to know. Is this all just for a story?'

'All what?'

'Hey, to coin an expression, you didn't gotta do all this, you know? You could have left me in the street. You didn't have to bring me back to your room.'

She put both hands to her breast. 'The kindness of my heart, Mikey.'

'Crap.'

'You don't think I got a heart?'

'I'll wait for the X-rays. Answer my question.'

'The truth. I'd tease a guy for a story. I wouldn't go to bed with him for one. I'm a bitch but I'm not a whore. There's a fine distinction.'

'Which paper do you work for, Amy?'

'*Bangkok Post.*'

424

'*Bangkok Post,*' he said, deadpan.

'None of the New York papers would have me. They said I was too pushy.'

'How can a reporter ever be too pushy?'

'Hey, I'm a woman. Editors didn't like me telling them their jobs, especially on the first day.'

He grinned. Yeah, he could imagine that.

'You get paid enough to live?'

'I write for other papers. They call me a stringer. Hired gun. That means they don't got to pay one of their own guys to sit here and sweat. If I come up with something they can use, they take it.'

'What other papers?'

She shrugged. '*Washington Post, New York Post, Far Eastern Economic Review.* Heavy duty. I'm not as dumb as I look, okay?'

'You know I can't help you.'

'You don't got to help me, Mike. Tell you a secret of my own, okay? The embassy here is just one big leak. How do you think the story of the B-52 raids on the PDJ got out so damned fast?'

'You aren't going to be helping anyone but the enemy with all this.'

'Thank you, Joe McCarthy. We got a whole war going down here, Mike, and no one back home ever heard of the place. If Congress didn't vote for it, whose fuckin' war is it? I mean, you know, that's democracy, right? We do live in a democracy, don't we? I mean, that's what we're telling everyone.'

'Sometimes you have to compromise.'

'Yeah, sure. But when you kick your principles out the loading door, what you got left to fly with, Mike?'

She's right, he thought. She's just saying back to me all the things I've been thinking ever since I got here. So why don't I want to hear it? 'We're fighting communism here.'

'What with? Fascism?'

'Somebody's got to fight this war, Amy.'

'Is that why you guys got into the drug business?'

'Are you printing that?'

'Oh, sure.' She rested her chin on her arms and watched him.

'You're crazy.'

'Hey, everyone knows Air America is moving dope. Flying high, right? You like Pepsi, Mike?'

'I'm more of a Coke man.'

'General Rattakone must like Pepsi. Five years ago he built a Pepsi factory right here in town. You know the place. Guess what? Vientiane's Pepsi generation is still waiting for their first bottle.'

'What's your point?'

'My point is, guy who manages the factory...' She turned around, fumbled on her desk for her ring pad notebook, flicked through the pages. '...Huu Tim Heng, is chiu chao Chinese. Along with the factory goes a licence to import chemicals. Like ether maybe, and acetic anhydride.' She looked up. 'You don't get it, do ya?'

'Get what?'

'They use that stuff to make heroin, pal.'

He stood up. 'This has got nothing to do with me.'

She leaned forward and rested her elbows on her knees. The weight of her breasts took the folds out of the shirt. This time he knew the effect was not premeditated. 'They fly it to Pakse, the Vietnamese Air Force flies it to Saigon. The Meo sell their opium, they get a good deal, they're gonna stay loyal, right? Rattakone sells it on to the Chinese, pays for his war. Somebody gotta pay for those bombs on the PDJ, Mikey.'

'I got to go, Amy.'

She stood up, and without warning slipped her arms around his shoulders. 'Jesus, you look a mess,' she whispered.

'Thanks.'

'What are you doing here?'

'In this room?'

'In Laos.'

'This isn't Viet Nam, Amy. God's on our side here.'

'Well, shit, maybe He understands this whole deal better than I do.' He felt the warmth of her body against his. 'You don't gotta go, Mikey.'

'Amy...'

She gave a little hop and wrapped her thighs around his hips. He had to grab her bottom with both hands or she would have broken his neck. She grinned at him. 'That ain't so bad, is it?'

'I can't help you with anything.'

She wriggled against him. 'Feels like you can.'

Oh, shit, Michael thought. This is it. I'm finished here. If Chad finds out about this, I'm out. They might as well find me in bed with Uncle Ho.

He thought about the black lace under the cotton drill shirt, saw her punching out the taxi driver who had run her off the road, remembered how she had stared down a room full of redneck pilots. Everything she did excited and confused him. My old man would really hate your guts, he remembered thinking as they fell on to the bed.

Michael woke in the middle of the night and lay awake for a long time, staring at the ceiling. Amy was nestled under his arm, her breathing soft and even. Finally he looked at the luminous dial of his watch and made his decision. He nudged her awake.

'Amy, wake up.'

He shook her roughly and she groaned.

'What time is it?' she said, into the pillow.

'It's quarter past three.'

'You gotta be kidding.'

'We have to get up.'

She rolled away from him. He tore back the mosquito netting, and lit the little kerosene lantern beside the bed. He started to dress.

'What are you doing?'

'You're right. I can help you.'

She sat up, hugging her knees to her body. Her thick hair fell over her face, and she pushed it back. Her eyes were hooded from sleep. 'It's the middle of the night.'

He sat on the edge of the bed. 'Got a deal for you.'

'Too early to deal, pal. I never do deals before midday, earliest.'

'You don't have any choice. You get one shot at this, Amy.'

She was awake now. 'I gotta get up for this, right?'

'Afraid so. We have to get out to the airfield and into the O-1 before anyone sees you.'

'What's the deal?'

'I'll show you the war, okay. Scoop. Biggest air base outside Viet Nam. That's what you want, isn't it?'

A moment of surprised hesitation. 'Is this dangerous?'

'Not for a tough New Yorker like you.'

'Wait a minute. Slow down. Why you doing this?'

'I get you there. You take your pictures or whatever you want. But the deal is this. When you do your piece, you don't talk about the drugs, okay? I show you the war, you sell it. This is a righteous fight, Amy. We're up against regular North Vietnamese troops who are trying to wipe out the Hmong.'

'Yeah, but who got those poor suckers involved in the first place?'

'Deal?'

'Jesus, Mike, what am I? Crusader Rabbit?'

'If you want me to help you, then you have to cut the deal.'

'Hey, what about my commitment to honest, uncompromising journalism.'

'It sucks.' He finished dressing and stood up. 'Ten seconds and I'm out of here, Amy. Make up your mind.'

'Okay.'

'There's more.'

'I just sold you my principles. What else you want, pal?'

'Soon as you get your story, I want you to go to Saigon for me. I want you to look for a little girl.'

'Any little girl, Mike, or does she have to be good-looking?'

'I'll tell you the story on the way to the airport. Come on, Amy, this is your big chance. The story's got to come out soon, you might as well have it.'

She jumped out of bed and gathered scraps of her clothes. 'Okay. But you're still not getting your room back.'

94

They took off from Wattay with the dirty orange border of dawn flung about the plain. The O-1 was not carrying its normal pay load of phosphorus rockets so Michael calculated the journey would take a little over half an hour. The cloud ceiling was a thousand feet and the mountains to the north were lost in another burn-off haze, plumes of brown smoke drifting across the jungle. A lousy day for flying.

Perfect.

'Come on, you bitch, get your nose up.'

Amy tapped him on the shoulder from her position in the back seat. 'Are you talking to me?'

'No, I was talking to the plane.'

'How is it,' she shouted at him over the noise of the engine, 'how is it an aeroplane has to be a woman?'

'You'd have to fly one to understand.'

'So where are we going, fly boy? Padoung? Kiou Cacham?'

'Lima Twenty. Sam Thong.'

'Sam Thong? Shit! I been to Sam Thong! I did one of Pop Buell's guided tours! Everybody's goes to Sam Thong!'

'Mike Dale's guided tour is better.'

He radioed ahead to Long Tieng, told them the weather was too bad to land, and said he was diverting to Sam Thong.

Sam Thong was the busiest dirt airstrip anywhere in the world, one hundred take offs and landings every day. Edgar 'Pop' Buell, an IVS worker, used the village as his headquarters, organising rice drops to the beleaguered Hmong in the surrounding mountains. If Esterhazy had been telling the truth, it was where Air America organised a lot of other drops too.

But the most important thing about Sam Thong was its value as a public relations showpiece. Amy, like every other journalist, had been brought up here in an Air America Huey when she first arrived in Laos. She had listened to Pop Buell talk about his rice drops and toured the two hundred-bed hospital and the USAID schools.

The airfield was on all the maps and had been designated Lima 20. There were no secrets at Sam Thong. The strip itself was nestled in the valley, surrounded by tall pinnacles of rock that were forever shrouded in mist, like some Chinese feather and ink painting. As Michael dropped into the valley Pop Buell's mountain city came into view; maintenance hangars, operations buildings, and billets clustered around the air strip, the village beyond, many of the buildings badly damaged in the recent fighting.

Michael taxied the O-1 to the edge of the dirt strip and jumped out. Amy scrambled down beside him, clutching her shoulder bag and cameras. 'What the hell we doing here?'

'We have to walk the rest of the way.'

'Rest of the way where?'

'Lima Twenty Alpha. Sam Thong's Alternate landing strip.'

'What?'

'Great idea, isn't it? You nominate your most important strip as an alternative landing area. Your story, Amy, is just on the other side of those mountains.'

The hour after dawn was rush hour on the mountain landing strips of Laos and Cessnas and STOLs and Air America choppers roared over their heads. They were not challenged as they walked through the village. Journalists were a common sight in Sam Thong.

They reached the outskirts and started to trudge up the road towards Long Tieng.

'I'll walk with you to the crest, then you're on your own,' Michael said.

430

'What are you going to do?'

'I'm going to get back in my Bird Dog and fly off into the sunset.'

'It's only just dawn.'

'Well, I'll point the other way and fly off into the dawn. Whatever.'

The morning mist muted every sound, the valley like a green tunnel under a milky shroud of cloud and smoke. Amy hefted her camera bag over her shoulder, breathing hard as they laboured up the dirt track. It was already sticky hot.

'You need to get into training, Miss Duke.'

'It's okay for you, pal, you come from San Francisco.'

'You'd be one of those wimps that takes the cable car.'

'Betcha ass.'

An AA Pilatus Porter took off below them and disappeared into the white ceiling of cloud, its engine whining like an angry bee.

'You didn't answer my question.'

'What question?'

'Why you doing this?' she said.

'I'm not sure.'

'Hey, great reason.'

'Okay, I guess it's this. We're losing this war, and I don't want to lose. I like these people. They've been sold a crock. I say, let's have a shit or get off the pot.'

'Nice line. Can I quote that?'

They reached the crest of the ridge. The sun broke through the haze for a moment and sparkled like dew on thousands of corrugated aluminium roofs. Antennae rose into the air like strands of silver trees. A silver Royal Lao T-28 raced along a black ribbon of macadam and climbed into the air.

Amy dropped on to her haunches and gaped.

'Sam Thong's alternative landing strip,' Michael said.

'Jesus H.'

'Largest city in Laos outside of Vientiane. The mountains over there are called Skyline Ridge. A week ago there were North Vietnamese mortars and rockets all along it. The two little mounds next to the runway are called the Titty Karst. For obvious reasons.'

'Unbelievable.'

'Just don't get too close, okay? If they find you, it's my ass in a sling as well.'

She nodded. 'I know the score.'

'I'm holding you to our deal.'

'I won't let you down.'

'If you do, I've got your co-ordinates. I'll call in a pair of Phantoms right on your hotel room.'

She nodded, her eyes fixed on the panorama in front of her.

'I gotta go,' he said.

'Hey, Mike.'

'Yeah?'

'Thanks.'

'Take it easy. I'll see you later.'

He headed back down the ridge hoping he had done the right thing, wondering what his father would say. He knew he would never betray his country to the communists. He just never believed he would have to haul down Old Glory for one of his own people.

A woman, at that.

Michael landed at Long Tieng half an hour later, and the Bird Dog he brought in was quickly configured for combat, armed with white phosphorus marker rockets. He took off again immediately and spent the next eight hours in the air directing Phantom strikes against North Vietnamese positions on the edge of the Plain of Jars.

When he landed for the final time late that afternoon a jeep pulled up on the ramp next to his plane. The man behind the wheel waved to him and indicated that he should get in beside him. Michael had never seen him before. He looked like a typical CAS man; they all dressed as if they were on their way to a game of golf. This one wore broad-checked pants, a short-sleeved yellow nylon shirt and aviator sunglasses.

After ensuring the O-1's wings were properly tied down and secured, Michael wandered over.

'Hi. Michael, isn't it?' the man said, too friendly. 'Came to talk to you about a friend of yours. Amy Duke.'

'Where is she?'

'Better get in,' the man said.

In the circumstances, Michael decided he did not have much choice.

95

He had never been inside the CAS compound, although some of the inhabitants sometimes visited the bar. He was taken to a small room inside the shack, and invited to sit at a table in the middle of the room. The man in the yellow sports shirt closed the door and sat down opposite him.

'Who are you?' Michael asked him.

'Just call me Uncle Dan.'

'Is that your real name?'

'Does it matter?'

Michael waited in resigned silence. They had found Amy.

'So, tell me, I'm interested. What did you think you were doing, Mike?'

'What have you done with Miss Duke?'

'Let me ask the questions.'

'You can ask all you want. But I'm not answering anything until you've told me what you've done with Miss Duke.'

'We're debriefing her, Mike. Like we're debriefing you. Cigarette?'

'Don't smoke.'

'Good for you. Do you mind?' Gerry Gates didn't wait for a reply. He lit a Lucky Strike and tapped the Dunhill lighter on the table top. 'Pretty stupid thing to do, Mike.'

'Just showing Miss Duke the sights.'

'Why?'

'She asked me.'

'You doing this for a bit of pussy, Mike? Is that it? Tell me it ain't so. You can get pussy anywhere over here, right?'

'I did it for my country, Dan. How do you like that?'

434

Gates stopped smiling. 'How does betraying your country's secrets help the United States, Mike?'

'Depends whether you think it should be a secret or not.'

'So you make those decisions do you, Mike? You're the government now?'

Michael sighed and sat back in his chair. 'Look, can we abbreviate this process a little. You're pissing me off.'

'You're pissing me off. too, Mike. More than you could ever know.'

Michael wondered what he meant by that. I'm not scared of you, he thought. I don't care what you do to me.

He thought about his father. Did he know what was going on here? Was this the crusade he had been on for the last fifteen years?

'Michael, I thought you loved your country.'

'Funny. I thought I did, too.'

Gates shook his head, as if this was the saddest moment in his life. 'I looked up your file. Your old man has a long and distinguished history of service to his country. How do you think he's going to feel when he hears about this?'

'I don't know. Why don't you call him up and ask him?'

Gates shook his head. 'You've got yourself a lot of trouble, Mike. You think your old man's going to buy you out of this? Is that what you think?'

'I'd like to see Miss Duke.'

'They flew me up from Vientiane for this little party, you know that, Michael? That's how serious this is.'

'I'm impressed.'

Gates dragged on the cigarette, Michael heard the crackle of the tobacco. 'She shopped you, Michael. We didn't even lean on her. She just fell to pieces and babbled out the whole story. Jesus.'

Michael leaned forward. 'Dan. Something I should tell you.'

Gates leaned forward, attentively.

'Fuck you.'

Gates got up and stamped out of the room.

'We want them disposed of!'

Gates smiled and shook his head.

Colonel Lee Lor slammed his fist on the table. 'They are spies! General Vang Pao will be furious when he hears of this!'

'We can't just take them outside and shoot them,' Gates said, reasonably. 'They're American citizens.'

'They are in a war zone. We can blame the enemy!'

Gates thought about Jonathan Dale. He had been his colleague once, and this was the man's son they were talking about. And as for the girl ... once you started killing reporters you bought yourself a whole bagload of trouble in his experience. But Lee Lor had made his point. This *was* a war zone.

'I don't know about this, Colonel.'

Lee Lor pulled his revolver from the holster on his belt. 'I will do it myself!'

Gates restrained him with a hand laid gently on his arm. 'That may not be the best way. Look, just leave this to me. I promise you, this story won't get out.'

Jesus. The things he did for his country.

Gates unlocked the door and held it open. He smiled cheerfully. 'Come on, Michael. Time to go.'

'Where to?'

'Vientiane,' Gates said, as if the answer was obvious.

'What's at Vientiane?'

'More trouble, Michael. Miss Duke is going with you. I guess the government will rescind her visa and send her back to the States. As for you, consider yourself under arrest. You're going back to Saigon, they can figure out what to do with you there. If it was up to me I'd put you up against a wall.'

Michael followed Gates out of the shack. A jeep was waiting. Amy Duke was sitting in the back, a Royal Lao soldier behind the wheel in front.

Amy had been crying. She would not look at him.

He got in beside her. 'It's okay,' he said to her.

'Goodbye, Michael,' Gates said.

'Uncle Dan's not coming along for the ride?'

'Not this time. Maybe I'll see you in Vientiane.'

He turned away and walked back into the shack.

*   *   *

436

Instead of driving across the airstrip, the driver headed up the winding mountain track to Sam Thong.

'Where the hell's he going?' Michael said aloud.

Amy leaned forward and questioned the soldier sharply in broken Lao and in French but he kept his eyes fixed straight ahead and ignored her. They bounced over pot-holes and rocks.

'Why the hell are we going to Sam Thong?' Michael repeated, and felt the first stirring of alarm.

Amy closed her eyes. 'It don't matter now, Mikey.'

'It doesn't make sense.' He thought about jumping out of the jeep. And going where? he asked himself.

'I'm sorry, Michael,' Amy said. 'I guess I let you down.'

The valley closed in around them. It was a primeval landscape, the lower slopes covered with thousands of white and red poppies and sunflowers as tall as a man. The higher crags were bare and wind-bitten limestone karst, dripping with moss and green slime. Trees grew from the cracks, roots groping along the sides of the mountains like talons. The high valley was shrouded in fog. It was late afternoon and the shadows were lengthening.

They crossed the ridgeline, out of sight of the base.

'I got so scared,' Amy said. 'I ratted on you, pal. How's that for a tough little New Yorker, huh?'

He squeezed her hand. 'It doesn't matter, Amy.'

It was the last thing they ever said to each other.

96

Michael did not remember hearing anything. It felt like something kicked him very hard in the right shoulder and slammed him back in the seat. The driver slumped over the wheel and a crimson stain blossomed over the back of his shirt. Looks like a poppy, he remembered thinking. Then the jeep swerved off the road into a tree and he saw the ground coming towards him and that was all.

A jumble of images, half remembered.

He was in the dormitory of his boarding school. He experienced a sudden and devastating loneliness. It ached in his gut, hollow and cold. It felt like baggage, and he looked for somewhere to put it down. The cold turned to fire and he knew he was dying, but he wouldn't cry out. Wouldn't give them the satisfaction.

He was in Amy's room in the Bungalow and the lemon dawn was creeping across the floor. He reached out for her but his arm would not move and there was a terrible throbbing pain in his head and in his shoulder. He whispered her name over and over but she did not hear him and he realised she must still be asleep. So he tried to get out of bed. He had to get to Wattay airport to take his O-1 to Alternate but there were people screaming at him and they held him down and he felt a sharp pain in his arm and then it was black again.

He was lying in his bunk in the Air Force Academy in Colorado and he was staring at the ceiling and trying to come to terms with the fact that he would never fly jets. He was listening to the excited chatter of a couple of the boys who had made it, and though they were once his friends, they were now somehow set apart from him. He wondered what his father would say when he knew he had failed.

A white figure moved across his vision, blurred like a ghost, silent on rubber-soled shoes. There were white spirits in the room, moaning and crying. Other spirits were bent over him and he had to strain to hear what they said over the terrible pounding in his head.

And then he heard another voice, strangely familiar, and knew he should recognise it. It was his father's. The voice kept telling him he was going to be all right and he was going back home.

Michael tried hard to remember where home was, but all he could think of was that they were sending him back to the dormitory again, and he cried out and told them he didn't want to go. He wanted to be in bed with Amy.

Then one day he was awake and there was a nurse leaning over the bed. He stared at the tubes that fed into his arm and his groin without comprehension.

'Hello, Michael,' the nurse was saying. 'You had us very worried. You've been a very sick young man.'

And he stared at her and tried to remember if he knew her.

And then he must have dozed off. And when he woke the nurse was there again and she was squeezing his hand. 'Can you hear me, Michael?'

'Where's Amy?'

'You're going to be all right.'

He looked around, realised for the first time there were other people in the ward, and that explained the moaning and crying he had heard. 'Where's Amy?' he said again.

'You're going to be all right,' she said. 'They're sending you back home.'

'Where's Amy?'

'Who's Amy, Michael?'

'Amy Duke.'

'Michael, I don't want you to worry about that now. You're going home.'

And that's when he knew: Amy Duke was dead.

*   *   *

439

He arrived at Travis Air Force Base in San Francisco. His hair was shaved to a stubble, a stitched blue scar extending from his temple to an inch above his right ear. His right arm was in a cast and his left hand held a cane. But he was in uniform. For the first time in months he was again wearing the uniform of an officer in the United States Air Force.

A colonel at the base shook his head and frowned. 'I wouldn't wear that downtown, son,' he said. 'Feelings are running pretty high back here.'

97

Susan wept when she saw him. His father's face was set like stone. He embraced Michael, stiffly, and helped him with his bags up to the house. They were surprisingly formal with each other, Michael thought. Perhaps a certain intimacy with death did that to people.

Susan had prepared a special dinner, just the three of them. They asked him about his wounds, but carefully avoided the subject of how they had been caused; they spoke in careful whispers, like mourners at a wake. Several times he caught his mother staring in horrified fascination at the scar on his skull. She appeared remote; she had felt the disgusting breath of grief too close, and now she wanted to distance herself from him.

'Where's Jen?' he said at one point.

He saw them exchange a glance. 'She'll be along later,' Susan said brightly.

A low grey blanket of cloud obscured the bay and the Oakland Bridge. The wind moaned, and rattled the window panes. By evening it had picked up and they could hear the waves slapping against the rocks. The lights of the city were blurred by the rain weeping down the windows.

Michael realised they had exhausted their repertoire of small talk. 'I think I'll go to bed,' he said. 'I'm tired.'

They put him in his old room. The pennants and the posters from his adolescence were still there on the wall; the Giants, Raquel Welch, a blown up photograph of a Cessna 195. It was as if he had stepped back five years in time.

Dale and Susan had pinned a map of South East Asia to the wall, with little American flags attached to Pleiku, Saigon, Vientiane, alongside all the photographs he had sent home; a grainy black and white of himself next to an O-1, a holster on his hip; a group shot of the Ravens outside the hootch; one of Ly May in a Giant's cap.

Wherever she was now.

He sat down on his bed. His father carried his bag from downstairs and set it down on the floor. He closed the door gently behind him and sat down at the old study desk.

'Your mother took it hard,' he said.

Michael nodded, unsure what to say.

'When we got the telegram, she just assumed...'

'I was lucky.'

Dale tapped his temple at the level of Michael's scar. 'How is it?' he asked for the fourth time that afternoon.

'Hey, I'll be all right.'

'So. You want to tell me what happened, Mike?'

'What did they tell you?'

'They said it was an ambush. You were in a jeep somewhere.'

'Well, there's not much more to tell.' Not unless I opt to tell you the truth, Michael thought. It seemed the Air Force had reverted to damage control. They had given him a Purple Heart and an honourable discharge. No further mention was made of the incident at Long Tieng. That had been buried in a file somewhere.

Amy Duke had been buried by her family in New York.

'Took a while to get home tonight,' Michael said. 'Got caught up in a demonstration. People really don't want this war, huh?'

'Forget all that. You did a great job, Michael. All of you boys over there, you did a great job.'

'A great job.' He closed his eyes.

'Jenny was supposed to be here tonight,' Dale said. Michael watched his father's face crumple. The disintegration was as sudden as it was unexpected. 'I did the best I could,' he said, and put his head in his hands.

Jenny had moved off campus, had not finished her degree. Dale was no longer sure where she was living, but she was working in a coffee shop in North Beach. Michael took the ferry across the bay the next morning, the address scribbled on a piece of paper in the back pocket of his jeans.

442

The trolley car dropped him two blocks from the café, but it took him almost half an hour to walk there. He could only walk with the aid of a cane, which he held in his left hand, his right arm still held against his chest in a cast and sling. Hills were not ideal for a man with a cast on his leg, and any exertion at all made his chest ache like fire. But they told him he would get back almost all movement eventually. Physiotherapy, Michael. Exercise.

He found the address Dale had given him. Formica tables sprawled over the sidewalk. Inside the café customers warmed themselves behind the glass, smoking and reading newspapers. He saw Jennifer balancing two espressos, wearing a long-sleeved brown jersey and brown skirt, her hair tied back in a severe pony tail.

He watched her through the window, shocked by her appearance. She had lost a lot of weight and there were hollow rings under her eyes.

He pushed open the door and went in. People looked up and stared. I guess I don't look a whole lot better, he thought.

Jennifer almost dropped her order pad. There was a hurried conversation in whispers to a grey-haired Latin behind the espresso machine and then she came over. 'I can only get five minutes,' she said.

He shrugged.

'Espresso?'

'Yeah, fine. Whatever.'

He sat down. It was a difficult process, balancing on his right leg, steadying himself with the left hand, swinging his whole body weight around as he eased himself down. He was still getting his breath back from his walk when Jennifer returned with the espressos. 'Jesus, look at you,' she said.

'I was about to say the same thing.'

Her nose was wet. She wiped at it with the back of her hand and lit a cigarette. Suddenly, impulsively, she threw her arm around his neck and kissed him. She drew away before he could respond.

'What did they do to you, Michael?'

He was sensitive about the scar, his shaved hair had not yet

443

grown back to cover it. He ran his hand across the bristles self-consciously.

'Rifle grenade.'

'You forgot to go to work in your airplane?'

He smiled. 'I guess.'

'If I'd known what they were going to do to my baby brother over there, I wouldn't have let you go.'

He sipped his espresso and waited for her to talk.

She looked at her watch, more sniffing. 'I only got five minutes,' she repeated. 'The boss doesn't like me doing this.'

'I'm a returning war hero.'

'Not in this town, Michael.' She rubbed her forehead. Her hands were shaking. 'I didn't want you to see me like this.'

'Dad said you're on the methadone program.'

She fought back tears.

'I thought you were clean.'

'Don't lecture me, okay?'

'I just don't understand.'

'I can't talk about this here. It's complicated, Michael. I didn't mean for it to happen.'

'Is it this boyfriend of yours?'

'No, Michael! If it wasn't for Scott ... he helped me get through this.'

Michael reached out and took her hand. Skin and bone. 'Dad's a mess.'

'I can't help that,' she said, and pulled her hand away. She lowered her voice. 'I don't want to talk about this here.'

'You promised him, Jenny.'

She swallowed hard, fighting back tears. Then her pride took over, and her expression changed suddenly from grief to defiance. 'He can't run my life. Where was he when we needed him, huh, Michael?' She looked up. 'Oh, Jesus.'

Michael looked up, saw a tall, baby-faced man wearing a grandfather shirt and jeans. There was a silver peace symbol around his neck, and he had a small goatee beard. He looked soft and serene.

Jennifer's tone was apologetic. 'Hi, Scott. This is my brother, Michael.'

Scott held out his hand. It was cool and smooth, like a

woman's. Michael's attention was still focused on his sister. She had the cringing look of a beaten dog, and he felt himself getting angry. She jumped up suddenly and went to fetch Scott an espresso.

'What happened to you, Michael?' Scott asked him.

'I fell off a ladder.'

'Jenny said you were in Viet Nam.'

'Over it more than I was in it.'

Scott glanced at the scar on his head, and raised an eyebrow. 'Just got back, huh?'

'That's right.'

'How many Vietnamese did you kill over there?'

Michael had seen it coming, was ready for it. 'Lost count after a while, you know how it is. So then you just count the ones under twelve. I must have got at least forty of those.'

'You have the same sense of humour as your father,' Scott said and turned away, his lips drawn in a thin white line of contempt.

Jennifer hurried back to the table. 'I've got to get back to work, Michael.'

'How about we get together for lunch or something?'

Jennifer looked at Scott before shaking her head. 'I'll call you, okay?'

'We're all worried about you, Jenny.'

'I just need some time on my own to sort things out, okay?' Sniff.

Michael looked at Scott. 'You better look after her.'

'Big war hero's threatening me,' he said to Jennifer.

Michael grabbed him by the hair. Everyone in the café stopped what they were doing and stared. 'Don't fuck with me,' Michael hissed.

Scott did not react. 'Peace, man,' he whispered.

Michael knew he was making a fool of himself. A one armed, one legged man trying to start a fight. Jennifer was staring at the floor, ashamed. He released his grip and struggled to his feet. Hard to retreat with pride when your ankle's in three pieces, he thought.

He limped out into the street as fast as he could, embarrassed and confused. It hurt him to realise that after all those years under the same roof he and Jenny had nothing in common. Their whole family had grown up in units of one. Susan without a husband, them without a father, he and Jennifer thinking of themselves as only children. But she was still his sister, damn it, and he did not want to see her hurt.

But perhaps it was too late for all such pious hopes.

When Jennifer got back to the apartment that evening, Scott was waiting for her in the bedroom. He was lying on the bed, wearing just a pair of jeans. There was a strap and a syringe lying on the floor next to the bed.

She stood in the doorway, watching him with hungry eyes. 'Did you score?'

'Maybe,' Scott said.

'Please,' she said.

'You gotta do something for me first, remember?'

He got up and unbuttoned his jeans. She knelt in front of him and closed her mouth over his soft penis.

'Come on, babe. You're going to have to work hard for your daddy,' he whispered. 'Work real hard for me.'

98

As soon as he was able to walk without the cane Michael bought a ticket on a civilian Pan Am flight to Saigon. For two weeks he walked round the military hospitals and the orphanages with his photograph of Ly May in her Giants baseball cap, and his story of a wounded refugee who had been brought to Saigon from Udorn. He tried everywhere, from the military hospital at Cong Hoa to the Nhi Dong Children's Hospital in Cholon.

But he did not find Ly May.

Finally, he was reduced to walking the streets. When he left his hotel in the morning, he would spend the entire day looking into the faces of every *bui doi* he saw, searching for her among the armies of bootblacks and beggars on the sidewalks, the street kids hawking Capstans and Juicy Fruit and garlands of flowers from paper bags outside the Caravelle. At nights he wandered aimlessly along the Tu Do and the Truong Minh Gian, mingled with the GIs who prowled the neon-lit bars, always wondering if he turned just one more corner whether he would find her squatting in the shadows, her eyes sightless, her hand outstretched.

But he did not find her. Perhaps she had died in hospital. In the end it might be a better fate. But he would never know for sure, and he knew that uncertainty would haunt him for the rest of his life.

99

Continental Hotel, Saigon

Rivelini's breath smelled of the vermouth cassis he had had with lunch, and of the foul Russian cheroots he liked to smoke. It also carried the taint of something else: death. The flesh had fallen off the cheek bones, leaving his eyes sunken in his head. He reminded Baptiste of an emaciated owl. His expensive suit hung off his frame as if it was two sizes too large.

Baptiste tried not to allow his shock to register on his face. 'Marcel!'

Rivelini raised a languid hand in greeting and did not get up.

'How are you, *mon vieux*?'

'How do you think?'

'You've lost a bit of weight. Been sick?'

'I'm dying,' he said, his voice flat, and nodded to the white-uniformed waiter for another drink. 'What are you having?' he asked.

'A pastis.'

When the waiter had gone, Rivelini took out his cheroots and lit one. As he inhaled, he erupted into a fit of coughing. When the spasm was over, he sighed and sat back in his chair.

Baptiste stared at him. 'Dying?'

'Lung cancer.' He held up the cheroot. 'Doctor said it's these fucking things. What does he know?'

Baptiste's first thought was of Rivelini's position in the chain that led to the *Union Corse* in Marseille. His second thought was: Poor Marcel. 'I'm sorry.'

'What are you sorry about? It's not you that's dying.'

There was a hoot of laughter from the lobby. A crowd of Texan engineers in Hawaiian shirts were standing around, their voices carrying clearly on to the terrace. Americans. The war was going badly for them but their confidence never seemed to diminish.

Another waiter manoeuvred a linen-covered trolley through the potted palms, its shelves filled with baskets of sweet rolls and croissants. Baptiste waved him away. Rivelini's death sentence had made him nauseous. It was not from any sense of personal grief, of course; it was just the proximity of death itself that scared him.

Rivelini seemed unnaturally sanguine. 'This is good news for you,' he was saying. 'The way things are going in Saigon, I suppose you'll be thinking about establishing yourself in Bangkok in my place.'

'Let's not talk about it now, Marcel. This is terrible news.'

'Oh, fuck you, Baptiste. Don't patronise me.'

There was a long and tense silence. 'How long does the doctor say you have?' Baptiste asked him finally.

'Three months. Is that too long to wait?' Ah, here was the bitterness, the anger, at last. 'There's a queue, you know.'

'A queue?'

'Remember Mittard? Of course you do. You tried to kill him once.'

'How am I supposed to remember everyone I've tried to murder?' Baptiste said, deadpan.

'He tried to take over your territory in Laos. He's still at it. In more ways than one.'

'What do you mean by that?'

'I heard he's seeing Noelle.'

Baptiste felt himself tense. The smile on Rivelini's haunted face told him it was the reaction he was looking for.

'I don't know if he's sleeping with her,' Rivelini went on, 'but you know his reputation.'

The waiter arrived with their drinks. Baptiste swallowed his quickly. He felt as if he'd just bitten down on something foul. Rivelini broke into another coughing fit, and when it was done he looked pale and exhausted. He flicked the butt of his cheroot into one of the flower boxes that lined the terrace.

The sky erupted, the monsoon clouds that had been building all morning burst into the street. The Tu Do quickly flooded, the drains unable to cope with the deluge, and the road was soon ankle deep in water.

Rivelini had to raise his voice over the hammering of the rain. 'You still want her back, don't you?'

'I've never let her go.'

'That is funny.'

Rivelini, the dead man, was jeering at him. Baptiste wanted to throttle him. 'What's funny?'

'When you're a ghost the whole world seems funny. And futile. You think you are going to live for ever, Baptiste? I tell you, when you are about to leave all this...' He waved a hand that encompassed the hotel, the street, the whole bloody battlefield of Viet Nam. 'When you are going to leave it all behind, it just seems pointless. What were we doing it all for? Perhaps the *bonzes* are right. Life is just the soul's journey of learning.'

'There is no soul – we die and that's it.'

'You hope.'

Rivelini lit another cheroot.

'Why don't you give those things up?' snapped Baptiste.

'Why? It's the only consolation I have left. I can smoke as much as I want now and it isn't going to make one fucking bit of difference.' He raised his glass. '*Salut!*'

100

Bangkok

She was put on this world to break my heart, Baptiste thought as he watched her cross the terrace of the Alliance Française. She wore a silk blouse of pale mauve that accentuated the violet of her eyes, and the slit black skirt was sheath tight. Her body was still as slim and svelte as he remembered, and her walk had the grace of a fashion model and the assurance of a princess.

They greeted each other formally, and for a while discussed their lives with the measured politeness of former enemies. Noelle had begun her own business, importing fashion direct from Paris, and had opened two new shops in arcades at the Indira Regent and the Dusit Thani. They discussed Lucien and his schooling at length.

The afternoon was sticky warm, an afternoon thunderstorm building over the South China Sea. A fetid wind gusted over the city, and in the distance they could see kites flying over the Sanam Luang. The river twitched, thick and heavy from the tropic rains. An endless traffic of sampans scurried by, loaded with rice from the Central Plains.

'So, what are you doing in Bangkok?' Noelle asked him finally. 'Are you spying on me?'

'I am looking for somewhere to live.'

Noelle's face set like stone. 'Why?'

'The situation in Saigon is uncertain. I will have to find another home. Bangkok is the logical choice. But there is another, more pressing reason. Marcel Rivelini is dying.'

'You're ambulance chasing?'

'I would not have put it so indelicately.'

She shook her head. 'How much has this to do with Marcel and how much has it to do with me?'

'You know I still love you.'

'Yes, I know. It just doesn't matter to me any more.'

He ignored the barb, and leaned forward. 'There is something else that disturbs me. I have heard rumours that you have been seeing Christian Mittard.'

Noelle stiffened. 'What business is it of yours?'

'You are still my wife.'

'In name only.'

'He is using you. How can you be so stupid? This is just revenge.'

He cursed himself as soon as the words had left his mouth. He saw the triumph in her eyes at this implicit admission of guilt. 'And why would he want revenge, Baptiste?'

'You know he has always thought I was the one responsible ... for the loss of his aircraft.'

'Which your friend happened to be flying at the time.'

'Please, let us not drag this up again.'

'I can imagine it must be painful for you.'

'Just tell me,' he hissed. 'Have you slept with him?'

'I cannot believe your presumption!'

'Have you?'

'I have no intention of answering that question, for two reasons. One, because it is none of your damned business.'

'And two?'

'Because not knowing will drive you crazy.'

For a moment he was too furious to speak. Let him stew, she thought. Of course she had not slept with Christian Mittard, she could not tolerate the man. But the French community in Bangkok was small and parochial, and she could not stop him pursuing her. She had no doubt Mittard would like to sleep with her, if she let him. She also knew that his interest in her was more than carnal. Of course she knew. What kind of an idiot did Baptiste think she was?

'Come back to me,' he whispered. 'This craziness has gone on long enough.'

She looked into her glass. 'Does vermouth burn?'

'Is that your answer?'

'Yes. Yes it is. You were the love of my life, Baptiste. I will never love another man the way I loved you, if that is any consolation. But you have become something else, and I want no part of it now. I may not be happy, but I am at peace. And please remember, I will choose my lovers and not you.' She looked at her watch. 'I think I must go now. Thank you for the drink.'

Baptiste watched her walk away. He angrily lit a cheroot, then remembering Rivelini, snatched it out of his mouth and flicked it over the side of the terrace.

To a man of Christian Mittard's jaded appetites, Hue Hue was a revelation. He had hired her for his nightclub in Patpong, but he made it a rule to break in all his girls personally before putting them to work. Hue Hue had been trained at an exclusive massage parlour in Chiang Mai owned by Marcel Rivelini, and came with his personal recommendation.

She was a small, cat-like girl with almond eyes and short-cropped glossy hair. She wore a black, backless napa leather leotard that clung to her vulva, and exposed the dark aureoles of her nipples. Seamed black stockings, ankle boots, a silver ankle chain and fingerless leather gloves completed the erotic costume.

She was not pliant, like some of the others, and for his own amusement he allowed her to take control. She turned off all the lights and lit scented candles around the room. Then she led him to the bed, and took off his clothes.

She massaged him with warm oil; his thighs, then his torso and his chest, then concentrated her attention not on his groin but on his nipples, as if he were a woman. He tried to touch her, but she pushed his hands away. After an hour of this, he was begging her to do something.

Finally she straddled him on the bed, but still she would not remove her clothes. Instead she pulled the crutch of her leotard to one side and guided him inside her. Again he tried to fondle her, but she pinned his hands above his head, leaning forward so that her small breasts grazed his chest. Her tongue darted over his eyes, his throat, his shoulders, in quick, butterfly movements.

Instead of moving her body in rhythm with him, she stroked

and squeezed him with her own contractions. His spasm came quickly and violently and left him drained and spent.

She fetched a warm cloth from the bathroom and dried him. Then she began her ministrations again, this time with her mouth. Mittard was not such a young man any more, and he felt sure it would be hours before he was able to climax again, but she was expert in her art. He felt the tension building again, the sensations even more intense than before. As one of the candles gutted and died, he groaned and spasmed a second time.

'I must rest now,' he said. Hue Hue nodded and fetched his opium pipe. It bubbled softly, the rain beat on the roof. He drifted into a sated and drugged sleep.

Hue Hue showered off the residue of their lovemaking, and sat down on the edge of the bed to watch him sleep. There was an expression of genuine regret on her face. She took the syringe and the packet of white powder from her shoulder bag and prepared the injection as Baptiste had shown her. And then, knowing it would be his last time, she poured the rest of the warm oil over her naked body and lay down on the bed next to him. It was an extravagance, but when you are about to kill a man it does not hurt to take him to the gods one final time.

The vivid colours of reality and the roseate world of his dreams blended into one. It could have been a hundred bodies, or just one; he could feel and hear the pulsing of blood and the stretching of muscle, sensations so exquisite and acute that the pleasure became almost a pain. It went on for hours, every movement, every sound, exaggerated by the drug; the night breeze that cooled their entwined bodies was as cold as liquid helium, the murmur of the fan the roaring of a hurricane, the final rush a torrent that drained him like a geyser of boiling lava. Through it all he did not utter a sound or open his eyes, and the hours were actually just a handful of minutes. He sank into dreamless sleep, sated and at peace, and that was how he died.

Two of Mittard's bodyguards were alerted by screams from the master bedroom. When they entered they found Hue Hue kneeling on the bed beside him, hysterical. His face was already turning blue. One of the men tried to resuscitate him, while the other rang for a doctor.

The story quickly circulated in the French community that he had died of a massive heart attack while making love with his Asian mistress. By the time the autopsy belatedly revealed the small puncture mark on a vein on his left ankle, and cause of death was established as a massive overdose of ninety-nine per cent pure heroin, Hue Hue had disappeared from Bangkok.

She was in the apartment Baptiste Crocé had bought for her in Saigon.

PART THREE

The Drugs Bazaar

'He who will fight the Devil with his own weapons must not wonder if he finds him an overmatch.'
— Robert South

101

Gulf of Thailand, June 1978

The horizon see-sawed from sky to sea, sky to sea, as the boat pitched and rolled. Ly May wretched again, painfully, but there was nothing left in her stomach but bile. The sun was so hot it burned the skin like a scald where the salt water had eaten away the seams of her black pyjamas. She held a scrap of cloth over her head to protect her blistered face.

They had been at sea for eight days, had run out of water two days ago. The night before there had been rain and they had collected all they could in cans and tins and their cupped hands but it had not lasted the next sweltering day.

Already the babies had died, and two of the old people. Now there were just six of them left. They were clear of Vietnamese waters by now, but none of them knew if the winds and currents had carried them east to the Philippines or west towards Thailand or south to Malaysia. Either way lay freedom.

If they lived.

They had all helped to build the crude raft, two dozen empty oil drums lashed together with chains to form two hulls, old gunny sacks tied to the drums to protect their skins from the hot metal. It had taken months to complete, cycling to the creek whenever they could get away from the camp, following the vague track that led through the tall reeds and mangroves, to where the raft lay hidden in a muddy inlet. Bringing the diesel fuel for the ancient outboard motor was the hardest part, ferrying it a few cans at a time in a *xe loi*, a small cart they attached to their bicycles. They piled fruit and vegetables on top of the cans to hide them.

459

They had all escaped together one night but on the second day the motor had broken down and they had been forced to dump the fuel they had risked so much to obtain. The old couple had died during the night and they had made a sail from the shirt and the black pyjamas they stripped from the corpses. But two days ago the wind had died, and the raft had since wallowed on a long, heaving swell. Ly May sucked on the pulpy remains of a cusan fruit, trying to squeeze out a little moisture. She handed it to another woman, old Phuong, but she was too weak to accept it.

Great banks of cumulus broiled on the horizon, taunting them. They all knew they would be dead if the storm did not break over them soon.

'Look!' someone shouted. It was Bich, one of the young men.

There was a boat churning towards them, a moustache of water on the bow wave. It was a fishing vessel, three-masted, its sails furled, but they could hear the throb of its engines.

'Have they seen us?' Bich said.

'They must have done,' Ly May answered. It was difficult to speak, her lips cracked, her tongue huge and gummy in her mouth.

'It's over then,' Bich said.

Ly May wanted to feel happy. She wanted to stand up and wave with the others, but there was no strength in her body, and a part of her could no longer anticipate happiness. It was a distant memory of childhood, a shadow in a dark room. For so long there had only been survival.

The boat was close now, just a few hundred metres. It was wooden-hulled, it looked shabby and the paintwork was peeling. Already she could smell it, diesel and fish and wood rot. The fishermen were ranged along the deck, most of them just in shorts, some wearing sarongs.

Ly May saw the glint of a knife blade and she was suddenly afraid.

'I shall light a thousand incense to Buddha,' Phuong said.

The others were still cheering.

The fishing boat was alongside now, towering over the tiny raft. One of the fishermen – the one with the curved knife glinting in his sarong – climbed down a rope ladder and lashed the raft to the side of the boat.

Then he drew the machete from his sarong, shouted something in a language none of them understood and pushed Bich towards the rope ladder.

'What's he doing?' Bich said.

'Do as he says!' Ly May shouted.

Ly May could sense the fear now, in herself, in the others. Their jubilation had evaporated.

Ly May followed the others up the ladder onto the deck.

'Pirates,' Bich muttered to her.

There were perhaps a dozen of them. They looked like ordinary fishermen to Ly May, except they all had knives tucked in scabbards on their shorts or their sarongs. Their faces were hard, their eyes greedy and watchful.

One of the men gave an order, but none of them understood. So he stepped towards Phuong and started to rip at her clothes. She screamed and he slapped her hard, knocking her on to the deck. He kept tearing at her clothes, till her shirt, rotten with salt, came away in his hands. He emptied the pockets, searching for money.

Now Ly May understood.

Phuong lay on the deck, sobbing. He started to tear at her pyjama trousers, and two of the other men helped him. Her body was wrinkled and nut brown. The men laughed, at her age and her terror.

The one with the moustache saw a ring on her finger and roughly pulled it off. He examined it carefully then contemptuously tossed it into the sea as worthless.

Ly May saw another of the fishermen move towards her. She knew what he wanted. She quickly stripped off her pyjamas, and threw them at him. She saw the way the men were looking at her and tried to cover herself with her hands. Even in her terror her cheeks burned with shame.

Bich and the other men stripped too.

The fisherman with the moustache was shouting angrily, perhaps because there was no money or gold. What did they expect? They had spent the last two years in a Zone. Then he looked at Ly May and said something to the other

461

fishermen which made them laugh. He grabbed her arm and pulled her towards the wheelhouse.

Ly May thought he was going to kill her. She fought to get away and felt a clubbing blow to the side of her head and suddenly there was no more strength in her legs. She fell.

She felt his weight on top of her. He smelled terrible, of fish and sweat and tobacco. She tried to push him off but he pinned her arms above her head. There was a sudden tearing pain between her legs. She heard herself screaming.

It ended as quickly as it had begun. Suddenly he stood up and walked out of the wheelhouse, shouting to one of the other men, jerking his thumb over his shoulder at her. Ly May rolled on to her side, clutching her hands between her leg. She looked down at her fingers, and they were smeared with blood and the man's seed. It felt as if her bottom had been torn apart.

Then another grinning face appeared above her and rolled her on to her back once more. She fought harder this time but then there was another numbing blow to her head and she almost blacked out.

She felt numb for long seconds, and couldn't focus. The man's grinning, bearded face swam in and out of her vision as he tore into her again and again. She begged him to stop in every language she knew, in Vietnamese, in English and in French, but that just made him laugh even louder. He hit her again and the world went black.

When she recovered from the blow, the man was standing over her, wrapping his sarong around himself. She heard shouts from the deck and then Bich's voice: 'Ly May! Run! Run!'

She dragged herself on her knees to the corner of the wheelhouse. There was blood all over the deck. Phuong lay on her back with her throat cut, gurgling out her life. The fishermen were thrashing at the others with knives. She saw Bich break free and jump from the gunwale.

One of the other fishermen saw Ly May, and came towards her. She scrambled to her feet. The blood on the deck was slippery and she stumbled and fell. The man grabbed her arm.

She turned and raked his face with her nails, hating him more than she had ever hated anyone. He threw his hands up to his eyes and staggered back.

462

She jumped. She couldn't swim, and knew she was about to drown. Better that, better the embrace of the sea than these butchers. I'll choose the way it's going to end, she decided.

And then she was under the surface, the screams were lost to the silence of the water, and her body twisted in the agony of drowning.

It was Bich who pulled her to the surface. 'Don't struggle!' he hissed in her ear. 'I can't hold you if you struggle!'

She felt his arm around her shoulders and did as he told her. She felt no gratitude that he had saved her; she was past all emotion. In her head was a jumble of nightmare images and sounds with only one thought: Why had she struggled so fiercely in the water? Why was it so hard to die?

Water choked her lungs, sending spasms of racking pain through her chest. She heard the throb of a motor and realised that the fishermen were leaving. Why fight? she wanted to say to Bich. Without the raft we are going to drown anyway. What difference does it make? An hour, perhaps less if the sharks came? Their fate was written on their forehead. There was nothing to be done.

Then she saw the raft, realised the fishermen had cut it free before they started the slaughter with their knives. Bich was swimming towards it, across the current, making slow, painful progress. They were still a hundred metres away.

He would do it quicker without me, she thought.

By the time they reached the raft Bich was too tired to haul himself up, so they clung on with their fingers. Ly May retched up the seawater she had swallowed. The spasms left her so weak she could barely hold on to the raft.

A body floated past them on the current, leaving a bloody slick behind it. The sharks would come any time for the feast, Ly May realised. Soon she would have to make the decision to live or to die.

Through sheer effort of will she hauled herself up on to the raft and lay for a long time on the rotten sacking, lost to pain and exhaustion. Her groin felt like an open wound, and the sun burned her naked skin and there was nothing she could do. She was too weak to tear off some of the sacking to protect her body.

She did not know how long she lay that way but when she finally stirred and looked around Bich was gone.

Flying fish scudded across the rolling purple valleys of water. Black cumulus clouds broiled up the sky, turning the western sky the colour of lemon and lead. The sea began to lurch beneath her. Like riding an angry buffalo, she thought. She wrapped the crook of her elbow around the mast, pulled down the scrap of sail and wrapped the sodden rags around her body against the sudden chill. The sky turned black and rain stung her face, the waves sending gouts of seawater splashing over her.

She started to shiver.

One by one the stars were blotted out. Ly May knew that soon she would have to make another decision, the decision to battle for life during the coming storm. It would be so easy to let go, to drop away into the dark water...

She was not shocked by what the fishermen had done. Life was cruel, people were cruel, they only wanted what they could get for themselves. It was the little kindnesses that were perplexing, the great ones even more so. Like Bich. He had given up his strength and his own chance to survive in order to save her. Why? All he had done was keep her alive for the next torment.

What he had done was a mystery, and it made her want to hold on. She could curse him for that.

She prayed to the *phi* who lived in the water, to Buddha, to God's virgin mother. She prayed for the strength to endure a little longer. Because of Bich. Because of the little puzzling kindnesses she had witnessed in her life.

As the night closed around her, her body shook from the cold. She drew her knees up to her chest, and shut her eyes tight, until there was just a dim awareness of the maelstrom breaking around her. The raft bucked and tossed, the rain stung like needles, the sea slammed over her, leaving her gasping for breath between each wave. The *phi* roared and crackled and shot their thunderbolts across the sky, while she clung like a shellfish under the breaking seas.

I will survive.

I cling. I hold on.

102

There was no warning.

All she heard was the sound of metal being ripped apart, felt the raft tip underneath her. She knew she was falling, but did not release her grip on the mast. Instead it was wrenched from her with such violence she thought she must have dislocated both her arms. When she hit the water all the breath was jarred out of her, and then she was rolling over and over in the breakers, and knew that she was drowning. This time there was no Bich to save her, all her stubborn defiance of her fate had been for nothing.

She thought she saw her ancestor spirits in their dark blue robes, floating in the water, pointing the way home.

'I want to go back to the mountains,' she said.

'This way,' they said.

She reached out her hand, knowing they would take her back. Another huge breaker picked her up and rolled her cartwheeling up the strand and bumped her like driftwood on the sucking sand. Suddenly she was on her hands and knees, her chest a shrieking agony as it sucked in the air, working on its own, independent of her. She retched, seawater streaming from her mouth and nose in violent spasms, staring in dumb astonishment at a distant row of lights.

The water was ankle deep in the black streets and twice she stumbled headlong into pot-holes. The rain and wind were physical forces that buffeted her like a boxer chasing a staggering opponent around the ring, trying to make him fall. Ly May was no longer aware of her surroundings. She saw a light, and veered towards it.

It was a two-storey house, raised on stilts, with wooden steps leading up to a door at the back. She dragged herself up the steps and slumped into the shelter of the doorway.

A face appeared, silhouetted by the yellow light inside. A voice spoke in a language she did not understand.

'*Cun toi voi,*' Ly May whispered. Help me!

The girl shouted out again in the strange language and then bent down beside her. Ly May heard her gasp.

Then, in Vietnamese: 'Who are you?'

'*Toi là Nguoi Viet Nam.*' I am from Vietnam.

And then she passed out. She spent the next three days in the vivid, fevered world of delirium.

It was a bright morning when she finally recovered.

They were all gathered around her bed, dressed in simple *patungs*, their faces white death masks. Ly May thought: I am dead. But why are my ancestors all young women? Or are these ghosts, devils from hell, come to torment me for my evil doings like the Sisters in Saigon promised?

Her whole body seemed to be on fire, and her mouth was gummy and dry. Someone put a cup of cool water to her mouth and she drank gratefully. She looked around. She was lying in a bamboo cot, her body covered with a white cotton sheet. She looked down at her arms and saw there were bandages on them.

One of the women, a tiny Chinese wearing a cheongsam, stepped forward. She looked much older than the others, and Ly May assumed she must be in charge. She said something in the strange language which one of the girls repeated in Vietnamese. Ly May recognised this girl. It was the face she had seen on the night of the storm.

'She wants to know if you're feeling better?'

'Is she my great-grandmother?' asked Ly May.

The Vietnamese girl repeated this and all the death's heads laughed except the great-grandmother, who scowled and shot back a reply. The women, Ly May realised, were not ghosts. They were wearing face powder.

The young girl leaned forward. 'My name is Noi,' she said. 'What's yours?'

467

'Ly May.'

'How did you get here, Ly May?'

'On a boat.'

She repeated this to the great-grandmother who nodded as if this explained everything. The girls all twittered like sparrows.

'Mama-san says the fishermen found oil drums on the beach.'

'That was the remains of our raft.'

'But where are the others?'

'All dead.'

Noi repeated this and the girls sighed and made clucking noises with their tongues.

Ly May tried to move, but the pain was too bad. Finally she succeeded in raising the sheet a little. She looked down at her body. It was covered with cuts that had been smeared with a red dye that looked like betel juice.

'It's medicine,' Noi said. 'We called the doctor.'

'Thank you.'

'Please do not thank. We are just happy you are well again.'

'Where am I?'

'Ranchoi,' Noi said. 'Thailand.'

The one Noi called mama-san said something else and all the girls seemed to speak at once. The mama-san shouted at them and they all fell silent and looked back at Ly May. The old lady yanked back the sheet and examined her as if she was a fish in the market.

She said something and cackled with laughter. All the girls laughed too, except one of the older ones, who looked very angry.

'What did she say?' Ly May asked Noi.

'She said you have nice, firm little fruit. Not as droopy as Naree's. She also wants to know if you are a cherry girl.'

Ly May remembered the men on the boat, but she was too ashamed to tell anyone about them. 'Of course,' she said.

The mama-san sat down on the edge of the bed and squeezed one of her small breasts as if it was a watermelon she was testing for quality. Then, before Ly May could stop her, she leaned forward and kissed her on the mouth.

The girls giggled, even Noi.

When the mama-san stood up her voice sounded cross but the girls laughed at what she said and then everyone was grinning at her, even the mama-san. 'She said you can stay,' Noi said.

'Thank you,' Ly May answered, but she had no idea why they were all laughing.

It was later that Noi explained to her that it was a brothel. But it was not a bad place, she added; the mama-san was good to all her girls and Ly May had no need to worry. She would not force her to do anything before she was ready. She would be well looked after.

Ly May was not sure what to make of this news. She had very distinct ideas of what a brothel was like but the mama-san's establishment conformed to none of them. The girls seemed happy, and well nourished, not like the girls she had seen in Saigon before the end of the war. But the thought of becoming a prostitute herself appalled her. Still, for the time being, there was nothing else she could do but wait and watch and see how things turned out.

After all that had happened to her in the last week, just being alive seemed miraculous.

That night she lay in her cot and watched the girls get ready for their work. They applied their face powder and lip gloss with elaborate care, then changed out of their peasant's *patungs* into short frilly nylon dresses of electric pink, lime green and brilliant orange. Noi had a black leather skirt that barely covered her crotch, a cut-away top in black silk and knee-high patent leather boots. As the sun set they all smiled at Ly May and giggled and waved as they tottered out of the door on their high heels. She was left alone to listen to the thump of the music from the bar downstairs and later still, the theatrical squeals of her new friends and the thumping of the cots against the thin walls in the cubicles next door.

For almost a week Ly May stayed in the dormitory while the

coral abrasions healed. Through Noi she began to learn the other girls' names; there was Naree, who had a sick baby that she cared for in another room; there was Menai who had painful periods and cried every night for her village in the hills; and there was Pim who told funny and ribald stories. One night she described how she persuaded her customers to reveal their secret fantasies to her and then pretended to be so disgusted that they lost their erections or reached their sublime moment before they were ready.

'There was this rice farmer last night. And I said to him, "Okay, I do anything you want." And he says to me,' (here Pim theatrically lowered her voice), '"Could you, you know, turn over, on your, you know, front, so that, you know..." And I says to him: "You want me to do what? That's the most disgusting thing I ever heard. And I hear really disgusting things all the time!" And he was so ashamed he begged me not to tell the mama-san and paid me my money and I didn't have to do anything!'

All the girls liked that. Noi translated it for her, and the girls waited for her to laugh but Ly May was too appalled and could only stare at Pim in utter astonishment. The other girls mistook her outrage for embarrassment and giggled, and Noi said she was a proper cherry girl and she would have customers falling over each other to pay for her, as if that was a good thing.

One morning Noi showed her the rest of the building. On the ground floor there was a bar and restaurant, open to the street, where the girls could sit and talk with the customers. There were curtained cubicles upstairs where she had heard the girls at work that first night.

The mama-san gave Ly May strict instructions not to go near the bar, especially at night. Not until she was 'ready'.

Ly May had no intention of every being 'ready'; she had already made the decision to run away. She could not stay in a brothel. She had done many bad things already in her life, but she had always promised herself she would never do *that*. But then she wondered where she would run to. She had no money, no job, no papers, she could not even speak the language. Here she had a place to sleep, plenty to eat, companionship, and a friend and translator and teacher in

470

Noi. In fact, Noi reminded her of her big sister, before the American jets had chopped her down.

But if she stayed, she would have to become a prostitute like the others. Her ancestors would be shamed, she would go to hell or come back as a pig or a goat and every good Buddhist would look at her as if she was dirt.

She felt as if there were many people inside her, wrestling in her heart to be heard; there was Buddha and the Virgin Mary and even Mai Koo, the American from the sky; there was also a filthy little *bui doi*, as well as the half-drowned girl who had clung so stubbornly to a creaking raft of oil drums. They all fought desperately inside, screaming to make their own needs heard over the tumult.

That evening, against the mama-san's instructions, she crept downstairs to watch.

There was an olive green jeep outside, spattered with ochre mud, and the bar was full of men in beige uniforms with heavy hand guns on their hips. Noi and Pim were dancing next to the juke box; Naree was sitting on a soldier's lap, and the other men at the table were laughing. Naree stood up and led him towards the stairs.

Ly May ducked behind one of the curtains.

When she peered out again there was a young *farang* standing there, grinning at her. He must have seen her watching. He had a faded white T-shirt and a dirty blond beard. He had been drinking too many Singha beers and his eyes were glassy.

'Look at you, sweet baby, just out of school.'

Ly May pretended not to understand his English.

'You got the cutest little ass, kitten.' She felt his hand hitch up her *patung* and grab at her bottom. 'I could just tear you up,' he whispered.

She screamed.

Immediately the mama-san turned and saw. Her face turned purple with rage and she let go with a long diatribe in Thai and pushed the American away. He tripped and fell. The soldiers started to laugh.

The mama-san chased the *farang* down the stairs. She grabbed his T-shirt and propelled him into the muddy street.

'Fuck you!' the American yelled at Ly May.

'And fuck you too, you son of a bitch lump of cat's gristle!' Ly May yelled back, and ran.

The whole bar fell quiet. The mama-san slammed her fist on the juke box and it stopped.

Ly May lay crying on her bed.

She smelt Noi's perfume as she leaned over her. 'Mama-san says you mustn't let the men see you. She says you are still too much of a cherry girl and she doesn't want to torment them so much.'

Noi lay down on the bed and put her arms around her. 'Mama-san also wants to know where you learned to speak English.'

'In Saigon,' Ly May said, which was partly true.

'Mama-san says it could be very useful to you in your future career.'

My future career, Ly May thought. The idea of becoming a prostitute did not please her any more than it had before. But she could not run away now. In Noi, in the mama-san, she had found herself a family. This was somewhere she could belong. It was not freedom. But in many ways, it was something like it.

103

Noi took Ly May under her wing.

She taught her to speak Thai, and gave her clothes to wear, and taught her about life in a provincial brothel.

'The men who come here are just soldiers and policemen from the border,' she said one morning as they sipped rice soup together at breakfast. 'A few Chinese businessmen maybe. Sometimes there is some old rice farmer or fisherman who has saved up all year and then gets so excited he comes in your hand. All they want is a quick time. But you have to be careful of the *farangs*. They want to make you do all sorts of disgusting things. I tell them, if that's what you want, go to Bangkok.'

'You've been to Bangkok?'

'My parents went there when they got out of Saigon. My father had a big house once in Nguyen Du street, with servants and a Mercedes motor car. But he had to leave all his money behind. We came to Songhkla, my father's brother lived there.'

'What happened?'

'My father's brother had no money either. They tried to steal heroin over the border and the police caught them. Because they are not big guys, you know, they could not buy their way out of it. They put them in Bangkok and then they executed them.' Noi made a pantomime of a machine gun.

'So that's why you work here?'

'Someone has to support the family. I've got two little brothers and my mother cannot work, she is too soft now. She has lived in a house with servants too many years.'

'What will you do when you're too old for this?'

'Maybe I'll become a mama-san too,' she said, nodding to the old lady in her cheongsam who was waddling through the dormitory fussing over her charges like a hen with her chicks. 'She has made a big donation to the temple and bought her purity back. Now she is a respectable lady, a big businesswoman in Ranchoi.'

Ly May wondered if the Sisters in the orphanage would let her buy back her purity too.

'So where did you learn to speak English?' Noi asked her. 'The *farang* opened his mouth like a fish when he heard you talk English back at him.' Noi was impressed. Her family had fled Saigon when she was ten years old and she only remembered a few words of French.

'That was just a few bad words,' Ly May said.

'It still worked pretty good. Do you remember just bad words or do you know more?'

'I learned English in the orphan school.'

'You went to school?' Noi said surprised. She had imagined this skinny little creature had spent her whole life on the streets.

'My home was in the mountains,' Ly May said, for she still did not fully understand that she came from a different country. 'When I was little I had to go to the hospital in Saigon. When I was better they sent me to an orphanage, a Catholic place. There were nuns, some of them French, some Vietnamese. They taught us English and French.'

Noi was amazed. 'You speak three languages?'

Ly May nodded. Four really, she thought, but she did not know the name of the other language she had used when she was a child, was not even sure she could use it any more. It was so long since she had heard it spoken.

'What happened to you when the communists came?' Noi asked her.

'We had to leave. I don't know what happened to the nuns. For a little while we lived on the streets, begging and stealing, but I wasn't very good at it. One day the soldiers rounded us up and sent us to a camp.'

'You went to a Zone?' Noi said, wide-eyed now. She had heard about the special Economic Zones the communists had created. She had spoken to other Vietnamese who whispered about the Zones as others might whisper of the devil. 'Is it as bad as everyone says?'

474

'We had to confess we were an enemy of communism and deserved to be punished. I didn't even know what communism was. They made us learn slogans. "Our great president Uncle Ho lives in our hearts." And: "There is nothing more precious than independence and freedom." ' Ly May laughed. 'That's exactly what we all thought. That is why we left.'

Noi picked up one of Ly May's arms and pinched the muscle. 'You're all skin and bone. Did they starve you too?'

'They sent us rice. Everything else we had to grow. But the soil was just dust and all we had was hand tools, even for felling trees.'

'Did they beat you?'

'Sometimes.'

Noi touched the tiny puckered scar and the slightly drooping eyelid of her right eye. 'Is that how you got this?'

'That was another time,' Ly May said.

Noi sensed that the scar bothered her and she took her hand away quickly. 'You're lucky you got out, little Ly May,' Noi said.

'Getting out is easy. It's surviving the sea that's hard.'

Noi put her arms around her and held her and stroked her hair. 'You're all right now,' she said. 'We're your friends here. I'm going to take good care of you, little bird.'

Ly May closed her eyes. It had been so long since anyone had been kind to her. She wished they wouldn't. It only made it worse when life returned to normal.

Noi slept next to her in the dormitory. That night Ly May heard her get up and slip outside. There was something furtive about her that made Ly May curious. She got up too and tip-toed after her.

From the stairs she saw Noi squat in the shadows on the beach and put a needle in her arm. Ly May knew what she was doing, had heard about drugs even in the orphanage. The Sisters had warned them, of course, and some of the other children had talked about needles and a white powder called heroin.

She slipped back into the dormitory, and lay awake for a long time. Her new big sister was in trouble, and she wondered what she could do to help her.

The girls were getting dressed, fluttering between the bathroom and the dormitory, preening themselves in the long mirror on the end wall. It was early evening, the start of another long, monsoon night at Ranchoi. Ly May watched, fascinated at the way they put on their 'lipastick', how they powdered their faces, trimmed their pubic hair, examined their naked reflections in the mirror for faults and virtue.

The mama-san came in and her attention focused on Ly May. She looked her up and down and put her hands on her hips, a sign that she was about to make an announcement. 'Well, Ly May, do you think you are ready for your big night?'

Ly May had learned her lessons well in the past weeks, and she was able to carry on a conversation in Thai with any of the girls if they spoke slowly. She understood what the mama-san was asking of her. Her heart jumped in her chest and she felt herself go pale. 'Tonight, mama-san?'

'You can't be a cherry girl for ever. Someone has to pay for the food you eat and the bed you sleep in.'

All the girls were looking at her. Ly May nodded. 'Yes, I'm ready.'

The mama-san threw some clothes on the bed. Before Ly May could look at them, the other girls had surrounded her, holding up her new costume, debating, criticising, offering alternatives from their own wardrobe. It was like the Christmas party she remembered at the orphanage, everyone getting dressed up to play.

She put on a backless black top, bikini briefs, a pair of fish net stockings, and patent leather boots with high heels. The effect was startling. She had been enjoying regular meals for the first time in years, she had lost the scrawny, starved look of a child, and her bottom and hips had assumed a woman's curves. In fact she was even more beautiful than Noi, who was considered by the mama-san to be her best girl. Now Noi pleaded with Ly May to allow her to make up her face but Ly May resisted all cosmetics except for a little lip gloss.

'You look beautiful,' Noi whispered encouragingly.

Mama-san took Ly May's hand and led her downstairs to

the bar. As they appeared, the customers stopped talking and stared.

Mama-san slammed her fist on the juke box and silenced it. 'This is Ly May, my new cherry girl,' she announced. 'She is fourteen years old, and she has never even kissed a man before. So I can't let her go for just the normal price. Whoever she chooses will have to be clean and respectable and he'll also have to give me the highest bid.' Mama-san had waited for a night when the bar was full of police from the border. The police, as everyone knew, had plenty of money from taking bribes from the chiu chao who ran drugs across the border into Malaysia. They entered into the spirit of the occasion enthusiastically. The bidding got higher; one thousand baht, one thousand five hundred...

Then a man in a pale green uniform with a gun in a holster on his hip stood up, walked over to the mama-san and whispered something.

'My cherry girl has her first customer!' she cackled, and pulled Ly May towards the stairs.

'Who is he? What did he say?' Ly May asked her.

'He wants to pay three thousand baht for you! I have never had such a big price for a girl, never! He is a very important man in the police. You must be kind to him, all right?'

She led Ly May to one of the upstairs cubicles.

'I'm frightened,' Ly May said.

'There's nothing to be scared of. It only hurts a little the first time. I did it all my life and after the first two times I didn't feel a thing.'

'I'll try not to make too much fuss.'

Mama-san looked horrified. 'No! You must make as much fuss as possible! Scream! Yell out! Faint, if you're good at that sort of thing! Men enjoy it. Men are idiots.'

She went out, drawing the curtain behind her. The juke box started up again. American music. She stared at the narrow cot and waited.

The man joined his hands in a *wai*. '*Savaddhi krap*,' he said.

'*Savaddhi ka*,' Ly May whispered. Her mouth was dry and she felt her knees shaking. A real cherry girl. Well, she would not have to pretend very hard.

'I am at your disposal,' she said.

'What is your name?'

'Ly May.'

The man seemed nervous also. He took off his holster and put it on the chair by the bed. He looked at her, as if discomfited by her inexperience and probably awed by the amount of money he had just paid for her.

'Undress for me, please,' he said, rather formally.

Ly May obeyed with difficulty. She could not stop her hands trembling.

This is it, she thought. I am a whore. The Virgin Mary will strike me down on the spot, and I will be reincarnated as a snake.

She peeled off the body stocking, then removed her bikini briefs. She kept on her stockings and shoes as Noi had taught her. She crossed her arms across her chest and stared at the floor, her cheeks burning with embarrassment.

'Lie on the bed,' he said. His voice was hoarse.

He took off his clothes, tearing a button on his uniform shirt in his haste. As he stripped off his clothes Ly May thought: No, I don't want to do this!

But I can't run out. I will have to find some other way.

After he had gone, the mama-san ran into the bedroom, followed by Noi and the rest of the girls. They were giggling like school children, all talking at once. Ly May sat in the bed, the sheet pulled up to her neck, ashamed and elated.

'What happened?' every one was saying at once.

The mama-san, who did not allow her girls to drink during work hours, had brought a big bottle of Cola to celebrate. She shushed them all and sat down on the edge of the bed. 'Tell us all about it,' she said.

'It seemed so big when he took off his trousers.'

The mama-san cackled like a veteran. 'A real big one, hey?'

'I don't know,' Ly May said. 'But I told him it was. Like

478

Noi told me to. I said it was the biggest, most wonderful thing I had ever seen in my life, and I praised Buddha for giving me the opportunity to sacrifice myself to such a huge and wonderful thing of maleness.'

'You said that?' Noi said, giggling.

'And then I asked him if he would give me the honour of letting me touch it with my fingers.'

The mama-san exploded, delighted.

'And then?' Naree said.

'And then I told him it was as smooth as a piece of silk and hard as teak wood, and that if all men were like him then I was indeed fortunate that I had chosen such a career. I told him that I had never imagined holding a man in my hands in such a way would be such a pleasure for me.'

'And then?' the mama-san said, eagerly.

'And then I felt it jerk in my hands and it was all over. I think he was rather disappointed.'

The girls were silent for a few seconds and then they all laughed together.

'You mean,' the mama-san wheezed, 'you mean you are still a cherry girl?'

Ly May nodded.

Mama-san laughed so hard Ly May was afraid she must be having a fit. She slapped her knee. 'She's still a cherry girl!'

'Did I do something wrong?' Ly May asked her.

Mama-san hugged her. 'Do something wrong? Keep this up and I can sell that cherry a hundred times! Aiii-oy. *"May I touch it with my fingers?"*' And she broke into a fit of coughing and Noi had to fetch her some water.

104

For the first time Ly May realised she was no longer a victim of her own life. She had found a source of power, and that power was her own body. She knew instinctively that she had only discovered a small part of its potential. If a man would pay three thousand baht for just a half hour with her, how much more would he pay to have her with him whenever he chose?

For a smart girl, she reasoned, there has to be more to life than this.

After that night Ly May was just another of the girls. She slept and ate and gossiped with them, and every evening she changed into her bodysuit and her high-heeled shoes and danced in the bar-restaurant like they did. She learned what men wanted and what men liked and although she did not enjoy their hurried and furtive performances, she had to admit that her new life was better than starving in the Zone in Viet Nam.

She learned that Ranchoi was in the far south of Thailand, near Narathiwat. It was a simple fishing village, surrounded by rice *paddis*. Most of the people were poor, the mama-san's best customers were the police who patrolled the border and the chiu chao businessmen who occasionally came to town in their Mercedes motor cars to pay the policemen's bribes.

Ly May learned that she could choose which men she went with. If she did not like the look of a certain man, she would simply not return his stares. The local men knew that it would be impolite to try and buy a girl who had shown no interest in him. It was only the occasional *farang* who wandered into the bar that gave them trouble.

The girls lived an insular life, like the monotonous routine of an office worker. They slept late, spent the afternoons smoking and gossiping and attending to their nails, and worked every evening downstairs. They had three days off a month and if a girl had a family she would go to visit them. For Ly May holidays were meaningless. She chose to work instead and save her money.

The worst disaster that could happen to a girl was to get pregnant. Mama-san encouraged the girls to make the men wear condoms but of course they usually refused. Some of the girls also fitted a little rubber device inside them at the start of the evening and used a special cream that the mama-san bought for them at the local pharmacy. But these methods were not always successful, as Naree's baby attested.

After four months Ly May considered herself a veteran. The mama-san could no longer parade her as a cherry girl, but she was still able to place a higher price on her services than any of the other girls. After mama-san's share was deducted, she still made more in one month than most of the poor fishermen in the village made in a whole year. Mama-san even helped her open a bank account. She was always telling her they should save their money for 'wrinkle time'.

Ly May had lived half her life as a refugee, had survived the streets of Saigon, enforced labour in the communist Zones, and a week adrift in the Gulf of Thailand. Now, for the first time in her life, she had savings in the bank and a way to make a living. But every day, despite the forced gaiety of the girls and besides the little dramas of broken fingernails and snagged stockings, she lived with the greatest burden she had ever shouldered.

Shame.

All the girls noticed the change in Noi. She had become moody, and money began to disappear from the little boxes some of the girls kept under their beds in the dormitory. There were angry exchanges, even fights, and Noi was always involved. When Ly May asked her what was happening, she shrugged off her questions with silence and sullen stares. She had lost weight. Ly May watched her dress in the bath house. Her flesh used to have plump lustre to it. Now it was yellow and she could see her ribs.

Ly May knew Noi needed help, but she had no idea what she could do.

The palm trees bent like fishermen over the cool white sand, and the dawn breeze rustled in the casuarina trees. Ly May could not sleep so she slipped on a *patung* and crept quietly out of the dormitory.

Noi's bed was empty too.

Up close the beach was not as lovely as it seemed from the balcony of the house. The villagers left all sorts of rubbish behind them on the beach; plastic bags, rotting fish heads, discarded coconut shells. This morning the Gulf had even choked up a dead dog. The sun had only just started its journey up the sky, and Ly May hugged herself against the chill, feeling the gooseflesh on her bare shoulders.

She saw a silhouette against the bole of a coconut tree, and ventured closer. It was Noi, hunched and shivering, her face half in shadow.

'Noi? Are you all right?'

Noi jerked around, startled. She was trying to hide something in her *patung*. 'Ly May. I didn't hear you.'

'I couldn't sleep.'

'What have you got there?'

'Nothing. I haven't got anything.' Whatever is was, Noi had pushed it into the sand. Ly May flopped down next to her friend. Without warning she grabbed Noi's arm and turned it towards her. There were tiny ugly scabs along the inside.

Noi pulled her arm away.

'Everyone knows,' said Ly May.

Noi did not answer. She looked terrified. There was sweat on her cheeks.

'You wear dresses with long sleeves at night, and during the day you walk around with your arms crossed like you have a stomach pain. All the girls know what you're doing.'

'I don't care about them.'

'I thought you were sending your money to your family.'

'I don't have a family. They're all dead.'

'Is that true?'

'It's none of your business, all right?'

Ly May reached out and stroked her cheek. 'I love you, Noi.'

She twisted away. 'Just go.'

'Please.'

Noi's manner changed suddenly. 'Don't be little Miss Cherry with me!'

'You're going to get into trouble.'

'I'm not a child. Anyway, it makes this place bearable. Maybe you should try it too. You'll like it.'

Ly May shook her head.

'A little poppy in your veins will do you good.'

'I don't want it.'

'Little Miss Cherry,' Noi taunted her.

So, life is getting back to normal, thought Ly May. My friend is my enemy, my new family is just a sham. Noi's kindness was just a ruse to coax me from my shell and hurt me again.

'You have to stop,' she whispered.

'Go away, Cherry Girl!'

Ly May left her sister squatting in the shadows and ran back to the house.

105

It was Captain Fantastic who finally exposed her vulnerability and drove Ly May from her refuge.

He was the same drunken American she had seen that first time she had ventured down to the bar. The girls said he had a yacht, and appeared in Ranchoi perhaps three or four times a year. He got on well with the local policemen, and all the girls thought he must be smuggling drugs on his boat. They all hated him, and whenever they saw the yacht in the bay they all pretended they had their monthly sickness or a bad cold so they would not have to work in the bar.

He was not drunk this time, but his eyes had that same wild look she sometimes saw in Noi's after she came back from the beach. His hair had been bleached by salt and wind, and he wore a dirty white T-shirt with CAPTAIN FANTASTIC printed on one side, a curling wave and a surfer on the back.

He drove up to the bar on a rented Honda motor cycle, and swaggered into the bar, shouting a greeting to the three policemen who were drinking beer in a corner near the juke-box. Mama-san looked fearful and watched him like a mouse watching a snake.

Ly May was dancing by the juke box with Pim, trying to interest the policemen, but it was too early for them. Captain Fantastic saw her and shouted out: 'How much?' He rubbed the thumb and index finger of his hand together. '*Cao rai?*' he repeated in Thai to mama-san.

'To you?' Ly May said. 'Five thousand baht.'

It was outrageous, she knew.

His face split into an ugly grin. 'Bullshit,' he said.

Mama-san ran over. 'She cherry girl. You leave be, crazy man.'

Captain Fantastic laughed. He slapped one thousand baht on the bar. 'One thousand baht. Now you put that pussy of yourn on the table next to mah money and we'll see if that little sweet thang's a cherry.'

Ly May walked away.

He went after her, a rattan stool spilling on to the floor. Mama-san's face was pale with fear. The policemen were watching too. Would they intervene on behalf of a prostitute against an American? She doubted it.

Captain Fantastic waved his money in her face. 'One thousand baht, cherry girl.'

Ly May thought about it. If I don't do it, maybe he'll hurt me or mama-san. Perhaps I can be clever. We'll see if the bamboo can break the knife.

She took the money and put it inside her halter top. Then she jerked her head towards the stairs. His leather boots hammered on the wooden treads behind her.

He doesn't want an act of love, she thought. He wants an act of violence. He's like a ticking bomb.

She watched him as he leaned against the door, his thumbs in the belt of his jeans, smirking.

'You ain't no cherry girl,' he said.

'Sure am, Joe,' she said, in her best imitation of Noi's casual arrogance.

'I bet you ain't worth a thousand baht, neither.'

'And how much do you think you're worth, you monkey-faced piece of cat gristle?' Ly May said, in Vietnamese.

'What was that?'

'I said you are very handsome.'

His lips twisted into a snarl. He knew she was laughing at him. He came towards her, twisted her around and threw her face down on the bed. 'For one thousand baht I'm going to get mah money's worth. If you ain't a cherry one way, I bet you're a cherry another.'

She felt him rip down her briefs and tear into her. The pain just went on and on. She bit hard into the mattress to keep from crying out, and she knew this new family was just an illusion and their kindness was another aberration in a cold world. She would have to find some other way to survive.

When she woke up next morning, Noi was gone.

'Where is she?' she asked Naree.

'She's gone.' Naree slipped on her *patung* and reached for a cigarette. She coughed and spat out of the window, scratching irritably at her rump. If only mama-san's customers could see their temptresses of the night right now! Ly May thought.

'Gone where?'

'She had a big fight with mama-san last night. While you were with the American.'

'What about?'

She did not understand all of the reply. Although she had learned the new language quickly, Naree's northern accent was too fast for her. But from what she could make out it seemed that mama-san had found out that Noi had used her days off to smuggle drugs across the border to pay for her own addiction. A triad from Bangkok kidnapped or bought small babies, killed and gutted them, and stuffed their abdominal cavities with heroin. They had girls carry them across the border into Malaysia, pretending to be nursing mothers.

The mama-san, who was now in the habit of going to the temple every day, had told Noi that the spirits of the dead babies would bring bad luck down on all of them if she stayed, and ordered her out of the house.

'She didn't even say goodbye,' Ly May said.

'Go and say goodbye now,' Naree said, yawning. 'The bus to Bangkok doesn't leave till eight o'clock.'

'Noi slept all night at the bus station?' Ly May had been in so much pain when she came to bed the previous evening she did not even notice that Noi was not around.

'Who knows where she slept?' Naree said, clearly as indifferent now to her former friend's fate as the mama-san herself. She slumped into the bathroom, the cigarette still dangling from her lips.

Ly May wrapped her few possessions – the bikini briefs, a

486

nappa leather skirt, some halter tops – in a *patung*, and ran out of the door.

It was still dark, the dawn only a lemon glow in the east. Scrawny dogs nosed at piles of rubbish in the gutters; on the beach the fishermen laboured in the semi-darkness, preparing their nets for the day's fishing. Siclo drivers rode up and down the main street looking for customers. Ly May hired one of them to take her to the bus station. He seemed almost pathetically grateful for the fare.

The bus was already waiting, and Noi was huddled shivering on one of the hard narrow seats. When she saw Ly May she gaped at her in wooden surprise. 'What are you doing here?'

'I'm coming with you.'

Noi's face betrayed, guilt, surprise, relief, all mixed together. 'You're making a mistake.' she said.

Ly May settled beside her, her body close to hers for warmth. She put an arm around her friend's shoulders. To her surprise Noi started to cry.

'You're the best friend I have in the world,' Ly May whispered. She had made a bargain with herself. If this friend betrayed her, then she would never trust anyone else, ever again.

106

Bangkok

Le Palais was sandwiched between a Thai silk emporium and an obscure government office. It was a tall building with shuttered windows, in a lane linking Surawong and Silom Roads. It had a good reputation among the visiting clientele of Thai, Chinese and Japanese businessmen; the interior was plush and clean and the girls were some of the most beautiful on offer and were checked regularly by a doctor. For this, clients were happy to pay the higher prices.

There was an escalator between the street level and the first-floor reception area. Inside the door was a shop mannequin, wearing a high-collared jacket and a silk wrap, her neck and arms hung with floral wreaths, her hands together in the traditional *wai* of welcome. It was customary for clients to return the salutation as they rode the elevator.

Beyond the reception area about fifty young girls sat on tiers behind a screen of purple-tinted glass. They wore silk evening gowns of chartreuse and black and crimson, their faces heavily made up, blunt bangs hanging down on their forehead like China dolls. They all wore a numbered badge around their wrist, like entrants in a beauty pageant. Some, like Ly May and Noi, had the letter 'B' in front of their numbers, indicating that they were available for body massage.

A plump Chinese matron wearing a cheongsam that seemed about to burst along its seams moved among the bevy of businessmen, encouraging or suggesting a choice with a throaty chuckle.

One of the men, a Chinese Thai, whispered two numbers

to the samlore. He repeated them into a microphone, which was connected to a speaker on the other side of the glass screen. Ly May and Noi heard their numbers and rose to their feet. They emerged from a side door together and led their customer to one of the escalators.

They got out at the third floor. An old lady sat by a desk near the elevator. She gave Ly May some towels, soap, lubricants, shower caps and contraceptives. The two girls led their client down a well-lit passageway, similar to a hotel corridor, with numbered rooms on either side. Noi glanced at the key in her hand to check the number and unlocked one of the doors. As they went in, the red light above the door blinked on.

Inside the door was a tiled area with a bath and an air bed, surrounded by a carved wooden screen. Beyond the screen the room was carpeted and furnished with a television, a banquette, table and chairs. It was like a hotel room in any international hotel, except the bed was set in an alcove, with mirrored tiles fixed to the walls.

Noi and Ly May exchanged a glance that went unnoticed by their client. Already, the two girls had planned their tactics, the result of many months of experience. They knew they would have to work carefully if they were to make any extras.

Noi stripped off her clothes, put on her shower cap, and ran a bath while Ly May helped the man undress. Then, while Noi bathed him, Ly May stripped down to her bikini and worked up a rich lather in a plastic bowl, spreading the creamy suds over the airbed. But she had taken one precaution: she had used cold water. Thais, especially Thai Chinese, were notoriously stingy and came even faster than the Americans.

Noi helped the customer out of the bath and laid him face down on the airbed for the body massage. Ly May put some of the suds over the man's back and buttocks, and then took off her bikini. She took up a press up position over the man and began to move her body against him in a long, sinuous motion. It was strenuous and exhausting work and after a few minutes most girls were exhausted. It was also the most dangerous part of the whole performance; if the man enjoyed his cloud burst now, he would not pay them more to finish the job some other way. Normally they could earn an extra one thousand baht to help the man to the clouds and the rain with their fingers, or their mouths, or on the vibrating bed.

To make sure their customer did not get too stimulated too quickly, Noi kept on her shower cap, sat down on a chair in front of the water bed and began to file her nails, gossiping to Ly May the whole time. Ly May made jokes as she worked, and once, when she thought their customer was becoming too excited, despite their attempts to distract him, she got up and turned on the television.

Finally the man told them hoarsely to get on with the job and a suitable price was negotiated. They dried him, laid him on the bed, and Noi pressed the button on the console marked '*Sanjuk*' – 'Fun'. The bed began to vibrate and the two girls worked on him enthusiastically. After his cloudburst, they bathed him once more and sent him on his way. They stayed behind to clean up the room, like domestics.

It did not take long for they were experienced girls by now, and they had the routine down to a practised art.

For a while, when they first came to Bangkok, Noi had promised Ly May she would stop using heroin. That was almost six months ago, and Noi had kept to her word. The continual sniffing stopped, and so did the shivering and the night sweats. The scabs on her arms healed, her skin took on a healthier milk-coffee pallor, and even the shadowed hollows in her cheeks disappeared.

But one morning May woke up and found Noi curled on the bed, in a foetal position, her whole body shaking, covered in a cold, oily sweat. When May touched her she cried out, as if all her nerve ends were exposed and raw.

'Noi? What's the matter?'

She whimpered like a small, wounded animal.

'What's wrong? Are you sick?'

'Help me, May.'

'Do you want me to get a doctor?'

Noi shook her head. 'No good. Just help me. Please.'

Ly May went down to the little bath house at the end of the alley, soaked a cloth with water and hurried back to the room. She laid it on Noi's forehead.

'There's a fruit seller ... comes to the corner ... every morning ... You know the little stall? ... Go and tell him ... you want something for Noi ... please, May ...'

'Noi, you promised!'

'Please!'

Ly May wanted to weep with frustration. She had started the drugs again! All those months she said she was going to give up, and all the time she was craving for more, just pretending! If she started the heroin again, it would kill her.

Noi screamed and sat up, brushing frantically at her body with her hands, her eyes as wide as plates, spittle looping from her lips down her chin and her breasts. 'Get them off me!'

Ly May felt the tiny hairs rise along her spine. Some *phi* had invaded her friend's body, she knew. She was in the presence of a demon.

'GET THEM OFF ME!' Noi shrieked, slapping hysterically at her own body.

'What's wrong?'

'The spiders! Get them off me!'

Ly May helped Noi fight off the spiders, killed them all one by one, but then the snakes slithered down the walls, their bodies cold and rustling, and Noi went into a fit on the bed, her eyes bulging, her mouth rigid and blue and flecked with foam. When it was over, Ly May was too frightened to resist her pleas for help.

'The fruit seller ...' Noi said, her fingers bit into Ly May's arm like pincers. 'Please ...'

May slipped on a *patung* and took her money from the little hiding place under her mattress. She hurried out.

The fruit seller was a young, aggressive city boy, with the accent of a southern Chinese. He wore a faded blue T-shirt with a decal of the Wat Arun printed on the front. When he saw her, he picked up one of the rambutans and shoved it at her. 'Very good. You buy.'

May shook her head.

'You want melons. Here. Feel. Very good, very cheap.'

'I want something for Noi,' she stammered.

491

Immediately, his demeanour changed. He became furtive. If there was a policeman watching us he would know straight away, May thought. What a clown.

'Where is Noi? Why doesn't she come?'

'She's sick.'

The fruit seller gave a knowing grin. Ly May wanted to hurt him, kill him even, for bringing her friend back to this. But there was nothing she could do now. And besides, if it wasn't him, it would have been someone else.

He produced a little glassene packet from his trousers and shoved it into her hand. 'You give me one thousand baht.'

'One thousand?'

'Come on, quickly,' he hissed.

Ly May fumbled in her purse and gave him the money.

He seemed to relax then. He gave her what he must have thought was a charming smile. 'Some for you?'

May shook her head.

'Is nice. Make you feel warm inside. Come on, you buy, won't hurt you.'

'You rump-sniffing piece of dog business!' she hissed into the boy's astonished face, and hurried away.

Ly May sat on the bed and watched Noi perform the arcane ritual with trembling and urgent fingers. Noi had turned her back to her, ashamed even now. She fashioned a makeshift tourniquet out of one of her belts, and scoured her arm for a suitable vein, wiping the sweat from her eyes with the back of her arm. She plunged the needle in quickly, and when she released the tourniquet gasped with the sudden rush of heroin and then ran outside into the alley to vomit.

May followed her outside and when she had finished retching, dragged her down to the wash house. She stripped her and ladled the cool water over her with the dipper. Already Noi had become dreamy and unresponsive, and Ly May had to support her all the way back to their room. She laid her on the bed and covered her with a sheet.

'Are you all right?' she whispered.

Noi smiled at her, her eyes unnaturally bright. 'I feel wonderful,' she said.

May dressed quickly for work. There was nothing more she could do, and the feeling of dread would not leave her.

107

The girls sat on tiers, behind the one way glass, knitting, attending to their make-up, or watching a dubbed episode of *The Brady Bunch* on the television that had been placed against the glass wall. The door opened and Noi came to sit beside Ly May. Her face was almost white with powder and she had on too much mascara and lipstick.

Ly May had not expected to see her at all that day. 'Are you okay?' she asked her.

'Sure. Don't fuss over me.'

Business was slow. The girl next to Ly May had her number called and through the door Ly May saw her leave with a middle-aged *farang* couple. Such special arrangements were expensive for the customer, but the girl still got a good tip.

'You have to stop, Noi.'

Noi ignored her, lighting a cigarette.

'You promised me you'd stop.'

'I can handle it.'

Ly May didn't know how to answer her. Handle it? She had been sobbing and helpless like a child a few hours ago, fighting off phantom spiders. 'You have to give it up. Look what it's doing to you!'

'I'm all right. Sometimes I still need a little to get me through a bad day. Nothing wrong with that, is there?'

It was as if the morning had never happened. She's convinced herself, May thought, she's convinced herself she's back in control.

James was a Canadian. He had visited the parlour twice that week, and had asked for her each time. He was delighted that she could speak English. The third time he came he asked for her number again, and paid the samlore another two hundred baht to take her home with him after she finished her shift that evening.

James was tall and rangy, with a sparse blond beard and watery blue eyes behind his horn-rimmed glasses. He wore a cotton Indian shirt and faded jeans with holes at the knees. She wondered how he could afford to come back to a place like Le Palais again and again.

In the taxi back to his hotel, he told her he had taken a year off from university to travel round the world. He had only been away three months and already he had spent nearly all his money. If you spend every night at a massage parlour, I'm not surprised, she thought. But James seemed to find the notion of running out of money amusing.

But he was gentle for a *farang*. He did not try to touch her in the taxi. They arrived at his hotel, the Atlanta. Cheap place, she noted sourly. He's spending all his money on me.

May ignored the looks of the hotel staff as they walked through the lobby and got into the elevator. When they reached his room, she immediately stripped off to her bikini and went to the window. The swimming pool below was empty, and shimmered under the courtyard lights. As she stared into the blue water, she imagined she could see her own reflection in the water. Youth and beauty, she thought, looking at the young girl with the long raven hair and perfect coffee skin, youth and beauty are all I have. They keep me alive for now, but these few gifts also have to buy my rice when I am old and wrinkled. She wanted to plunge into the silent, cool water, down into the chill blue currents, no Bich to drag her back to the surface this time.

Stop it, she told herself. This is just business. Just surviving.

When she turned away from the window James was lying on his back on the floor, naked. He had his head under the glass-topped coffee table, his fist clasped around his erection.

'What are you doing?' she said.

'Shit on it,' he said.

She thought she had misunderstood his English. 'You want me to sit on the table?'

'No, not sit on it. Crap on it. Please,' he begged.

Ly May stared at him. Girls who had been up to the American base at Udorn had told her some of the disgusting fetishes the Americans liked, but this was something she had never heard of.

'Just crouch on the table,' he mumbled. Even he seemed embarrassed.

'Are you crazy?' she said.

'I'm paying,' he said.

'No,' she said. Ly May picked up her clothes from the bed and walked out, left the money lying on the bedside table. She heard James shout at her through the door but she ignored him. She dressed in the elevator on the way down to the foyer, disregarding the leers of two long-haired German boys.

I have standards, she told herself. There are some things I cannot do. Isn't it enough that they want me to sleep with them for money? Do I have to perform every kind of depravity? I am young, I am beautiful, I should have a young boy who loves me. Instead I wallow around in the gutter with all this sickness. I have to find another way to survive.

108

Noi sipped a coke while Ly May blew the steam from her rice soup. The little restaurant opened on to the street and the noisy tangle of *tuk-tuks* and motorbikes and buses crawled past in the heat and pollution on Soi Sukhumwit.

'Can you lend me some money?' Noi asked.

'What for?'

'I need two thousand baht, that's all.'

'I lent you some money last week. And the week before that. You still haven't paid me back.'

Noi looked ill, even worse than she had looked at Ranchoi. There were dark rings under her eyes like purple bruises, and her skin was a sickly yellow. She sniffed continually.

'You have to quit, Noi.'

'I will, I promise.'

'Not tomorrow, now.'

'Look, it's not so easy. This is a bad time for me. I promised you. What else do you want?'

It had been like this for weeks now. If she did not give her money Noi would get the sweats and then the pains would come and she would writhe on the bed as if someone was burning her with hot brands. There would be fits and hallucinations. So Ly May always gave in and bought her what she needed from the fruit seller.

'I can't keep giving you money.'

Noi lit another cigarette with shaking fingers. She coughed and spat on to the ground. 'How else am I going to stand this miserable life?'

'I thought you didn't mind.'

'Didn't mind? You like it, May? You like waking up in the

morning feeling like a gutter? That's what we are, little May, just a gutter where men squirt their seed. Yesterday a man made me turn over and he did it in my bottom. I didn't even get a tip.'

'You should just stick to body massage if you don't like it. You don't have to go back to their hotels.'

'I need the money.'

Ly May pushed her rice soup towards her. 'You should eat. You're looking thin.'

Noi shook her head and pushed the bowl away.

Ly May hesitated. 'When I left Ranchoi, Naree told me you had been smuggling heroin into Malaysia. In dead babies. Is it true, Noi?'

She drew on the cigarette and shrugged. 'Oh, don't look at me like that. Like you're still a little cherry girl.'

'They kill the babies. They buy them and they kill them. You know that?'

'Maybe they do them a favour.' She threw the cigarette into the street. 'I have to go to work.'

'It's our day off.'

'Not for me, I need the money. Especially if my friends won't help me out.'

'It's going to kill you, Noi.'

For a moment she looked scared, a young kid again. 'I know,' she said. She tottered away on her high heels. Ly May knew there was nothing else she could do.

She got a bus to Tatien pier. She walked past the sweating, noisy tangle of coolies and hawkers in the dimly lit hall of the big market, and went down to the water's edge. She sat on one of the wooden bollards to listen to the gentle rhythms of the river.

The Chao Phrya, the Mother of the Waters, was slow-moving and thick, the colour of milky coffee. Heavy sampans glided past, long lines of washing drying on their decks; there were smaller sampans too, loaded with rattan baskets of fruit, women in straw hats poling them through the shallows. On the Thonburi side, the ceramic- and porcelain-encrusted *chedi* of the Temple of the Dawn glinted in the morning sun.

A clump of grass, torn loose from a weeded bank further upriver, was carried past her on the current. I'm like that clump of grass, Ly May thought. As soon as I was torn away from my roots, I no longer had any control over where I was going. Life just carried me with it, tossed and eddied with the currents, no hope of turning and swimming my own way. And where would I go if I chose? She had no answer.

Later she walked back into the city, along Rama IV Road, a cacophony of screeching brakes and car horns. An ugly, dirty city, she thought. Distant memories stirred, half forgotten, of hazy mountains, the warm smell of animals sleeping under a bamboo floor, of drifting woodsmoke, of fields bright with poppies and great forests scorching with fire.

But that was another life. She knew she could not go back there now. It remained an icon, a vision of faith.

To amuse herself and to pass the time, she wandered through the arcade of the Dusit Thani Hotel. She stopped outside a jeweller's window and stared at a gold bracelet in the window, studded with twin rows of blackish-red Chantaburi rubies. She raised a finger to the glass. So close, I can almost touch it. What would it be like to own such a treasure? she wondered. It was impossible even to contemplate. She could never imagine having so much money.

'Do you want it?' a voice said. She whirled around.

He was tall for a Chinese, and his hair was carefully groomed, brushed back from his forehead in western fashion. But it was his clothes that set him apart; the pearl grey Cardin suit, a wine-coloured silk handkerchief in the breast pocket, matching tie, black crocodile skin loafers. He wore magenta-tinted sunglasses and on his wrist there was a chunky yellow gold Omega de Ville wristwatch. He could have been a business executive, except for his face, which was seamed with ancient scars.

Ly May could only stare.

'Do you want it?' he repeated, and without waiting for her reply he took her arm and led her inside the shop. He pointed to the bracelet in the window and the proprietor fetched his keys, took it from the showcase, and laid it on the counter top for her to inspect.

This can't be happening, Ly May thought.

'Try it on,' the stranger said.

The proprietor helped her fasten the clasp at her wrist. She felt the weight of it, turning her wrist so that the rubies caught the light. The stranger asked the price. Two thousand United States dollars, the proprietor told him.

'Do you still want it?' the man asked her.

Ly May knew what he wanted. He was buying her. Two thousand dollars was a ridiculous price, even if she slept with him every night for a week.

'You can't,' she said.

'I can do whatever I want,' he said. He reached into his wallet and almost contemptuously tossed a pile of notes on the glass counter. The proprietor bobbed his head in gratitude.

'Are you hungry?' asked the man.

Ly May checked her reflection in the mirror above the counter. A plain pink silk dress, to the knee, with a respectably high collar. Hardy any make-up. She revised her initial estimate; this man could not have guessed her profession. So what did he want?

'You want to take me to lunch?' she asked him.

'You can show off your new possession,' he said.

A white Mercedes Benz with smoked glass windows waited in the forecourt of the hotel. A uniformed chauffeur held the door open for her. The stranger got in beside her.

The car was air-conditioned, the atmosphere inside almost frigid, the engine so quiet the sound of the cooling fan drowned it out. Ly May gazed in awe at the street she had walked down just half an hour before. It was the same, but from in here it appeared utterly different. Now she was cocooned from the heat and the fumes and the roar of the traffic. For a moment her eyes locked with those of a coolie sitting beside a pile of broken rubble on the road, sipping soda from a plastic bag. An hour ago they had sweated together out there. Now she was a world away from him. This was how life could be, she thought, if you had money. It couldn't hurt you any more. From here, its misery could appear almost benign.

'What's your name?' he asked her.

'May.'

'May,' he repeated, slowly. 'My name is Douglas. Douglas Ho.'

Douglas. He seemed hesitant in her company, for all his wealth and assurance. As if it was a performance he felt compelled to carry through. His fingers tapped impatiently on the leather arm rest of his seat.

'What do you do, May?'

Well, body massage, mainly. 'I am a student at Thammarasat University.'

He appeared to accept this. His eyes, she noticed, were cold and empty. Not a lover's eyes. The eyes of a predator. She felt a little afraid. She turned her attention to the bracelet on her wrist. She wondered again: what sort of deal had she just made?

'You live with your parents, May?'

'I live with a girlfriend.' She suddenly felt compelled to lie. 'My parents are from Songhkla.'

'And what do they do?' he asked her, though he did not seem really interested.

'My father is a schoolteacher,' she said.

He told his chauffeur to drive them to a little restaurant on Tanon Suttisan. She had never seen any restaurant quite like it. It was built on stilts above a pond filled with plants. A narrow bridge led to a kitchen in the middle of the pond; other bridges led to islands where the diners sat, surrounded by the croaking of frogs.

It was one of the most beautiful meals she had ever eaten. He ordered two steamboats, one flavoured with chicken and lemon grass, the other with crayfish. There was rice in coconut milk with paw paw salad, beef with salad in oyster sauce, pork stir fried with garlic, and Chinese *gaoliang* to finish.

He spoke desultorily, as if it were a burden to him. After the meal was finished, he said to her: 'You're very beautiful.'

She lowered her eyes. What a performance, May! she thought. You still remember how to play the cherry girl. 'Thank you.'

'I like to surround myself with beautiful things.'

'You have been very kind.'

'I am not kind, May. Never think that. I don't trust kindness, do you?'

No, she thought. Never.

501

'Do you like it?' he said. He nodded at the bracelet on her wrist.

'It's wonderful.'

'Let me explain something to you. I am the closest thing you will ever find to a god on earth, May. Worship me, and I will grant you favours. Any favour you wish. But like any god, I demand that my followers be faithful. Do you understand?'

He's crazy, she thought. But he's also serious, and he may also be right. Perhaps he is the closest thing I have found to a god. 'If I did not understand,' she said, 'I would not have allowed you to buy me the bracelet.'

For the first time, he smiled. It was a smile of triumph, rather than humour. 'I have been sent here from Hong Kong. Business, you understand. I can be very generous to someone who gives me what I want.'

Ly May took a deep breath. She was frightened of him but fear, she knew from her own past, should not sway a decision. 'Perhaps you should show me what you want,' she said.

They went back to his suite in the Dusit Thani Hotel. He slouched in a chair, watching her. 'Undress,' he said.

May wondered what he expected. An innocent little Buddhist girl? She had played the part of the cherry girl before, but never like this. He had bought her beauty. Perhaps he should have a bonus for his money.

She took off everything except the bracelet, and stood in front of him. She pushed back her hair with her hands, and slowly turned around. Let him examine the merchandise thoroughly, she thought. Her heart was hammering now. Let this god show me favour, she thought. Take my sacrifice. In return he can make all my prayers come true.

He watched her with hard eyes. A bidder at an auction, settling on his price. 'Make me happy,' he said.

'Stand up,' she said.

He frowned but obeyed, rising slowly from the chair. She helped him out of his jacket and shirt, then dropped to her knees and undid the gold clasp of his belt. His body was a patchwork of scars, and there was a huge cicatrice on his thigh, a jagged, livid thing that extended from his hip to his knee. She traced the contours with her finger.

His eyes glittered in the darkness as he watched her reaction. But he said nothing.

When he was naked she coaxed him to arousal. As she worked she looked up once and saw him in the mirror. He was not watching her; he was watching himself, flexing the muscles of his arms and chest in time with the rhythm of her strokes.

Yes, a god, she thought. And like all gods, he is vain to the point of madness. What he is in love with is his own power. I am just his accessory.

Afterwards he walked from the room without a word and she heard him running a shower. She dressed and sat down in the chair opposite the door and waited.

He came back into the room naked, carrying a monogrammed towel, water dripping from his body onto the thick carpet. He leaned against the door, the towel around his neck. 'Your father's not a teacher, and you're not a student,' he said.

She shook her head.

'Who are you?'

'I can be whatever you want me to be.'

He was silent for a moment, thinking about this. 'Next month I am moving to Bangkok. I have business here. I will be buying a house and I need furniture.'

She realised he meant her. 'I understand.'

'Where do you live?' he asked her.

'Off Soi Sukhumwit. Near the Grace Hotel.'

'My driver will come with you to get your clothes. You will stay here in the hotel until I have completed my other arrangements. Understand this – you are my property now. From today you do not even look at another man. You will disappoint me at your own peril.'

Ly May almost drew back. She was tempted to run from the room. After all, she had the bracelet, not bad for an afternoon's work. You fled Viet Nam looking for freedom, she told herself, and now you want to sell yourself back into slavery?

But had she ever really been free? A refugee isn't free, nor is an orphan. Or a prostitute. Life is giving you a chance, she thought, the first real chance you have ever had. Take it.

She murmured her compliance. As she got up, she thought about Noi. She couldn't just abandon her.

She took a deep breath. 'I'll need some money.'

His face twisted into an expression she couldn't fathom. Was it anger or amusement. 'What for?' he said.

'For my family.'

'Your family,' he said, and it was apparent he thought she had a lover she wanted to pay off for the sake of her conscience. 'How much?'

'Just something to tide them over until the next time I see them.'

His jacket lay on the bed. He took out his wallet and counted out five one thousand-baht notes and tossed them carelessly on the bed. He went back into the bathroom to blow dry his hair.

But when Ly May got back to their room off Soi Sukhumwit, Noi was gone.

Ly May's few possessions, her clothes and her shoes, had disappeared too. Ly May thrust a hand into her secret hiding place in her mattress. Noi had taken all her savings.

Every last baht.

109

San Francisco, May 1981

Dale had arranged to meet Gerry Gates at a bayside café near the quay. The parking lot was filled with Ferraris and BMWs, the sun deck crowded with braying young men with Rolex Presidentials on their wrists. A $100,000 Cigarette throbbed towards the pier.

He had not seen Gates in over ten years. The last he had heard he was back in Asia, working for an acronym he had never heard of, training local paramilitaries in anti-drug and anti-terrorist activities.

When he arrived, Gates was sitting at a table overlooking the water, California casual; mirrored sunglasses, a powder blue polo shirt, tan slacks and Sperry topsiders. His hair was completely grey now, and he had shaved off his moustache so that he looked almost benign, like a retired stockbroker or lawyer. His smile flashed like a beacon when he saw Dale and he stood up to welcome him. 'Hey, Jack, good to see you again!'

He embraced him like a lost brother.

'Hello, Gerry,' Dale said, embarrassed at the unexpectedly effusive welcome.

'You're looking great.' It was said with so much enthusiasm that Dale realised he must be showing his age.

'So are you.'

'Good living and a clean conscience. Come and sit down. I got us a table in the sun. Christ I'd forgotten how cold it gets here in spring, even when the sun's shining.'

He ordered a large jug of white sangria, made with Grand Marnier. They both ordered crab burgers.

'So. How are things, Jack?'

Dale did not commit. He had developed a standard response to this question, a lie that slid easily off the tongue. 'Great. Looking forward to retirement.'

Gates was silent, the perfect interrogator. He let the silence hang.

'What about you, Gerry? What are you doing these days?'

'Still with the Company. Only it doesn't appear on the stationery.'

'Asia?'

He nodded. 'The game goes on, Jack.' The sangria arrived. Gates raised his glass. 'To old soldiers. May they never die.'

'Old soldiers never die, Gerry. Just young ones.'

Gates took a big swallow of his drink. 'Hey, that's good.'

'Hadn't heard from you in so long, I thought you must have gone native. Or maybe the bad guys had got you.'

'The bad guys won't get me, Jack.'

'So what's all this about? You just call me up for nostalgia, or is this leading to something?'

'We'll get too that,' Gates said easily. 'Tell me about things. I heard you had a few problems.'

Dale wondered how he had heard, but didn't press the point. 'Largely my own fault. Couple of years after I got back I invested my Air Force pension in a condo development up the coast. The major partner was one of Susan's brothers.'

'Susan?'

'My wife ... my ex-wife. A year later I found out he'd used most of the shareholders' money to pay off debts on another land deal near Sacramento. I took a bath. So did the old man.'

'You still with Daddy's firm?'

Dale suspected Gates already knew the answer to that. 'He died last year. To be frank, I never had much interest in the law. A few months ago, I let the partners buy me out. So I'm not broke. If I'm careful, and don't make the mistake of living to be a hundred, I'll get by.'

'I heard it was worse than that.'

'Yeah? What was it you heard?'

'I heard that this condo deal just about cleaned the family

out. I heard that after the divorce settlement, and the death duties, you were still down six figures. I also heard you inherited some of your old man's problems with the IRS. I was told it was so bad you had your house on the market.' Gates' tone was gentle, almost apologetic.

There was no point in denying it, Dale thought. Gates' sources were, of course, impeccable. 'Well, that's the way it crumbles, cookiewise,' he said.

'Yeah, well, maybe there's still a few more cookies in the tin, Jack. Hear what I'm saying?' Their burgers arrived, and Gates immediately bit into his. 'Damn, that's good. Great to eat some place where they remember to take the shells off.' Dale could feel Gates watching him. Like a specimen in a jar, he thought. 'Why did you get out, Jack?'

'That's ancient history now.'

'You never really explained.'

'I was sick of it. Sick of losing. Sick of having to play by rules that *guaranteed* we were going to lose. You don't win a football game if you can't throw the ball over the halfway line.'

'Didn't have anything to do with Jennifer?'

Dale knew that Gerry Gates was not the sort of man who remembered names for personal reasons. He must have found this in a file; and to find it, he must have been looking. He realised he was Gates' latest case file. And wondered why. 'It was part of it.'

'Hey. Kids,' said Gates, as if that just about explained everything.

'Yeah,' Dale said. 'Kids.'

'Heard she got herself a little drug problem?'

'She's better now,' he said, as if it was a disease. Perhaps it was.

'Kind of like getting hit by friendly fire, isn't it?'

'How's that?'

'Jack, let's face it. Where do most of this country's drugs go? Used to be the hippies, the Haight, that shit. Now they go straight into the black and Latino ghettoes. Their natural home. But good kids like Jennifer aren't supposed to get hurt.'

'Jennifer isn't a good kid. That's her problem.'

'She comes from a good family.'

'It doesn't seem to help much.'

They finished their jug of sangria and Gates ordered another. 'So what are you doing these days?'

'A little golf, a little reading. I watch the news. None of it's good.'

Gates leaned forward, and now his eyes were bright with fervour. 'You can't give up the game, Jack. The war's still going on. The battlefield's just changed a little, that's all.'

'I don't care about any of that any more,' he said. He had lost his ideals, his daughter, his wife, his mistress. Guilt and betrayal. After a while they both felt the same, heavy and numb, they sat in the gut like lead and you didn't know which of them was killing you.

It wasn't that he thought he could have saved the world from communism. Oh, once he had believed that, as fervently as any missionary. But not any more. The ground had shifted under him, and he had the feeling that someone, somewhere, had broken the rules. God was supposed to be on their side, the side of the good and the free, but they had lost just the same.

If it could have meant something, he thought, all these disasters, both personal and international, Jennifer, Vietnam, maybe I could have made some sense of my life. But now I just want to be left alone.

'What are you thinking, Jack?'

'That I made two mistakes in my life. Having children and having ideals.'

'This isn't like you. You sound like a quitter. You disappoint me.'

Dale offered a rare smile. 'Please. No more. I've got enough guilt to last me this lifetime.'

'You give up, you might as well be dead.'

'I've thought of that as well.'

The sangria arrived, and Gates poured two more glasses. Dale sipped his, watched a white-hulled yacht motor past the jetties towards the club. A blonde in a string bikini squealed with laughter, and there was the sound of a popping cork.

'Why did we lose Indochina, Jack?' Gates asked him. He didn't wait for Dale to answer. 'Because we didn't have the money and we didn't have the men. Right?'

'Well, that just about covers it, I guess.'

'Because we had to use our own soldiers, who didn't know the country. Because our military is only geared for fighting conventional wars. Because we had to fight on two fronts, Hamburger Hill and Capitol Hill. We had to beg for every dollar we needed from Congress. We were betrayed, Jack. By the hippies and the bleeding hearts. Am I right or am I right?'

'That was the way it seemed to me at the time.'

'How many good boys did we lose over there? Fifty thousand. That ain't going to happen again.'

'Because we're not getting involved in any more foreign wars.'

'Oh, sure we are. We're just fighting them a different way.' He leaned across the table. 'I always admired you, Jack. This thing you had going with the Meo – that was the way we should have gone. Train the local people to do the fighting. They know the terrain, how it's done. But to do that you need money, and you need support. That takes a different kind of organisation. Not the Army, for Christ's sake. They get rusted out and fucked up anywhere west of Nevada. We learned a lot from that war, Jack. We learned we should play it a little smarter from now on.'

'So what has all this got to do with me? I can't train mercenaries in jungles any more. I've got arthritis in my right knee.'

'He also serves who stays right here in California. Look, Jack, we need someone we can trust. An ex-Company man who knows a little bit about international banking laws. Guy's got to be discreet and committed to the cause. I suggested you.'

'Suggested me? To whom?'

Gates grinned. 'Come on, Jack.'

'What have you got in mind?'

'Deal cuts both ways. We could help you with your current fiscal problems. And you could help us. You're a former high-ranking officer in the United States Air Force, decorated in Asia, plus some experience in international law. You won't just look good on the stationery.'

509

'So?'

'So maybe we could use you.'

'In what capacity?'

'How would you like to be the director of an international brokerage house?'

'I've never given it much thought,' Dale said, deadpan, but the irony was lost on Gates.

'Our problem is the same as it's always been. Money. So we finally figured that instead of going to Congress, cap in hand, we'd put the principles of capitalism to good use. After all, that's what we're fighting for, right? So we've gone private.'

Dale felt the first stirrings of alarm. 'The Company? Or just you and a few friends?'

Gates looked wounded. 'Hey, Jack, okay I break the law now and then, but I wouldn't do anything against the interests of America.'

'So what have you got?'

'One of the traditional cash cows, along with gambling and prostitution. A bank.'

'A bank?'

'Well, kind of a bank. Suppose you're Mr X from Hong Kong, or Bangkok maybe. You've got a little extra cash you want to invest in the United States. But there's currency regulations. Now, the Company knows who you are, and what you do. In fact the Company knows you real well, because you're on the payroll, you're selling us information. Very sensitive information. Okay, the Company suggests that if you approach a certain brokerage house, they may be able to help you out. In return you pay a certain percentage in brokerage fees. It helps to keep the Company fluid.'

'These people involved with drugs?' Dale asked.

'Wait a minute, Jack, before you go off half-assed about this.' Gates held up his hands. 'Look. No shit on these. But you've got to face reality. This is the eighties. If we're going to influence policy in a third world country, we won't be getting into bed with virgins. If we get squeamish, we'll get our asses kicked all over again. Some of the people

510

we deal with are very legitimate, big corporations who just want to bend the rules a little. Well, okay. But sure, I admit, some of our other friends don't look good on paper. But most of our pals in Asia never did.'

'Maybe I'm getting old, Gerry, but I never thought it would all end this way.'

'Hey, I don't like it either. Just call me a realist. We've got to make a choice. Are we going to stop crime, or are we going to fight communism? If you read the papers, you know we're never going to stop crime. It's right here on our doorstep. One of Nixon's best buddies was a Mafiosi, for Christ's sake. Crime is an unavoidable by-product of a free society. Remember the twenties when they tried to stop people drinking? You can't do it, Jack. People will want to drink, they'll want to fuck whores, they'll want to take drugs. The only place maybe it doesn't happen is Russia and China because over there people don't have the choice. Freedom sometimes means the right to fuck yourself up.'

'What's my part in this?'

'All you have to do is put your name on a letterhead, sit in an office, and answer the phone occasionally.'

'You want me to front a brokerage house?'

'Right here in San Francisco. In return, we can help solve some of your problems, talk to the people down at the IRS. Plus you get some of the cream for a change. You deserve it. A man serves his country, he shouldn't be driving around in a Toyota, for Christ's sake.'

'Let me think about it.'

'Okay. But one more thing I have to know.'

'Am I working for the *Washington Post?*'

'Are you still with us? This thing with Jennifer, all that crap, it's a shitty thing to happen. Hey, we know this is fire we're playing with here. We're not dumb. Okay, so these people bring in a little stuff, it gets shot in the arms of a few boogaloos in Detroit, some wetbacks in LA, who gives a shit, right? But sometimes things go a little wrong when they're not meant to.'

'Yeah, right.'

Gates leaned forward and gripped Dale's arm. 'Some of

our Air Force jocks who got shot down during the war? When they came back from Hanoi they were almost card-carrying communists. If you lose it, then maybe it's better to ship out and go home. No harm done. Up to you, Jack. You want to fight the good fight again? It would be great to have you back on the team.'

'I don't know. I'm tired, Gerry. Like I said, I'll have to think about it. The only bunkers I see these days are on golf courses.'

'Have to give me a game before I fly back to Washington.'

'Sure. Are you going to tell me what you're doing back there now, or is it classified?'

Gates smiled and finished his drink. Down on the water the blonde in the string bikini was performing an impromptu strip tease for her companions on the deck. In the car park a light-haired man in a Lamborghini was punching his horn in appreciation.

Gates called for the check, left cash on the table. Then he picked up a napkin, took a Parker ball point from his shirt pocket and scribbled a number on it. 'I'll be here for the next two days. Call me, let me know what you decide.'

'I don't know . . .'

Gates nodded. 'Come back on the team, Jack. Believe me, this time we're going to win.'

As they were walking out to the car park, Gates asked casually: 'How's Michael?'

'He's okay.'

'I heard he's with the DEA in Thailand.'

'Yeah, three months ago. Kind of the enemy, isn't he?'

Gates thought that was funny. 'Practically the same department, Jack. You've been away from things too long.'

'He was different when he came back in '70. Something happened to him over there. But he won't talk about it.'

'I heard he got wounded.'

'Enemy ambush,' Dale said, wondering again how much Gates already knew.

'You don't sound convinced.'

'I heard he was somewhere he shouldn't have been, with

512

someone who shouldn't have been with him. It was pretty dumb. You'll have to meet him some time. You'd really hate each other.'

Gates grinned. 'I'll look forward to it,' he said. He got in his car – a rented Mercedes, Dale noted – and drove away.

110

Without children, without a wife, a house might as well be a hotel room. The housekeeper had been in that day and the old house had the ordered, precious quality of a display home. In the kitchen on a shelf above the sink, there were ceramic jars marked TEA, COFFEE, SUGAR, RICE, standing side by side, like soldiers on parade; in the living room, the latest issues of *Forbes* and the *Far Eastern Economic Review* lay on the coffee table unopened; the bed looked as if it had never been slept in.

And some nights it wasn't. It was just himself and Bernard Fall and two glasses of brandy – he was careful about drinking alone – and the leather sofa.

A storm had swept in from the Pacific during the afternoon, and it was too cold and wet to go out on the deck, so he retreated from the ordered intensity of the house into the den. The room, Susan had once remarked, looked as if he had tried to recreate his own mind. The walls were panelled in conservative oak, there was a glass-doored cabinet with crystal glassware and selected bottles of fine brandies and malt whiskies; the wall over the stone fireplace was hung with family portraits, placed in order of priority and importance, together with mementoes of the years he had spent in Asia. An Aka cap covered with ancient silver coins, most bearing the head of George VI; a Hmong hunting rifle in a glass case; a revolver taken from a dead Viet Cong; photographs of himself with Westmoreland, with Gerry Gates, with Cao Ky; a menu from the Continental Hotel from 1967; an antique map of South East Asia in a glass frame, bearing names like Siam and Cochin and Annam.

He poured himself a Jack Daniels, sat in the winged back leatherette by the fireplace and stared at the array of portraits.

Michael in his USAF uniform; Jennifer in her graduation gown; in the centre, a black and white photograph of four people: himself, Susan, a freckle-faced three year old Jennifer, and a baby in Susan's arms – Michael. An icon so ancient, he decided, it might as well be Lincoln's tomb.

It seemed to him that he had watched his children grow up through the changing procession of these photographs, kept in moulded wallets in the jungles of Asia, or preserved in cheap frames in hotel bedrooms in Saigon and Vientiane and Manila. Each stage of their lives was captured, not in his memory, but in a glossy Kodachrome that arrived in embassy mail.

I want to go back and start again, he thought, and the pain of that realisation was so sharp it hit him in the gut like an ulcer.

Tonight was going to be bad, he realised. The ghosts were going to walk.

A beautiful dark-haired woman holding a child sat down by the window. Her long raven hair was braided down her back, and her face was pale and proud and very beautiful. Noelle.

'I'm sorry,' he said. He closed his eyes, hoping she would go away. His obsession with her had been completely selfish, the impossibility of the relationship perhaps part of the attraction. Doesn't matter who you hurt, he thought. Just get what you want.

He opened his eyes and she was gone.

Noelle's phantom would not be the cause of today's torment. His haunting today would be Jennifer. He remembered the coolies he had seen in Hong Kong, staggering along narrow wooden planks with enormous loads balanced across their shoulders on bamboo poles, backs bent, their eyes glassy with pain, empty of anything except concentration on their load. That is my life, he thought. Bowed under the weight of regret.

He recalled a few months ago finding some of Jennifer's things stored in the attic. He had blown the dust off one of her old schoolbooks and it had opened in his hands to something she had written in first grade:

My dad is a hero. He is in the Air Force and works in
a place called Saigon. I see my dad at Christmas and

515

for summer holidays and he wears a uniform and brings back lots of presents. My dad will come home as soon as the war is over. I love my dad.

He had started to hyperventilate like a teenager.

Suddenly she was lying on the rug at his feet, writing a letter. Her hair was in a pony tail. 'When are you coming home, Dad?' she said.

'Soon as I can.'

'Michael says you're never coming home.'

'Don't listen to Michael.'

She returned her attention to the letter. She drew a picture of herself and Michael playing football in the back yard with their grandfather. He still had that drawing somewhere, he remembered. He got up and went to look for it in the bureau drawers. When he came back with it, she was gone.

'Where were you when I needed you?' a voice said.

He turned. She was sitting in his chair. Her hair was tied with a bandana, there were ugly scabs along the insides of her arms, and dark bruises under her eyes. The Haight days.

'What?'

'Where were you when I needed you?'

'I couldn't help it. There were things I had to do.'

'And we just got in the way.'

'I tried to keep you with me. But it was just too dangerous.'

'I needed a father. So did Michael.'

'I had a job to do! An important job!'

'And you failed. Was it so bad in the end? They won in Vietnam. They won in Iran. They won in Afghanistan. Was any of it worth it?'

'I'm not ashamed of my life,' he screamed at her. 'I'm not!'

And he stormed out, leaving her sitting there. She was right. He had failed, and none of it had been worth it, not in the end.

He found the number that Gerry Gates had given him and dialled.

111

The Hong Kong restaurant in Chinatown is a large box-like room, the mirrored back wall and tiled floors giving the restaurant the acoustics of a public swimming pool. Gates and Dale walked past the queues of people waiting for tables. Sammy Chen had a table in the far corner of the room. He beamed a welcome as they entered.

Dale had not see Sammy Chen since Cholon in 1967. It might have been yesterday. He seemed not to have aged at all, and might even have been wearing the same clothes; a dark suit with shiny patches at the elbows, an open-necked white cotton shirt. He rose and shook hands with Dale, his hand cold and soft, like dough. He was alone, but Dale noted that at the table directly behind four young men in zippered jackets and wrap-around sunglasses sat impassively watching the door.

Triads, Dale decided.

They ordered Chinese tea, and Sammy enquired politely after Dale's family and he reciprocated. Their previous dealings in Saigon were pointedly ignored. *Dim sum* trolleys passed between the tables, and Sammy concentrated his attention on these, eating rapidly and with great appetite. The dishes were removed by the waiters, but they were not hurried out, like the other patrons. Sammy sat back and lit a cigarette, and released the belt on his trousers to aid his comfort and digestion.

A fresh pot of green tea was brought, and Gates brought up the subject of business. It seemed that Sammy had previously told Gates that he was thinking of transferring his interests from Hong Kong to San Francisco.

Gates turned to Dale. 'Sammy is worried that he may have certain difficulties transferring some of his assets into the United States. I suggested we might be able to help him.'

Dale leaned forward. 'As Gerry's probably told you, I've just been made a director of International Pacific Commodities. The company is based in Hong Kong, but we have offices all over America, all independently incorporated. I've just opened a new branch here in San Francisco. I'm sure we could facilitate the process for you, Sammy.'

'Must be all okay, Mr Dale. Must not break laws, okay? No funny business.'

'As far as the United States government is concerned, it is all perfectly legitimate. You see, security companies like ours are not subject to reporting requirements. For example, you can purchase one million dollars in gold contracts, both for and against. Returns can be as high as three or four thousand per cent in six months. When the market moves, we just tear up the negative contract. It never appears on our books. You can make the contract in Hong Kong, and the profit appears as a credit on your account here.'

'And what fee you charge for such service, Mr Dale?'

'Six per cent.'

'That's a lot of money.'

'That's a lot of service.'

Sammy folded his hands across his belly and thought about this. 'Maybe you give me discount?'

Dale looked at Gates.

'We're always willing to negotiate, Sammy.' said Gates.

'Still have friends in Viet Nam, in Swatow, in police, in army. Know many people, in many place. Can give you much good information, okay?'

'As I said, Sammy, we're always willing to negotiate.'

Sammy thought about this for a long time. He chose a lotus seed bun with great care and deposited it in his mouth. He leaned forward as if he was about to divulge a great secret. 'I think I will like it here in your America, okay?'

* * *

As he drove back home that evening along Highway 101, Dale reviewed the conversation in his mind. He wondered what Michael would think if he knew his old man had just had lunch with someone like Sammy Chen. And he wondered how he would ever tell him.

112

Near kilometre mark 15, Thailand/Burma border

David Lee was a third-generation American-Chinese. He wore aviator glasses and a Yankees baseball cap, and spoke with a fast New York accent. He had been with the DEA in Chiang Mai for three years; long enough to understand the utter futility of his job. As he drove he kept one hand on the wheel of the jeep, the other drew pictures in the air. If anyone cut off his hands he would have been struck dumb.

'His name's Chang Chi-fu, but he likes to call himself Khun Sa. That means "Prince of Prosperity" in Burmese. He's half Chinese, half Shan, and he's the biggest narcotics operator of all time, even bigger than the British East India Company. He has his own army, the SUA – the Shan United Army – of fifteen thousand men. He likes to tell everyone he's fighting for Shan independence, but that's bullshit. He uses the arms our government gives him to force the Hmong to grow more opium. Any chiefs who defy him are publicly tortured. Now he grows and processes almost half the opium in the entire Golden Triangle.'

It was Michael's third month in Thailand. He experienced those same feelings of exhilaration and purposefulness he remembered from his first days in Vietnam. He felt he was doing something worthwhile, something his grandchildren would thank him for.

It had been a long time since he had sat behind the controls of an aircraft. When he got back from South East Asia he had tried to get a job as a commercial pilot, but the airlines and aviation companies were in recession, and there were just no vacancies. He met one former Raven in a supermarket. A year before he had been dodging anti-aircraft batteries on the Plain of Jars; now he was selling soap powder.

Michael's father had wanted him to go to law school, which was perhaps why he enrolled instead in the police academy. It seemed like a honest job with good pay, and it went some way to filling the yearning in his soul to be one of the good guys. On his first day as a patrolman he disarmed a man who had threatened to shoot his own wife and kids with an automatic pistol. After that, he was hooked.

He became one of the youngest detectives on the force, and in 1978 the Bureau of Narcotics invited him to a two-week school in Chicago. At the end of the course they offered him a job. In his first year as an undercover agent he made a case against a group of corrupt Vice Squad detectives. After their conviction he received a number of threatening phone calls so his boss asked him if he wanted to go to Thailand.

They pulled off the dirt road, plunged over a shallow stream and then up a steep hill, ploughing over thick vegetation. Lee stopped the jeep and jumped out. Their Hmong guide, Chao Cho, went ahead. Lee pulled an M-16 from the back seat and indicated that Michael should follow him.

'We walk from here.' Lee said.

The jungle was utterly silent. Michael understood how the traffickers could operate with impunity here. It would be impossible to get close to anyone in this cathedral hush without alerting them.

They followed Chao Cho for two hundred metres and suddenly Michael realised they were against the walls of a large building. The walls were made of split bamboo, scorched black by fire. They had been obscured by the undergrowth and shields of green bamboo. Lee found an entrance and led Michael inside.

There was no roof, but it was gloomy inside because of the overhanging trees and creepers. Broken glass, shattered beakers and twisted metal cauldrons littered the earth floor. Two black fifty-gallon drums lay skewed in one corner, the metal contorted like a torn sardine can.

'They used to make two hundred kilos of base here every day. We hit it just before you got here, just before the poppy harvest. They know it was us, but we told the embassy it was the KMT. We're not supposed to operate this side of the border.'

'This was one of Khun Sa's?'

He nodded. 'The whole of the fucking Shan states is like this. You blow one up, another one appears somewhere else. He's had heroin laboratories up here since 1974, moves them back and forward between Thailand and Burma, depending on who's applying the most pressure. There's around thirty of them now.'

'There's nothing we can do about this?'

'You can see for yourself, there's no border, no Checkpoint Charlie. The Burmese don't control this part of the Triangle, and most of the Thai government is on his payroll. This part of the Triangle's completely lawless. No, check that. Khun Sa is the law here. You should see his headquarters at Ban Hinn Taek. It's like a palace. There's a cinema, tennis courts, swimming pools, even shops selling leather furniture and booze. Costs two million dollars a month just in upkeep. And it's right in the middle of the jungle!'

They tramped up the winding paths for another hour, and Michael began to realise the full extent of the problem. The trail they were on was so narrow and overgrown that it could never be seen from the air, and besides, you could hear a rotor or aircraft engine long before it reached you. There were no airports, just two washed out roads. You could hide a hundred rebel armies in here, Dale thought. In fact, someone probably is.

Chao Cho put his finger to his lips to indicate they were close to the village they were looking for. Lee pointed through the trees and Michael saw it perched high on the far hillside, smoke rising from the thatched roofs. He heard the barking of the pi-dogs.

Lee pulled the binoculars from his pack and focused. After a few minutes he passed them to Michael. 'See the building right at the top of the ridge? There's three mules tethered outside. That's one of Khun Sa's trading posts. Inside there's three hundred kilos of number four heroin, packed in watertight bags.'

Michael shook his head. 'All I can see is the hut. Where's the X-ray switch on these things?'

Lee laughed. 'Trust me. A CI told us it's there. But the embassy says we have to wait for them to bring it across the border on to the Thai side before we make our move.'

A CI, Michael knew, was shorthand for Confidential Informant. 'A thousand things can go wrong between now and then. Why don't we just go in and get it?'

'Embassy says no.'

'For Christ's sake!'

'Welcome to the world of drug enforcement,' Lee grinned. 'Come on, we'd better get back. I've got the jeep on a meter.'

Chiang Mai

The DEA compound was in one of the poorer sections of the town, surrounded by a tall concrete wall with reinforced steel front gates. The perimeter was fitted with elaborate electronic security. These precautions were not unwarranted. Just the year before Joyce Powers, wife of one of the senior DEA agents, had been kidnapped off the street and murdered.

Once inside the gates the impression was of walking into a Hollywood film set. The compound was a Disney recreation of middle America, with two-storey gabled homes, manicured lawns, aquamarine swimming pools and tanned men and women in whites playing tennis on asphalt courts.

There was also a gymnasium fully equipped with the latest Nautilus equipment, and this was where Lee and Michael went to work out while Lee explained the intricacies of the job.

'That three hundred kilos is going to be hard to nail,' he said in between grunts from the bench press. 'Normally they come down the trails with a caravan of four hundred mules, fifty kilos of opium on each mule. Twenty tons at a time. And we still can't catch them. For three hundred kilos they'll only need half a dozen mules. They'll be faster and lighter. Or they'll run it in as part of a larger caravan.'

'What about the border patrols?'

Lee laughed so hard he had to replace the bar. 'There's another private army on the Thai side, the KMT, supposedly the remnants of the old Republican Chinese Army. These days they're just press-ganged tribesmen, like the Shans. The Thais give them arms to patrol the border. But what they do is use the guns to take a tax from the Shans, five dollars US a kilo on opium. Or they run opium themselves. It's a farce.'

'So how do we stop them?'

'If we have a good CI, we can contact the Thai Border Patrol Police. But if we do that, something usually goes wrong.'

Lee went to the exercise bike, and got on.

'You mean they're corrupt?'

'Everybody in Thailand's corrupt. What I mean is they're owned, body and soul, by the enemy.'

'The enemy?'

'The CIA. Only we don't call them that here. They're known as the Third Floor, because they're on the third floor of the embassy in Bangkok. They call themselves the Special Reporting Facility or SERF. They just love cryptonyms, those guys. There's no getting away from those assholes here. Hey, I go to the jungle, I shake a tree, a spook falls down. I scratch my ass, I find a miniature camera.'

'You're saying the CIA want to disrupt what we do here?'

'It's nothing personal, Mike. Don't take it to heart.'

He put down the weights and slumped on a bench. His T-shirt was drenched with sweat. 'But why?'

'You were in Laos during the war, weren't you, Mike?'

'For a few months.'

'You hear stories about Air America carrying dope?'

'Hear stories? I saw it with my own eyes.'

'It's the same deal. The Border Patrol are a counterinsurgency unit. When the students started making trouble at the university in Bangkok four years ago, they sent in the Border Patrol Police to kick ass. Down at the embassy they're not interested in drugs, they're only interested in politics. Reds under the bed, Mike. Somebody has to pay for all this. Besides, drug runners, as a group, are very right-wing, very conservative. Also they cross borders all the time. Spooks love those guys. They're worth a small fortune in intelligence.'

524

'Jesus.'

'I don't think he'll help us much either. Don't forget, he was into politics, too.' Lee laughed at his own joke.

'If the Border Patrol won't help us, why don't we grab these guys ourselves and then hand them over? Then they don't get a chance to screw us up.'

Lee started his warm down. 'Nice idea. But this isn't the States. We're not talking about some small-time hoods, this is a fucking army we're up against. Just one of these caravans has around three hundred soldiers, young Hmong or Lihsu who'd make your average mountain climber look like a couch potato. They got fifty-calibre machine guns, recoilless rifles and sixty-mill mortars for Christ's sake. Plus field radios to call for back up if that shit still ain't enough. Man, what we going to do? Jump out from behind a bit of bamboo with a badge and a revolver and shout, "Stop right there, you bastards, you're under arrest?" '

'So what the hell *do* we do?'

'Me, Mike? I do my best. I play with my kids in the morning for maybe an hour, then I go and do my job not knowing when, or if, I'm ever going to see them or my wife again. I get shot at, fucked with, and pissed on. I work with guys who drink too much, Thai cops who would sell me down the river for a digital watch, and guys in button down shirts from the embassy who I know, for a fact, are passing on everything I tell them to the other side. And I do it because I still tell myself that at the end of the day it's going to make some difference. Because I, almost alone of my generation, think that one key of heroin poses a bigger threat to America than Joe Stalin in a rocket launcher. Because I'm a pilgrim. Because I'm crazy. Because I will not give up on a lost cause.'

'And that's it? That's the job?'

'They never promised you a rose garden, Dale. Welcome to Chiang Mai.' He laughed like a madman, grabbed his towel, and walked off to the shower.

113

Chiang Mai is to drugs what Wall Street is to money, and the locals are not coy about the reason for the town's celebrity. Many of the local restaurants have wallpaper with poppy motifs, the place mats have poppy decals, the tourists who eat there have T-shirts emblazoned with logos of poppies. Opium scales can be bought anywhere.

The town is both a drugs bazaar and an intelligence market. The hotels and restaurants and nightclubs and coffee shops serve as meeting places and rumour mills for the transient armies of arms dealers, drugs czars, spies and mercenaries.

And the activity reaches a fever pitch each spring, just after the opium harvest.

David Lee put on his Dodgers cap and zippered jacket and took Michael into town, to the lobby of the absurdly named Welcome Inn, to watch the passing parade. The coffee shop was crowded with young Chinese in sharp suits, wearing Porsche wrap-around sunglasses and gold Rolexes on their wrists. A gang of young Thais in T-shirts and jeans stood at the door to discourage tourists and gawkers. They glared at Lee as he slouched in the banquette in the foyer. He grinned and winked back at them.

'Most of the guys in there are triads,' he said. 'Chinese gangsters, junior executive level. Look at the way they dress. It's a fucking uniform, those sunglasses. The other guys work either for General Li – he's the local KMT warlord – or Khun Sa. They're working out prices per kilo and degrees of risk. This is the start of the trail, Mike. Shit happens and it starts right here.'

'And there's nothing we can do?'

'And there's nothing we can do. Thailand has no conspiracy laws so they can sit in there and talk about drugs all they want. We eyeball them and they eyeball us, and it's all macho posturing and shit. Unless they get caught with the stuff in their pockets, they're not breaking any laws. Even if they do get caught in possession, they're protected right at the very top. If not by their side, then by ours.'

'The Third Floor?'

'Fucking A right. For now, we just hold the line, keep our shape. One day it's going to get so bad someone will have to do something. Then we'll get these pricks.'

They both turned their heads to look at a woman who had just stepped out of the elevator. She was a strikingly attractive Asian who seemed to glide across the foyer in a sheath-tight black silk cheongsam, slit to the thigh. Her jet hair fell loose around her shoulders.

'That's a woman, Mike,' whispered Lee. 'That's why chinee man think you all same big hairy barbarian. I don't see what all the fuss is about white women. These little Chinese girls, man! Float like a butterfly, sting like a bee.'

The girl stopped in the middle of the foyer and stared at Mike. Her gaze was so frank and intense that he was almost embarrassed by it.

'Oh, man,' Lee whispered to him. 'Is she looking at you or me? Please don't let it be me. I'm a married man.'

'What the hell's she looking at?'

'I think it's you, big boy. Must be checking out customers. No more than a thousand baht, Mike, tops. Any more and she's ripping you off.'

She turned and came towards them. As she drew closer Michael recognised the scent of jasmine.

'No thanks, I'm working right now,' he said.

'What?' the girl said, confused.

'Maybe some other time.'

'You don't recognise me.' It was a statement, not a question.

'Should I?'

For one crazy moment he thought she was about to cry.

Bizarre. Then she muttered something under her breath, turned and walked away.

'What did she say?'

'I think she called you a son of a bitch,' said Lee.

'What was all that about?'

'Shit, she don't look like no thousand baht hooker to me. Look at the ice on her wrist. That's not paste, Mike.'

'I have no idea who she is,' he said, and desperately searched his memory for some clue.

'Well, she sure thinks she knows you. I guess we'd better start making some enquiries.'

'Her name's May Wong. Mean anything to you?'

Michael shook his head.

They were in Lee's office in the DEA compound. Lee had his feet on the desk, and his hands behind his head. His citation for bravery from the Marines hung in a frame on the wall behind his chair.

'Well, it may not be her real name.'

'Who is she?' Michael asked him.

'She's not all that important by herself, Mike. It's her boyfriend. His name is Ho Kuan-ling, also known as Douglas Ho, aka Sharkfin. He's a Red Pole in the Fei Lung triad, and he's thought to be number two to a major drugs trafficker by the name of Sammy Chen. He's thirty-seven years old, and he's the most vicious little shit you're ever likely to meet. And for some reason his woman thinks she knows you.'

He leaned forward, both arms on the desk, and stared at Michael, waiting. Michael knew what he was thinking: Either I have a foot in the enemy camp or they have a foot in mine. Which is it?

'I've never seen her before in my life,' he said. 'Woman like that, I think I'd remember.'

'So what the hell's going on?'

'I don't know.'

'Then you're going to have to find out.'

Michael nodded. He had racked his brain for some answer, thought of all the girls he had known for the last five years. There had been a Vietnamese girl he had dated a few times in San Francisco, but apart from her there had been no Asian girls in his life. 'I think it's a case of mistaken identity,' he said. 'Perhaps I have a twin.'

'I don't care if you're a quadruplet. Find out who she thinks you are, and then you'd better learn to be that fucking guy. Because I want to know what's going on here, Mike.'

He nodded. 'Okay.'

114

The street was full of western-style boutiques; Roxy Music's *'Love is the Drug'* thumped from a cassette stall. Long-haired young men in dirty T-shirts and torn jeans wandered the street looking for scores. Hill people, many of them women with children in slings on their backs, made their way through the crowds to the night market.

The Mercedes stopped outside a brightly lit shop selling antique wood carvings and heavy teak furniture. The driver, a Chinese in a dark suit with a conspicuous bulge under the left arm of his jacket, jumped out and opened the rear passenger door. May got out and went inside. The driver leaned on the bonnet and took out a packet of cigarettes. He lit one and waited. His stance was casual. He hawked and spat in the road. He wasn't expecting trouble.

Michael parked his brown Toyota a little way up the street and followed her into the shop.

She was studying a heavy table of dark teak, while the proprietor hovered around her, trying to open a negotiation. Michael was careful not to approach her. He caught her eye, was impressed by her reaction.

There was none.

She turned away again, and tossed back her hair. He saw her look out into the street, check that her driver's back was towards her, and then walk quickly out of the shop, leaving the proprietor talking to himself. Michael followed her. She turned into an alley.

It was filled with hill people; Lihsu, Hmong and Black Tais, sitting on blankets selling opium pipes and hand-carved silver jewellery. Children hawked buckets of dried opium poppies to backpackers. Michael felt something tug at his leg, looked down and saw a young Akha woman, holding a deformed child, her hand held out piteously. The purple neon of the Golden Poppy nightclub threw a purple aura around her face. He dropped some coins in her lap and hurried after the girl.

'May,' he said.

She turned around. He could not see her face in the shadows. 'You remember?' She sounded breathless.

Oh shit, now what should I do? Michael thought. Who the hell do you think I am? 'Sure I remember.'

'It is ten monsoon, more. You are not change. I cannot believe when I see you.'

He did not know what to say. Give me some kind of clue! Something!

'Mai Koo,' she said.

Mai Koo. In what chapter of his history had someone called him that? That was way back. In Laos...

'You not remember?' she said.

Laos. This girl was in her early-twenties, perhaps younger. Laos was eleven years ago...

'You not even remember me.'

He tried to fathom her features in the darkness. The neon flashed on – off – on – off, a strip of electric purple illuminating her face, then throwing it back into shadow. He remembered a small child, sitting on the floor of the hootch at Long Tieng; playing baseball in the dirt in a Giants cap many sizes too big for her; a pathetic bundle of rags lying bandaged and bloody in the base hospital...

'Why you leave me in the hospital. Why you never come to see me?'

'Ly May,' he whispered.

'Why?'

Not that little girl, he thought. That little girl was dead in an American military hospital or on the streets of Saigon. That little girl is part of a nightmare past, something I tried to do right and screwed up. This beautiful and elegant young woman has absolutely no similarity to that little girl at all. Then in the flash of the neon, he saw the tiny puckered scar around her eye.

531

'Why you not come back for me?' she repeated.

'I couldn't,' he said.

There was a commotion in the street. May's bodyguard had realised his charge was missing and had charged into the alley like a wounded animal. Probably already beaten up the shop owner, Michael thought. It's all these guys know to do when something goes wrong.

'I go now,' she said.

'Wait,' Michael whispered, but she pushed past him and hurried back down the alley.

He took a step back and watched her from the shadows.

She was already at the end of the alley arguing with her muscle in Thai. He was telling her not to wander off on her own. She was telling him, in faultless Thai, to go and fuck himself.

Michael smiled. So much for the little Hmong girl who never spoke a word, whom he had scolded for learning to say 'Sumbich'. She had grown into a very eloquent young woman.

A jumble of emotions battled inside him for his attention. Astonishment. Excitement. Disappointment.

Ly May. May Wong. The little village girl had done well for herself, but she had also found some bad company along the way. Somehow the road had taken her from the mountains to the streets, and back to the drug bazaars of the north. She had endured, had found money and protection and an education. She had survived, against the odds.

The question was this: was he now prepared to do the American thing and place her future in jeopardy again, in order to exploit her some more?

115

Vincent Paderewski had the well-worn air of a man who had spent too long in a job that he believed could not be done. His tie was loose, and he was surrounded by a perpetual fug of cigarette smoke. An Italian-Pole, he had been known as The Pope around the DEA's Bangkok office ever since the election of John Paul II. He was the chief case officer in Bangkok, a job he considered second only to lavatory cleaner in Djakarta as an exercise in futility.

There was a photocopied inscription Scotch taped to the wood panelling behind his head:

President of the Mushroom Club:
Kept in the Dark and Fed on Bullshit.

On another wall was a whiteboard with a link analysis depicting relationships within Douglas Ho's organisation. Circles and squares were filled with Thai and Chinese names, a hopeless maze of intersecting lines that seemed to confuse more than illuminate.

'I'm told you have an in with Douglas Ho,' The Pope said.

Michael shrugged. He felt uncomfortable with this. He wasn't sure he wanted to go through with it.

'May Wong,' Paderewski prompted.

'It's an ancient association.'

'But David Lee thinks we might be able to exploit it.'

'Perhaps.'

The Pope picked up a manila folder three inches thick and tossed it across the desk. Michael caught it to prevent it toppling on to the floor. 'Look, I'm as sceptical as you are,

Mike. That's the file we have on Douglas Ho. He's untouchable. Protection goes all the way to the top of the Thai government. But what the fuck. We've got a job to do, right?'

'That's what I thought before I got here.'

'Hell, you only been here two months. Wait till you've been here six fucking years, like I have.' Paderewski spilled ash from his cigarette on his shirt. He ignored it. 'What do you know about the triads, Mike?'

'Not a great deal.'

'Yeah, well, no one in America does – yet. Maybe another ten years they'll start to wake the fuck up.'

'Douglas Ho is a triad, right?'

'That's like saying Cardinal Spellman's a practising Catholic. This guy is a senior official in the Fei Lung, with some very heavyweight connections in Hong Kong. We think he's a Red Pole, that's like a guy who takes care of the wet jobs. But he's not just a hitter, he's a thinker as well. The worst kind. A one man crime wave. He was sent here from Hong Kong about a year ago to take care of business.'

'And the girl?'

Paderewski shrugged. 'The girl's a girl. He gets them, keeps them for a year or two, throws 'em away. From what we know of him he doesn't have any particular vices. Even the women just come one at a time. The way I figure him, they're just for show anyway. I don't think sex is a big deal for him. I've met him once or twice. Last month he was presented with the Order of the White Elephant or some fucking thing by the King. For all his good works for charity. Last year he gave away a hundred thousand dollars to an anti-drugs campaign. Makes you want to puke, doesn't it?'

'You say you met him?'

'I went along representing the embassy. I wanted to meet the guy. I tell you, Mike, looking in his eyes is like looking into the ocean.'

'If we can't touch him, why are we doing this?'

'Beats me. But that's what they pay us to do. Right?'

I'm back in Vietnam, Michael thought. Back with the Romeos and the remfs and all the rest of the crap. Life doesn't change. It's just more of the damned same.

'So what good is this going to do?'

The Pope's tone changed. His voice suddenly had a harder edge to it. 'Because somebody has to give a shit, Michael. Because it's bad now, but if it wasn't for us guys in the white hats, it would get a whole lot worse. We get a line on Douglas Ho, we can make him hurt for a while. Maybe we can get a few of the bad guys in America. Or maybe he'll make a mistake and walk on to American soil and we'll arrest his ass too. Does that make you happier, Mike?'

He nodded. That much he agreed with. Somebody had to care.

'Before you get real involved in this, maybe you better understand a little about the triads. A little history lesson for you.'

'Okay.'

'The first thing you've got to understand about the triads, is that they've been around for fucking ever. You know how it is. You get two Brits together, you got a club. You get two Irishmen together, you got a fight. You get two Chinese together, you got a triad.' The Pope sat back in his chair, warming to his favourite subject. He lit a Winston, but was too involved in his subject to put it to his lips. As he talked ash spilled down the front of his shirt. 'The triads started off as a rebel sect, like the IRA or the PLO, fighting against an unpopular government. Except there was a lot of mumbo jumbo went with it, to ensure secrecy and loyalty. A bit like the Freemasons. They first showed up in Hong Kong in numbers in the 1850s when they ran there to escape a crackdown by the Manchus. Over the years they started to use their muscle more for crime than politics, and in Hong Kong they managed to infiltrate the government and the police. The watershed was 1912.

'That was the year the old Manchu dynasty was kicked out and Sun Yat Sen declared China a republic. He was a triad, so if you wanted to get to the top in China, membership was essential. The political imperative disappeared, but the triads continued. By then they made up a number of very powerful crime syndicates, and they all but owned Hong Kong.

'The thing you have to understand about the triads, Mike, is they're cannibals. They eat their own.'

535

'Wanchai in Hong Kong, for instance. If you're a coolie, you have to go to the triad to get work. In return they take half your wages, maybe more. The firm you go to work for is triad-run. The tenement you pay rent to is triad-owned. The hawker you buy your food from has inflated prices because he's being squeezed by triad thugs. You're so poor you have to steal to get by, and whatever you steal you have to fence to the triads. If you want sex, the prostitute pays your money to the triad. If you want to smoke some dope to forget the cruddy life you've got, you go to a triad opium den. They own your ass, boy. In this life and the next. The only way out is to become a triad, if they'll have you, and do the job on someone else.

'But to join you have to be sponsored by an existing member, and that's going to cost you money too. You're checked out thoroughly by a triad official, usually the recruiting officer who's called the Vanguard. The initiation ceremony itself used to take three days, but these days the young kids coming through can't be bothered with tradition, and it's just a simple blood oath.

'Here in Thailand the Chinese have been around so long it's hard to distinguish them from the pure blood Thais. They have a stranglehold on commercial life, much like the Jews in Europe before the war, and most of the city's commerce is controlled by chiu chao speakers. Bangkok, Hong Kong, any large Chinese city, you'll find the triads. It's unspoken a lot of it, like the Brits with their old boy network. It's why they're so damned difficult to stop. They have a saying: "Armies protect the Emperor, secret societies protect the people." Unfortunately, it's not true.

'But that's what we're dealing with here, Mike. Not just a syndicate, but a whole fucking way of life.'

'And May's our way in?'

'Sent from Heaven, if you believe in God.' Another cigarette, more ash down the shirt. 'Can you turn her for us, Mike?'

'I'll try. But I don't know if it will work.'

'Well, if it doesn't work, you're back to Drug City, and getting jungle rot in your boots. But we're due for a break.'

'I need to get her alone, talk to her.'

'Won't be easy. Douglas Ho has muscle watching his women every minute of the day. My guess he has someone squatting down at the end of the bed with a .357 even when he's screwing. He's a cautious guy.'

'So what do we do?'

'We wait. And we watch. The opportunity will come. We have time on our side. Anyway, we don't have any other way to get this guy.'

116

Douglas Ho's villa nestled discreetly behind a forest of banana trees, near the Belgian Embassy, in one of the city's finest residential neighbourhoods. The gate was topped with iron spikes and the walls were strung with razor wire. The bars on the gate were backed with a bullet proof steel sheet that blocked any view into the house from the street. Two ragged fishtail palms rose from behind the walls, their fronds bowed and frowsy in the midday heat, like two old ladies snoozing in the sun.

'We can't get in,' Michael said. 'So we'll have to wait until she comes out.'

The Pope hammered the air conditioner vent with the palm of his hand. Broken. He loosened his tie and flicked a droplet of sweat from his neck. 'We need to get her away from Bangkok. Too many eyes. But initially you'll have to wait until she leaves the villa, perhaps on one of her shopping expeditions. Like you did in Chiang Mai. Slip her a note, make a rendezvous for somewhere outside the city. See if she takes the bait.'

Michael nodded. He kept thinking of the little girl he remembered, in Long Tieng; blowing gum, playing baseball, sleeping under his chair in the hootch. Now she was about to be thrown to the lions. Expendable. Again.

All for a good cause.

Again.

It was late-evening. The gate opened suddenly and the white Mercedes drove quickly through. The windows were smoked glass so it was impossible to know if she was inside. They followed anyway, at a discreet distance.

Their brown Toyota was unremarkable, and anyway, The Pope had told him, it was not hard to follow any car in

Bangkok. It never got too far ahead of you. During the upheavals of the seventies the Thais had always joked that Bangkok would never be invaded. The Vietnamese would get stalled on Rama IV Road and would give up and go home before they made the city.

The Mercedes stopped outside the Dusit Thani Hotel. The muscle ran around the car to open the door, and May stepped out and went inside. The Toyota was stalled in traffic so The Pope did not have to pull over. Michael jumped out, weaved through the tangle of trucks and buses and followed her into the foyer. He looked back through the glass doors. The muscle was back behind the wheel of the Mercedes, scowling at the doormen.

May had turned into the shopping arcade. By the time he caught up with her, she was in a jeweller's, comparing jade bracelets.

Michael went in.

She must have sensed him for she looked around without warning, and this time the surprise registered on her face. Then she recovered and returned her attention to the bracelets.

Michael stood close to her, so close he could feel the heat of her body, the static charge from the fine golden hairs on her arms. He pretended to study the array of Burmese jade and Chantaburi star sapphires.

One of the salesmen approached and asked Michael if he could help him. His tone suggested that he had summed him up by his sports shirt and casual slacks as a remote prospect.

He took a business card from his shirt pocket, held it between his thumb and index finger, and tapped on the glass showcase, indicating a jade pendant. The salesman unlocked the glass cabinet and placed the piece on the counter top for Michael to inspect.

He knew she was watching. He tapped again on the glass and shook his head. 'Thanks,' he said, and went out, leaving the card behind.

He looked over his shoulder quickly, as he left the shop. The card was gone.

Golden Nine lived in a crumbling wooden shophouse off the Soi

Saladaeng. An old grandmother with a sticky black queue and a high, shiny forehead showed May into the parlour. Golden Nine was sitting with his leg tucked underneath his stool, sipping tea. He was very old, with rheumy yellow eyes set in great folds of skin, and his mouth had hardly any teeth. There was a large mole on his left cheek and three long white hairs sprouted from it. He fingered them constantly. He wore a blue silk gown with gold thread stitched into the cloth. It made it appear as if he had a golden aura.

The tools of the geomancer's craft were laid out in front of him: a hand-painted chart with the twelve signs of the Zodiac laid out on a wheel; a set of astrological charts; a small porcelain Buddha; a lacquered vase with sticks of smouldering incense.

'Hello, Grandfather,' May greeted him respectfully.

He nodded and smiled, pointing to the wooden stool opposite. She sat down.

Golden Nine reached for the pot on the table beside him and poured some green tea into a cracked cup and invited her to drink. Despite his age he still had beautiful hands, she noticed, with long, tapering nails, the cuticles perfect white half moons. The nails on the little fingers had been allowed to grow, like talons, and they were about an inch long.

'You are May Wong,' he said, his voice cracked and sibilant like the hinges of an old door. 'You live with the Dragon in the big house.'

'The Dragon?' she asked him.

'The Dragon as a man,' he said, and she realised he meant Douglas. 'I have seen you with him,' His tone was disapproving. Perhaps if he can see the future, he can also see my past, she thought, and felt her cheeks flush with shame.

'What is it you want to know?'

'My future.'

'Has something made you wonder about your future?'

'Yes, it has.' May thought about the card Michael had passed to her, asking her to meet him in Ayoddhya.

He nodded. 'Your future is carved on your forehead the day you are born. There is nothing you can do to change it.' He reached out and took her head in his hands. They were dry and surprisingly strong, and his fingers explored the

540

contours of her forehead and her skull, and then moved down her face, her eyebrows, lips and jaw. Then he picked up her hands, holding them towards the window as if they were translucent, and minutely examined her knuckles and fingernails, rubbing the lines on her palms with his fingers. When he was satisfied he dropped her hands back into her lap, closed his eyes and seemed to fall into a trance.

The sun filtered into the room through the shuttered window, and May could see the joss dust floating in the shafts of soft, yellow light. The crimson paper dragons that hung from the ceiling were stirred by a soft breeze.

Golden Nine opened his eyes once more, indicated she should finish her tea, then examined the leaves that lay in the bottom of the cup.

'You are indeed fortunate, Dragon Lady. Your future has two roads. One leads to the Dragon's mouth, the other leads to the mountain top. One leads to pain, the other to happiness. It is for you to decide.'

'What must I do, Grandfather?'

'You must make a choice. Not today. When the roads break. You will know that day. But when that hour comes you must stay away from the Dragon. You must run as far and as fast as you can. Run one second too soon, or one second too late, and he will consume you.'

'Do you see anyone else?' she asked him.

Golden Nine nodded slowly.

'Who do you see?'

'I do not have to tell you that. He is the reason you came here.'

'Do you see him written on my forehead, Grandfather?'

'There are two names written on your forehead, Dragon Lady. Either of them is your destiny.'

May dropped her money on to the floor and hurried out.

117

Michael sat in his room in the Holiday Inn, staring at the seething, sulphurous Bangkok afternoon through the thick glass of his hotel window. He got up and padded the room like a caged tiger. He wanted to get this over, get this done; but more than anything else he wanted to see her again. If only my pretext was more honest. She thinks I want to see her but I am just here to use her.

Ly May. In his memory that nine-year-old child had never grown up; she had remained a child for all these eleven years past. It was impossible to equate those haunting memories with the reality of this startling young woman. What am I going to say to her? What am I going to say?

He was torn between conflicting emotions: relief that she had survived; an eagerness to explain to her what had happened, that he had not abandoned her; disgust at what she had become. For that was what he also had to face: the little Hmong girl with the runny nose and the dirty feet and the innocent smile had become a triad's woman. Her journey from Eden was complete.

He picked up one of the magazines lying on the smoked glass coffee table: *Far Eastern Economic Review*. He turned the pages listlessly, found himself looking at a photograph of his own father, smiling back at him from a full-page advertisement:

FORMER WAR HERO COMMANDS PRIVATE BANK:
NEW COMMODITIES HOUSE

When Major Jonathan Dale exchanged his colonel's bars for a banker's pin stripes, he brought with him the management experience of a man who had been responsible for the lives of thousands, and the financial expertise of one who once controlled multi-million dollar budgets and programs. Like all good bank executives he intends to see his new clients on their own ground, face to face, to help them find solutions to the complex problems of international finance. As the new General Manager of Pacific International Investments in San Francisco, Major Jonathan Dale expects to see himself at the forefront of Asian-American business in the next decade . . .

He looked at the date on the magazine. Jesus! It was nearly a month old. A month, and his father had not mentioned this to him. Michael had spoken to him twice on the phone since then, and he had not breathed a word about it; he had said he was doing some freelance consultancy work.

Two months ago the name Pacific International Investments would have meant nothing to Michael. He had first run across them in Chiang Mai; they had an office in the same building as the DEA. When he had asked Lee about them, he had grinned and said: 'That's the Drugs Bank. Run by the Third Floor.'

He picked up the phone and punched the code for international dialling. He was halfway through his father's number when he slammed the receiver back on its cradle.

He threw the magazine across the room.

'Jesus!'

The Pope was right. It was getting harder to find anyone who gave a shit. Especially in your own family.

There was a queue of people waiting to join the boat to Ayoddhya, a narrow sampan with seats for about fifty passengers. She was just ahead of him in the queue, the protection beside her, looking bored and grim in his black sharkskin suit and inevitable wrap-around sunglasses. He was shorter than her, with the truculent look of a nightclub bouncer. Beside him May looked fragile and beautiful, in a pale lemon silk blouse, and a tight black skirt. Nobody could ever mistake them for a couple, he thought.

Michael had dressed for the occasion; the loudest Hawaiian

543

shirt he could find, bright orange pineapples and emerald green coconut trees. He had a Pentax slung over his shoulder and was wearing voluminous white shorts. Hardly sinister, he thought. His strategy was simple. I cannot hide in a small crowd, so I'll make myself look so absurd they will not suspect me later.

May sat under the awning on the shaded side of the boat; Michael took up a position in the stern and busied himself with taking photographs. The boat motored slowly upriver, stopping off at schools and temples where passengers waited in small *sala*. Houses of reddish-grey teak rose out of the water on stilts, women squatted on steps beside the river washing clothes, naked children jumped from the banks waving and screaming to the stupid *farang* in the ridiculous clothes.

After a while Michael tired of the charade, put away the camera and sat on the stern watching the back of her head. He wondered what the hell he was going to say to her.

The restaurant in the hotel was air conditioned, waiters in black jackets and bow-ties fussed around the handful of patrons, mainly holidaying Thais. Michael did not look up when May entered with her protection, who seemed sulky and bored. He made a point of asking, in the broadest mid-western accent he could manufacture, if they had any steak or hamburgers, playing his role to the hilt.

He ordered lobster. As he ate he studied a tourist guide and drank three bottles of beer very quickly. He stumbled as he got up and as he passed May's table, he almost fell in the protection's prawns. The muscle leaped to his feet, furious, and Michael read the hate in his eyes.

Michael apologised profusely, and offered to pay for the spilt drinks, while May restrained her companion, smiling graciously. Michael weaved out of the restaurant and across the foyer.

Well, it was done now. For better or worse. Here we go, little May. The United States is back in town. Now let's drop you in the shit.

The Bang Pa Inn had been built by King Chulalongkorn in memory of his wife who had drowned when her boat capsized on the lake. The beautiful pavilion had been constructed

544

right into the water, a *sala* of filigree wood on a pillared platform of semi-precious stone.

She was already waiting there early next morning when Michael arrived from Ayoddhya in a *tuk-tuk*. She did not appear to have seen him, was lost in thought, gazing at the water. He stood looking at her for a long time.

A finger of mist stretched across the lake.

She is so beautiful, he thought. Hard to think of her as the same Ly May, impossible to comprehend how a little peasant girl with dirt between her toes can grown into a scented woman with silk stockings and diamonds at her throat.

As he watched she blew a bubble of gum that spattered across her nose. He laughed and she turned around.

She smiled too. 'You teach me this trick.'

She had known he was there the whole time. 'Ly May,' he said.

She crossed her arms and put her head on one side. 'How you do this, how you arrange, okay?'

He shrugged, as if he didn't quite understand.

'Prenom says he has a fire in his stomach, cannot sleep, screams like he is dying all night. You put bad *phi* in him.'

'When I bumped into your table, I put something in his beer. He'll be all right. He won't die.'

'Where is very nice pineapple shirt?'

He grinned. Yesterday's tourist costume had been replaced by jeans and a white cotton shirt. 'You like it? You can have it.'

His collar was unbuttoned and her eyes fell on the little jade Buddha he wore at his throat. The original leather thong had long ago been replaced by a silver chain. She touched it lightly with her fingers. 'This bring you good luck?'

'So far.'

She suddenly became serious. 'We walk, okay?'

They followed a path beside the lake. She kept her distance, he noticed, treating him with caution.

'So many questions,' he said.

'Me too.'

'I remember ... I remember a big-eyed little girl who never spoke. I remember she had dirt under her fingernails and wore the same little raggedy-ass black dress every day.'

545

'What else you remember?'

'I remember seeing her with a blood-soaked bandage over her face in some nowhere hospital. I remember this pilot breaking all the rules so he could get her to Udorn for me.'

She was furiously biting her lip, in the grip of her emotions. But she would not look at him.

'I remember the guy got killed and I didn't know where they sent her. Then a few weeks later I was wounded and I ended up back in the States. I came back to Saigon to look for you, Ly May.'

She stopped and stared at him. I want to believe you, her face said. But I need proof. He bent closer and pushed back his hair so she could see the jagged white scar that followed his hairline. 'War wound.'

She touched the scar with her fingertips. He could feel her trembling. Finally she pulled away.

'I'm sorry,' he said.

There it was. Proof. Vindication. Redemption. Whatever.

'You save my seeing, Mai Koo. But when you don't come back, I die, never mind. Here inside. Imagine with your heart how I feel. I am just a little girl, then, I not understand this. I hate you then, so much.'

He didn't know what to say to her.

'Well, I guess things turned out all right in the end,' he said, knowing it was not true.

He reached out for her, and she started when his fingers brushed her cheek. He turned her face towards him. There was the faintest puckering of flesh above the eyelid where the shrapnel had torn into her eye.

'The doctors they save one,' she said. 'Other one, the seeing not so good. Like misted glass, okay? But can see.'

'How did you get here, Ly May?' He touched the diamond at her throat. 'How did this happen?'

'Beautiful girl always get beautiful thing, okay?'

'Where did you learn to speak English? And Thai? How did you get out of Saigon?'

She shook her head and pushed his hand away. 'I have good luck.' She walked on, and he followed her. It felt as if there was a band around his chest. He wasn't sure he could do this.

546

'I practise this ten thousand thousand times,' she was saying. 'I think always I will see you again, and you will know me straight away. Instead you just think I am some cheap stuff looking for business.' She looked up at him for confirmation. He said nothing. 'I burn joss for you, I say rosary for you to Virgin, just want to see you one time more, don't know why. You look just the same, Mai Koo.' They walked in silence for a while. 'So, now you tell me why you are in Chiang Mai.'

'I work there.'

'You are pilot no more, I think.'

'No, not a pilot.'

She turned and stared at him. Her face underwent a transformation. 'Douglas.'

He just stared at her.

'Don't look at me like I am fortune teller man. I have brain, not empty-headed cheap stuff! Until Prenom is so sick, I think you follow me because you want to see Ly May, find out she is okay. I think I want to see you also. I love you too bad, Mai Koo, still love you too bad, silly country girl! But when Prenom is so much sick, I think this is all too clever. So why you in Chiang Mai, why you in Bangkok? Not sure. Now I figure.'

Michael ploughed on, unwilling to try and dignify his mission with justifications. 'Do you know who this man is?' he asked her.

'Yes, I know. It doesn't mind. World is full of badness. Girl must live, must eat.'

'Not this way.'

'Why not this way, okay? Easy for you, never been starving, never sleep in dirt, never do dirty stuff for money. When you ever hungry, Mai Koo?'

'This man sells misery.'

'Don't sell it to me! Don't sell it to Ly May! I just look pretty for him and give him dirty stuff when he want. For this he give me gold like this one on my arm, so when I have wrinkle time I don't beg like all the old mothers selling little wood things and rambutan in the street! Don't you say to me misery! Misery I don't have now!'

'My sister destroyed her life with heroin. Twice she nearly died.'

'Then I am sorry for you. But I am more sorry for me. I never chase the dragon and maybe I have more bad stuff in my life than her.'

Michael felt the world spinning. She was telling him his sister was partly to blame. The suggestion rocked him. 'My sister ...'

But the words would not come.

Michael knew he had lost control of this. 'If you help us, you'll never starve again.'

'I not starve anyway.' She held out her wrist. She was wearing a gold Piaget, set with tiny diamonds.

He knew there was no point in saying more to her.

'This is why you make sweet eyes at me, Mai Koo? You want me to be spy for you?'

'No,' he said, 'it wasn't just that.'

He could see by her face that she did not believe him. She didn't even say goodbye. She just turned and walked away.

118

When May got back from Ayoddhya, Douglas took her to an exclusive restaurant off Suriwongse Road. There were caged bears and a snakepit in the middle of the room. When they arrived a mongoose and a cobra were involved in a fight to the death.

They had a table overlooking the snakepit. Douglas ordered a cognac. 'Did you enjoy yourself while I was away?' he asked her.

May knew he never asked a question without a reason, and she was immediately wary. 'I went shopping. I spent a day at Ayoddhya.'

Douglas smiled, but his eyes glittered without humour. May was accustomed to his moods, but they still frightened her. She had spent the last two years of her life with Douglas Ho, and she was no closer to understanding the essence of the man.

He nodded to a waiter who fetched a pair of steel clamps and grabbed a five foot cobra from a pit near the bear cage. With a swift and practised motion he grabbed the snake's head with one hand and with the other slit its body with a sharp razor, from the throat to the tail. He squeezed the blood into a large cup, which Douglas drank. Fresh cobra blood was a guaranteed aphrodisiac.

The waiter then sliced out the bladder and cut the remainder of the snake's body into bite-sized pieces which he fried right there at the table.

'Prenom said you went off alone in Ayoddhya.'

'He got sick. You would rather I sat in my hotel listening to the disgusting noises coming from his toilet?'

'I told you never to go anywhere alone.'

'I was bored.'

'Prenom said you have been making a habit of wandering off alone.'

May remembered Chiang Mai. 'Perhaps you should find me protection that is a little more efficient in their job.'

'I think that idea has some merit.'

May pretended to look unconcerned. She looked down into the snakepit. The mongoose had made a mistake. It had ventured too close to the cobra and the fangs had pierced the fur. The mongoose was shivering and convulsing.

Douglas leaned forward. 'A word of warning, little May. Don't ever betray my trust.'

'Why would I want to do that?'

'Why would you?' he repeated. He sipped his Hennessy brandy. 'If you ever do, I'll slit you up the middle like that cobra and eat your bladder.' And he popped the snake's innards into his mouth.

A little of the bloody juice leaked on to his chin.

119

Hong Kong

Sammy Chen's lair was high on the Peak, on Mount Davis Road – *Moh Sing Ling To* to the Chinese – *The hill from which we can touch the stars*. It was a mock Ming Dynasty palace with upturned eaves and rococco curlicues, hidden away behind high walls. The glazed blue and green tiles shimmered in the early-morning sun as if they had been freshly coated with ice.

There were two wrought iron gates, elaborately carved dragons chasing each other along the fretwork. A burly thick-set Chinese in a dark suit was on duty. When he saw Douglas he immediately swung open the gates and Douglas drove through.

Sammy Chen was in his study, a room as large as an ordinary house. The furnishings were both eclectic and awesomely expensive; two oils by Andrew Wyeth, a statue of Ganesha, as tall as a man and carved from a single piece of mahogany; a bronze Shiva head stolen from a temple in India. A heavy rosewood desk was set back from a smoked glass window that took up one entire wall. Beyond the window a balcony looked out over a kidney-shaped pool and, in the hazy distance, the sprawl of white towers in Kowloon.

Sammy had his back to him, his black silk dressing gown embroidered in scarlet silk with two warring dragons. He was sprinkling fish food into an aquarium. A huge goldfish hovered lazily in the water, its mouth pressed against the glass.

'Douglas.'

'Kee Lung,' he said, with careful respect.

'I wanted to talk to you. I have come to a decision about America.'

Douglas felt a surge of excitement. At last. For almost two years they had been contemplating moving their base of operations to San Francisco. Douglas welcomed the move; it had the potential to vastly increase their heroin profits. They already had their own courier networks, with international air freight companies and baggage handlers and flight crews on their payroll, as well as freighter captains who could transport bulk shipments to Vancouver and San Francisco. If they established themselves on the west coast of America they would be able to handle the wholesaling of the product and be able to launder the profits into secure investments. Two of Sammy Chen's sons were already living in San Francisco, and had quietly established branches of the Fei Lung in Chinatown, running nightclubs and mah-jong parlours. They paid a percentage to Henry Wing, to show 'respect', but Douglas had always assumed that when the time came they would fly in soldiers from Hong Kong to challenge the Chuen Chung Wa on the street.

Sammy wandered on to the balcony. Tendrils of jasmine, wet with dew, wound around the wrought ironwork. The hills of the New Territories were partly obscured by swirling clouds of white mist, focusing the eye on the harbour, already busy with sampans and junks and the tubby green and white Star ferries.

'Look at this, Douglas. In twenty years the communists will have it all. Some functionary from Peking will use this as his summer house.'

'Twenty years is a long time.'

'To a businessman twenty years is tomorrow.' Sammy fell silent, his face turned towards the city. The morning light did not flatter him. It revealed the pouches under his eyes and the fleshy dewlap that hung from his chin. 'We have been discussing this move to America for a long time. At the last meeting, you spoke out against any accommodation with our Hung Mun brothers in San Francisco. You also wanted us to take a more aggressive attitude towards the Italians.'

'Why not? We have the connections, we already supply Miami and San Francisco with number four. If we wanted we could throw the Italians out of the business.'

'That's right, Douglas, it's a business, not a war. If we put blood on the streets we'll have American police breathing down our necks. There is enough for everyone.'

'Why should we co-operate with them? We supply their number four and they get rich at our expense. Everyone knows it is the distributors who make all the profits.'

'We are businessmen not soldiers. You want us to fight the Chuen Chung Wa *and* the Mafia?' The Chuen Chung Wa were the most dominant triad in San Francisco's Chinatown.

'We could defeat them separately. Besides, we have the heroin. They come to us, we don't go to them.'

'They can get it somewhere else. You're too greedy.'

'We would not be here if we were not a little greedy.'

'No, it was not greed. We saw business opportunities, we took them. We have always made accommodations for everyone, that is how we grew strong. When I was in Saigon, I paid my dues to the Vietnamese government and the VC. In Bangkok now we pay our respects to the Thais. That is the way we do business.'

'With the government, yes, not with our competition.'

'There are other considerations.'

Douglas was silent and said nothing.

'Wars are expensive. The victor is often the loser. A big gang war will only attract the interest of the newspapers, and the police will have to act. The politicians, too. What happens to our protection then? We operate best in darkness, in anonymity. Even if we won the battle, we might lose the war.' Sammy turned around and stared at Douglas. 'Sometimes it is better to compromise a little.'

He fought to keep the anger and disgust from his face. He had suspected Sammy would go this way. He was getting old and soft. He wanted to leave their business to accountants and lawyers.

'I am leaving for San Francisco next week,' Sammy went on. 'I am having a settlement talk with the 489 of the Chuen Chung Wa, Henry Wing. I will also have meetings with the Trincas. There will be no war.'

'Yes, Kee Lung,' Douglas said. He knew it would be unwise

to argue further. Sammy would not change his mind once he was set on his course, and to confront him would only forewarn him of his intentions.

'You are disappointed.'

'But I bow to your greater wisdom in these matters, Kee Lung.'

'You are foremost a warrior, Douglas. That is your strength, but also your weakness.' He turned back to the panorama of the morning. 'You will assume responsibility for my affairs here in Hong Kong until I return.'

'Thank you, Kee Lung.'

Kee Lung! Fearless Dragon! You are a dragon without teeth, without claws, and all San Francisco will know it! He knew what would be the result of these settlement talks! Henry Wing would demand a percentage from them as respect, and they would lose all face. If we go to America we must go there with knives in our fists or not go there at all! You are selling out to Henry Wing and that barbarian Trinca and they will laugh at us and know we are weak, and one day they will swallow us all!

A solitary kite hovered over the Peak. It spotted something in the scrub below, a mouse perhaps, or a small lizard, and dropped like a stone. A few seconds later it rose again, screaming in triumph, its prey wriggling in its beak. An omen for you, Douglas thought. This is how I will destroy you.

'May good fortune smile on your endeavours,' he said, and left, raging.

120

Bangkok

Noelle came in from the terrace, dripping, leaving wet footprints on the dark teak. The bathing suit was embarrassingly sparse, in Lucien's opinion, and revealed far too much of her chest, which was heaving with the exertion of the forty laps she had just swum in the pool. Tiny droplets of water gleamed on her skin like a dusting of diamonds. Lucien was aware of his friend, Jean-Claude, watching her as she went to the bar in the corner and splashed some Mekong whisky into a glass with soda water. Her bikini briefs clung to her like a second skin and Jean-Claude could not take his eyes away.

Lucien cleared his throat, hoping to remind both of them of their manners, without success.

'*Bonjour, Jean-Claude, ça va?*'

'*Oui, ça va,*' he said, and his voice sounded hoarse and strange. Noelle had been to dinner with Jean-Claude's father, an attaché at the French Embassy, on several occasions. Lucien could imagine what he was thinking. Sometimes, he thought, my family and my friends are equally disgusting.

'What are you boys doing?'

'Jean-Claude is just getting ready to leave,' said Lucien.

Jean-Claude's cheeks were flushed. He has the guilty look of a boy caught fingering underwear in a lingerie shop, Lucien thought. I should throw him in the pool to cool him off.

'Yeah, I'd better be getting home,' he mumbled.

'I'll see you out,' Lucien said.

When he came back Noelle had wrapped a towel around her, and was sitting on a sun chair by the pool with her drink.

There was a frangipani bloom in her gleaming black hair.

'I wish you wouldn't do that, *Maman*.'

'Do what?' Noelle asked sweetly.

'You're over forty years old, for God's sake. You're my mother.'

'What have I done wrong now? I only went for a swim.'

'You know what you did! Don't pretend you don't.'

She grinned at him and he wanted to throttle her. 'So I flaunt a little. What's so bad about that? It's good for my ego. I'm not so bad for an old woman, am I?'

'You should be ashamed of yourself.'

'You would be happy if I was fat and ugly, and when I jumped in the pool all the water jumped out?'

'I would be happy if you put on the towel before you came in to talk to my friends.' She made him feel as if he was a hundred years old. How did she manage that? At his age she was supposed to be scolding *him* for his excesses.

'You will not have to worry about me next year,' she said. 'You'll be in Paris. I won't be able to embarrass you any more.'

'What will you do with your time then?'

'I'll call all your friends and have a really big party here on my own.' She stood up, and then saw his expression. 'Oh, Luc, don't look so cross. I'm only teasing.'

'You're too beautiful for your own good.'

Her cheeks flushed with pleasure. 'Oh, Luc. You always know the right things to say to your mother!' And she gave him a torchy laugh, and went inside to shower.

As the afternoon faded to evening the gilded spires of the stupas glinted in the last sunlight like gold coins in dirty water. The dipping sun was a rusted orange behind the milky haze of heat and rush hour exhaust fumes. The red roofs of the city and the tall white towers of the hotels faded quickly into the hot night, and the chirruping of insects joined with the roar of traffic on Sukhumwit Road.

Half an hour later Noelle reappeared, bringing with her the scent of Balmain. Dressed to kill, Lucien decided, dressed for revenge. A little black number, one of her own imported lines, a Patou or Givenchy and very expensive. There was

556

gold at her wrists and a cabochon-cut Burmese ruby at her throat. She was right, not so bad for an old lady. There were faint lines around her eyes, he noticed, and if you looked very, very carefully, you might find a fleck of grey in the ebullient black curls. But they only seemed to add to her allure. Jean-Claude certainly seemed to think so.

'Have you forgotten, Luc? We're meeting your father for dinner.'

'I'm ready,' he said. He had on the cotton short-sleeved shirt and jeans he had worn all afternoon.

'They won't let you in looking like that, even in Calvin Kleins.'

'Then I won't go.'

'It's your birthday. I know you're a teenager but try to be pleasant.'

'You know what it's going to be like.'

'He's your father, Luc. I don't like him, I don't trust him, I would rather throw myself on electrified barbed wire than be near him, but he's your father and we're going.'

'Did you always feel this way about him, or have you just warmed to him over the years?'

'Please go and get ready.' When Lucien did not budge, she said: 'Please go and get ready or I shall ring Jean-Claude and ask him to accompany me.'

He slouched off to the bedroom. When he returned he was wearing a blazer, slacks and even, *merde alors*, a tie. 'Well, that's better,' Noelle beamed.

'Don't forget, don't sit with your back to any doors tonight. We don't want to get caught in any crossfire.'

'I never forget that,' she said.

Baptiste Crocé was an impressive man to have as a father, Lucien had to admit; the eye patch, the grey wings of hair, the powder white smile – he could imagine how easily his mother had once fallen in love with him. Lucien himself had once made the mistake of introducing a girlfriend to him; she had fawned over Baptiste the rest of the night, hanging on his every word, ignoring Lucien. She was just seventeen years old. Baptiste was old enough to be her father, and also old enough to have had the

557

sense and decency to discourage her, which he did not do.

But then, everyone was charmed by his father's imposing Gallic looks and easy charm when they first met him. You had to know him really well to understand how even poison can be coated in rich dark chocolate.

He was already waiting when they arrived at the restaurant, dressed in blazer, flannels and black silk shirt. A rope of gold glistened in the black and silver hairs at his throat. He was, thankfully, alone. He had at least had the good grace not to bring one of his mistresses to his son's birthday.

Well, almost alone. Lucien noted the two men sitting moody and silent at the next table, their sombre but beautifully tailored suits not quite able to disguise the unsightly bulges under their armpits. Either a glandular disease or 9-millimetre Berettas, he decided.

Baptiste rose to greet them, and Noelle allowed him to embrace her briefly. After all, it was a special occasion. Then he gripped Lucien's hand in his own and crushed him to his chest. Lucien disentangled himself as quickly as he could.

'Happy Birthday, Lucien.' Baptiste beamed at him. When they were all seated he reached into his jacket pocket and produced a rectangular black box. 'Here, I got you a present.'

Lucien opened it. Inside was a Rolex Oyster Presidential, the face inlaid with diamonds. Five figures at least, in US dollars. One of his father's typically underplayed gestures. Lucien looked at his mother, but she had her head in the leather bound menu. 'Thanks, Baptiste,' he said.

'Thanks? That's it?'

'I'm just a bit overwhelmed.'

His father looked irritated. 'You're just like your mother. I could never please her either. No matter what I did.' He looked for a reaction from Noelle, but she pointedly ignored him.

'Well, that must be some sort of record,' Lucien said. 'Thirty-eight seconds and you've already got your first shot in at *Maman*.'

'That's unofficial timing,' Noelle said, from behind the menu. 'With the Presidential you can get that down to one hundredths of a second.'

The waiter brought a bottle of Taitinger Brut de Brut.

558

He poured the sparkling golden champagne into three flutes and Baptiste raised his glass. 'I ordered some champagne to celebrate. What did you get the boy for his birthday, Noelle?'

'A pair of socks.'

He gave her a cold stare, knowing she was mocking him.

'And a Lear jet,' she added.

'Please,' said Lucien. 'Can we just drink the champagne?'

They touched glasses. He knew it now. It was going to be one of those nights.

The restaurant was cool, heavy with the scents of spice and ginger. The window overlooked the dark ribbon of the Chao Phrya, the yellow glow of the urban sprawl beyond. The lights of the sampans and teak barges on the river looked like fireflies.

'So, Lucien, what are you going to do now you have left school?' his father asked.

'I have been accepted at the Sorbonne.'

'The Sorbonne. And what are you going to study?'

'Business.'

Baptiste raised an eyebrow and looked at Noelle. 'You should have sent him to me. I could have taught him everything he will ever need to know about business.'

'Especially the drug business.'

'Don't preach morals at me, Noelle. It's not a nice world, if you hadn't noticed. Your neighbour, Colonel Pramual, for instance. As a policeman he earns two hundred and fifty US dollars a month. Yet the houses in your exclusive little street are all worth a hundred thousand dollars each and I happen to know the good Colonel has a Swiss bank account with a seven-figure sum in it. There's no difference between me and anyone else in Thailand.'

'I don't want my son peddling dope.'

'You demean me. I don't peddle it. I move it in container loads. Besides, I learned everything I know from Rocco.'

At the mention of her father, Noelle flushed and lapsed into silence. Baptiste smiled, knowing he had made his point.

'So how have you been, Noelle? How is the world of fashion?' There was distaste in his voice whenever he spoke about her business. Lucien had the impression that his father would prefer to see her bankrupt and begging on the street. Even though he declared he still loved her.

'Last month I opened another store in the Indra Regent. Life has been good to me. Lately.'

He let that one pass. 'Any men in your life?'

'Do you want their names and addresses?'

'Just their names, I can find out their addresses for myself.' He smiled, but Lucien wondered if it really was a joke.

Noelle ate a spiced prawn. Lucien watched the way she savoured it. Everything about her was sensual. 'I have a few close friends, Baptiste, and some ongoing social engagements. But I don't fall in love any more. I tried it twice and I didn't like it.'

'Twice,' he said, and it was as if he had a mouthful of ash.

'You would have thought once was enough.'

There was a centrepiece of flowers on the table. Baptiste took one of the blooms, held it between his thumb and forefinger. 'Bleeding hearts,' he said. 'Do you know the legend, Lucien? A young woman, abandoned by her lover cried her tears on this flower and left these marks. Abandonment. An appropriate theme for this evening.'

Noelle pushed her plate away. 'Please, *chéri*, you're going to have the whole restaurant in tears in a moment.'

'I mean it. It is how I feel. Abandoned.'

Noelle leaned closer to him and lowered her voice. 'I loved you once, Baptiste. I loved you more than I loved my own life. You had your chances. But there were other white flowers that you loved more than me.' She excused herself and headed for the ladies' room.

He lit a cheroot and sat back in his chair, watching the smoke curl towards the ceiling.

'You handled that well,' said Lucien.

'If you know a good way to handle your mother, Lucien, please tell me. I have been searching for the right way all my life.'

He shrugged.

'I do not know why we do this. Meet like this. It is always so distressing for me.'

'I know what you mean, Papa.'

'You should come and see me sometimes. Without her.'

'What for?'

Baptiste fixed him with his single dark eye. The intensity of the look made Lucien turn away. 'You don't want to see your own father?'

Lucien took the easy way out. 'You're never in town long enough. I never know where you are.'

'Well, there is a lot of business I have to take care of. I could probably do with a little help.'

'A secretary, maybe?'

Baptiste leaned forward. 'Let's stop playing games here.' He put a hand on his son's wrist. 'What are you doing with your life? Is that what you want – university? A big education? Huh? What can they teach you in university? Business! I'll tell you about business. You cut off the other man's balls before he cuts off yours. There. That's business. I just saved you three years of your life.'

'Great, Papa. Do I get a diploma?'

'I can give you something better than a diploma. I can give you anything you want. What do you like son, huh? Tell me. You like girls? You like to gamble? You like fast cars? Or maybe you just like to play chess with people, like to play the game?'

'I don't want to play the games you play.'

'Why not? What do you know about me, huh? What does she tell you?'

Lucien felt uncomfortable. 'She hasn't told me anything.'

'I sit on the board at a bank. I have interests in shopping departments and hotels and mining companies and shipping fleets. I know the King of Thailand. I have government ministers to my house for dinner. Did she ever tell you that?' He closed his fist and held it out, palm upwards, to Lucien. 'Did she ever tell you that you are the heir apparent. All you have to do is say that you want it. I can give you everything you ever wanted, every secret desire.' He unclenched his fist. 'What is it you want? Take it.'

Lucien felt a moustache of sweat form on his upper lip. 'I just want to have my own life,' he said.

Baptiste raised an eyebrow in sardonic amusement. 'You're

nineteen years old. You know nothing about life. Yours, or anyone else's.'

At that moment Noelle reappeared and Baptiste stood up to hold out her chair for her. Always the perfect gentleman, thought Lucien.

Noelle sat down. 'Thank you, Baptiste. What were you boys talking about while I was gone?'

'I was trying to teach him the facts of life.'

'A father and son talk?' Noelle gave Lucien a proprietary glance.

'Papa thinks that rather than go to university I would be better advised to get practical experience in an established business.'

Noelle's eyes flashed in anger. 'You never give up do you?' she said to Baptiste.

'Not with you. Not with him. Not ever.'

'I won't have him corrupted. I don't want to see greed do to him what it did to you.'

'You can't avoid corruption, *chérie*. It's what happens to you after you're born.'

'We'll see,' said Noelle, but there was something else behind the determination in her eyes.

Fear.

After dinner, Baptiste took a mother of pearl cigarette case from his breast pocket and lit another of his filterless Russian cigarettes, beckoning the waiter. 'Would you like a liqueur, Noelle? I would suggest a cognac, but in the circumstances I think perhaps something a little less flammable might be better.'

'Shit doesn't burn, Baptiste,' she said, sweetly.

He grinned. 'Bitch.'

'Does that mean it's nearly time to go?' asked Lucien.

Noelle got to her feet. Baptiste stood also and turned to Lucien. 'Remember what I told you. And don't forget to take your birthday present.'

'I can't.'

'You can't what?'

'Take it.'

'Why not? It's just a toy.'

562

Noelle put a hand on Lucien's arm. 'He is saying no because I told him not to let you get your hooks into him.'

'What a thing for a mother to say.'

'Thank you for dinner, Baptiste. It's been a wonderful evening.'

'Why do you hate me so much? This I have never understood.'

'It's not personal.'

He banged his fist on the table. An appalled silence. Around the restaurant conversation stopped and heads turned; the women in their diamonds and Givenchy gowns, the tanned and elegant Westerners who escorted them, Chinese and Thai and Japanese businessmen in expensive and sombre suits. In Thailand, public displays of anger were considered an appalling breach of protocol.

Baptiste reined in his temper. When he spoke his voice was so low barely anyone at the other tables heard. *'Tu es con!* I did it all for you!'

'It must have seemed like a good idea at the time,' Noelle said. 'Now we really must leave. Unlike you, I detest scenes.'

She walked out and Lucien hurried after her. She jumped in the passenger seat of the Mercedes and Lucien drove her home through the tangle of Bangkok's night traffic. They hardly spoke. He looked around at her once, and saw that her eyes were shining and her mascara had smeared her cheeks.

He reached out and squeezed her hand. He wondered if he would ever know the full truth of what had passed between his parents. He was almost sure he did not want to.

As he turned into the alleyway behind their villa he did not notice the black Toyota that followed them. Its headlights were switched off, and it stalked them like a panther in the dark.

121

A child leaped out in front of the car and Lucien plunged his foot on to the brakes. The child brought up a spray bottle and squirted detergent on the windscreen. He waved a rag at them and then shouted that for one baht he would wipe it off. It was not an uncommon ploy among the street kids of Bangkok.

But outside their own villa, at this time of night...

'*Petit salaud!*' Noelle hissed. The evening had exhausted her reserves of patience. She threw open the passenger door to chase the child away. Lucien saw a shadow run across the alley in his rear vision mirror and tried to shout a warning.

After that everything happened very quickly.

Noelle felt a hand go around her throat and screamed. Her first thoughts were of rape. It did not occur to her in those first few moments that she was not the target. Her assailant pushed her into the wall, she hit her head and blacked out.

When she recovered she saw Lucien struggling with two men. One of them had climbed in the passenger side door, the other had reached in through the driver's side and was trying to pull Lucien out from behind the wheel. The engine was still running and the car suddenly lurched forward and careened into the wall on the other side of the alley, with a crash of metal and glass. The man on Lucien's side cursed and jumped clear.

He shouted something to his colleague. Noelle recognised the dialect: chiu chao Chinese.

She realised it was Lucien they were after, not her, and all fear left her. They were not going to harm her son. Whatever they wanted, whoever they were, she would not let them hurt Lucien.

Noelle stumbled to her feet, and aimed a kick at the man struggling with Lucien through the passenger door. It found its mark, the pointed toe of her shoe arcing up between his legs. He gave a shrill cry of pain and dropped to the ground. Noelle hesitated, looking for her next target. The shadows blurred by her right shoulder, she felt a flurry of movement, and something hit her very hard on the right temple.

She had no idea how long she had been unconscious. Someone was shaking her by the shoulder, and asking her in Thai what had happened. She tried to raise her head, couldn't. She rolled on her side and retched.

'What happened?' the man said again. He was shining a torch right in her face, and Noelle pushed it away.

She suddenly remembered how two men had tried to drag her son from the car. 'Lucien,' she said, but her tongue seemed to be twice its normal size and what came out was no more than a mumbled cough.

The man swung the torch towards the Mercedes, its fender crumpled against the wall, the alley littered with glass. The passenger door yawned open. The car appeared to be empty.

'Lucien,' Noelle said again, and she knew she had lost him.

122

Noelle lived two blocks from Sukhumwit Road, on Soi Sapphankwai. It was an old Thai house, nestled discreetly behind a forest of banana trees and a carefully tended garden of lavender and boungainvillea. An ancient Chinese amah ushered him in.

Baptiste looked around. It was a riot of greenery; orchids hung in slatted wooden boxes, there were tapioca trees in dragon pots, fragile monkey tails and fragrant frangipani. The teak floors were scattered with Chinese silk rugs and against the windows were armchairs upholstered in cream silk. It was the first time he had ever been allowed inside her Bangkok home; he recognised her touch.

Noelle was in the bedroom. She was sitting on the bed in a red silk dressing gown, propped on pillows, an ice pack against the side of her head. He would not have recognised the same woman who'd sat down to dinner with him just the previous evening. On the side of her head was a swelling the size of a baseball, and one eye was swollen shut. She was deathly pale and looked as fragile as a child's china doll thrown carelessly on the bed.

'They took my son,' she said.

'I'll get him back.'

'Why? Why did they take him?'

'I don't know,' he said. 'But I will find out. And I'll bring him back.'

'Is this you?' she said. 'Is it you that's involved him in this?'

Baptiste shook his head. 'I swear to you, I don't know what's going on. Do you think I would knowingly put my own son at risk?' He sat on the edge of the bed and picked up her hand. It was cold and limp. 'Are you all right?'

'I have concussion. Mild. The doctor wants to send me to the hospital. I told him I won't go.'

'It would be better for you. I am sure he knows what's best.'

'When have I ever done what's best for me, Baptiste?'

He took out his cigarettes, changed his mind, put them back in his pocket. 'Tell me what happened.'

'We had just turned into the alley. A little boy ran in front of the car, squirted something on the windscreen. As I got out to shout at him, a man came up behind me, put his arm around my throat. I thought they wanted me, or perhaps our money, our car. But I never thought...' She stopped, took a moment to compose herself. 'They threw me out and wrestled with Lucien. He was still in the car. I tried to help him... I don't remember then. One of them hit me. I remember waking up. Colonel Pramual was there with a torch and his revolver. The car was empty. He'd gone.'

'Did you see who these men were?'

'It was too dark, I didn't see their faces. But I heard them talking to each other. They were chiu chao, Baptiste. Chinese.'

'Chinese?' he said. Surely some young triad soldiers who had gone rogue. No triad leader in Bangkok would have had reason to sanction this.

'The police say they will do everything they can,' said Noelle.

'The police! The Thais couldn't find a wild elephant in a duck pond. There is only one way we are going to get our son back.'

Baptiste tried to reason this out. He knew this was no coincidence. Lucien had been taken because he was Baptiste Crocé's son. But why? If they were chiu chao they could be from any one of a number of syndicates that operated in Bangkok. So far no one had contacted him with a ransom demand.

He just hoped that the men who had taken Lucien were professionals. By the blood of God I'll make them pay if they harm him. I'll tear out their guts with my bare hands!

'Do you want me to stay here tonight?'

'What for, Baptiste?'

'Protection. Comfort.'

'I don't need any protection and you're no comfort. Just find my boy.'

He had hoped their grief might unite them, if only for a few days. But Noelle was as remote in her sorrow as she had been all her life. There was nothing else he could do here.

He went out, closing the door gently behind him.

123

San Francisco

For Jennifer's birthday, Jonathan Dale had booked a table in one of San Francisco's most exclusive restaurants, L'Etoile in the Huntingdon Hotel. Crystal chandeliers, a grand piano, hushed conversation. Dale was on his second dry martini when Jennifer made her appearance. She tottered after the maître d', weaved, almost barged into a marble pedestal and toppled a potted fern. Heads turned and disapproving glances followed her across the room to the copper-coloured banquette where Dale was waiting.

She was wearing a shapeless and crumpled cotton dress, a knitted shawl, gold slave bracelet on her upper arm, junk jewellery and lace-up boots. She looked like a gypsy fortune teller at a circus. Hey eyes were pink and streaming, and she reeked of stale sweat.

It was a miracle they had let her in.

Dale rose to greet her. They embraced briefly and she slumped onto the banquette. She was stoned, he realised. Or perhaps coming off.

'Christ, Jennifer, what have you done to yourself?'

'Hey, I'm fine.'

'You're stoned.'

Jennifer gave a theatrical sigh and raised her eyebrows. 'Don't start on me, okay? I just got here.'

'You promised me you were off this time.'

'Hey, it was only a little grass.'

Only a little grass.

There had been so many promises, and they had always been broken. But he'd really thought that this time it was going to be different. For three months she had stayed clean; no more frantic messages from the police station to be bailed out, no more calls from the hospital to inform him she was in emergency being treated for an overdose and could he come down immediately? Once she had gashed her heel on a piece of broken glass on the sidewalk, and then trod in some dog excrement; she had been too stoned to notice. That time she nearly lost her foot.

There had been the methadone programs for her heroin addiction, and drug rehabilitation centres, and compulsory government programs, so many psychiatrists he couldn't remember all their names. After each attempt to save her, she had promised that she had had enough, that this time she was going to quit drugs and get on with her life. This time he thought she had actually made it.

And now here she was, stoned again. It was the uncertainty that hurt him the most, the expectations followed by crushing disappointment. He suspected she knew that; sometimes she seemed to play him like a professional torturer.

She rubbed her nose with her sleeve.

'Why, Jenny?'

'Hey, it doesn't hurt. It's not like smack or anything.'

'But it always starts this way.'

'It helps me to relax.'

'You need to be relaxed to have dinner with me?'

Jenny looked around the restaurant, scowling, her eyes heavy-lidded and inflamed. 'What a fucking tight-ass place! Did we have to come here? Why couldn't we go to Taco Bell or McDonalds?'

'It's your birthday. I wanted to do something special.'

'Whooo! Special! I don't recall ever being special before.'

Oh, no, not that old route again. The waiter approached. Dale was a regular in L'Etoile, and the man knew him well. 'Would you like me to take your order now, Mr Dale?'

'I'll have the sole, thanks, Roger.'

Jennifer tried to focus on the menu. She sniffed and tossed it on the table. 'Got a burger?'

'No, we don't, I'm afraid, Miss Dale. If you like steak, you might like to try the châteaubriand.'

'Does it come in a bun?'

570

Roger looked confused. He looked to Dale for clarification. 'Two Dover sole,' Dale said. Roger nodded and moved away.

'What is this? No one asks my opinion? What am I, a little kid?'

'Only if you insist on behaving like one.'

'Well, excuse me.' She leaned her head against the banquette, her eyes heavy. Her ash blonde hair had turned mousy and was stringy from lack of attention. Her skin had a greyish tinge. She was still a young woman and middle age had taken her already.

'Have you seen Susan?' he asked her.

'Sure. Mom's been around. She didn't take me to a fancy restaurant though.'

'I thought this would just be...'

'...special, right. Hey, I got a new stepfather. You heard?'

'I heard Susan is planning to marry again, yes. That hardly amounts to a new stepfather. Not at your age.'

She ignored him. 'Sure hope he's better than the last one.'

Dale was getting tired of this. He had not brought her here for another of her Oscar performances. She was now leaning on her elbows and staring at a grey-haired man two tables away, lasciviously tracing her lips with her tongue. The man flushed angrily and turned away.

'What the hell are you doing?'

'He was staring at me.'

'If you don't want people to stare at you, you could maybe think about wearing something a little more restrained.'

'I wear what I want.'

'Sure you do.'

The sommelier appeared. Dale shook his head. He didn't think his daughter needed any more substances in her system right now.

'If you want to keep behaving like this, we're leaving.'

'Any time you want.'

They lapsed into silence. Jennifer sniffed continuously. I can't do this any more, Dale thought. For almost thirteen years my child has held me to ransom for the mistakes of the past. It started off as a game but now the game has got her. I can't endure this any more; I can't.

571

Their food came, but Dale discovered he had no appetite. This was meant to be a celebration; her birthday, as well as the longest period she had stayed clean in almost ten years. Now they were back in the old cycle, the rat trap they had played out so many times before. She would go straight; after a while she might do a little dope, just to relax her, now that she had proved she could stay off. Then one night she would visit one of her old friends, Scott perhaps, and she would smoke some heroin or even mainline because like an alcoholic she could not bear to be in the presence of her addiction and not submit. And then she would be off on the slow spiral down once more, and it would be left to Dale and the doctors to save her. At the last she would pull back from the brink and the cycle of suffering would be complete. Until the next time.

In his mind Dale remembered the mountains of Laos, saw the poppy fields blazing in the morning, the Hmong women bent over the petals with their blades, as peaceful and as beautiful a scene as he had ever witnessed. He wondered how so much misery could come from a field of flowers.

He watched her devour her lunch, Dover sole in a pinot noir sauce, as if it was a plate of beans. He sipped a Perrier water.

'You still have a job?' he asked her.

'What's so great about having a job? That's all you care about, isn't it? I got to have a job, be a good American citizen. It's not what your country can do for you, it's what you can do for your country. Right?'

'I didn't want a lecture on leftist politics. I just asked if you still had a job.'

'Yeah, I still got a job.'

A job. A waitress in a North Beach café. The full circle, the same sort of job she had been doing at university. After Berkeley she had worked for McGovern's doomed election campaign against Nixon, then worked in welfare, taking care of other people's problems, the supreme irony. She had lost that job for absenteeism. There followed a series of increasingly futile dead ends, boyfriends, therapists, menial jobs in law offices, a long period of volunteer work when she had convinced herself she was doing something useful with her life while Dale paid her bills and she took refuge from herself in heroin.

'Well, you've still got a job,' he said. 'That's something.'

'It's not anything.'

'Yeah, I guess you're right.' And perhaps the expression on his face really wounded her, because she turned away at once.

'I got the munchies. What else they got to eat in this place?' She saw Roger at a nearby table. 'Hey, dickhead. Get your ass over here.'

Dale jumped to his feet. 'That's enough.'

'Hey, what's up? I do something wrong?'

'We're leaving.'

'I don't want to fuckin' go. This was your idea.'

He grabbed her by the arm and jerked her to her feet. He had played into her hands, he realised. She was going to put him over the wheel of embarrassment in his own restaurant. Oh, she plays me like a tune. Why don't I ever see it coming?

'Out. Move it.'

He threw some money on the table and dragged her outside; he could feel eyes on them the whole way. When they were on the street she pulled herself free.

'I'll drive you home,' he said.

'I don't need this bullshit.'

'Neither do I.'

'Well then, just get the fuck out of my face.'

'I intend to. I can't be the kicking post for every damned thing that's gone wrong for you. While I'm around, you'll never take responsibility for your own life.'

'Oh, sure. You never cared about me anyway.'

People walked around them on the sidewalk. A woman walking a small dog stopped to listen. Dale no longer gave a damn. 'If that's what you choose to believe.'

'It's what I know.'

'How many times do I have to say I'm sorry?'

'I don't know, I haven't been counting.'

'That's it. That-is-it.' He walked away. He realised it now; if she ever gave up destroying herself, it would mean she had forgiven him for the past. And she would not let go of the past; she was too proud for that and she hated him too much. They were locked together in their mutual misery; he couldn't forgive himself until she did.

And she just wouldn't.

She walked in the opposite direction along California, not heading anywhere, just away from him. Well, that had a certain symmetry to it. She realised people were walking around her as if she was a leper, mén in suits, women with Nieman Marcus shopping bags. They were all idiots, pain in the ass straights, limp dicks and tight ass matrons. She didn't know that twice she stopped to shout these very words right in the faces of the passers-by. The separations between thought and voice had become blurred. The world was a maelstrom of confusing sounds and images. A bad trip. A bummer.

She hated her old man. He was always on her case. *You promised me you were off this time*. And that hangdog look he always had. Well, sure, she had tried to give up. Her whole life was about trying to give up. But without drugs life was drag ass and colourless, she felt as lonely and as unwanted and desperate as she always did. So what the hell was the point?

The point was carrying, the point was using, and not just for the high, the mellow. All her friends did drugs, and they depended on her to get them their fixes. When she was straight everyone hated her and looked at her snake-eyes, and nobody loved her. Like they had her whole life. But when she was holding they loved her, they needed her.

It was nice to feel needed.

You couldn't carry, and not use a little now and then. Christ, you'd have to be superwoman.

So thanks, Dad. For everything.

If she had had a regular father she'd be straight.

It was all his fault.

124

Chinatown

From the outside, the headquarters of the San Francisco Chinese Benevolent Society looked like any other brownstone. From the second-storey windows came a jumble of Cantonese and chiu chao and Mandarin and the rapid fire clack-clack-clack of mah-jong tiles. This was not the tourist Chinatown; on one side of the building was a sweatshop, and on the other a rundown tenement where Chinese lived and slept in the same overcrowding as the worst slums of Hong Kong.

On the steps of the brownstone an old man, his trousers rolled up to his knee, was reading a Chinese language newspaper, through spectacles with pebbled lenses. Four young Chinese piled down the steps past him, wearing sneakers, designer jeans and wrap-around sunglasses. They deliberately jostled him on the way, knocking the newspaper out of his hands.

The gulf between the three generations of immigrant Chinese could not have been wider.

On the top floor of the building Henry Wing sat at a long, stained teak table under a photograph of Sun Yat Sen. On the walls hung a Republican flag, and the banners of the Chuen Chung Wa.

Henry Wing was in his seventies now. He wore an ill-fitting grey suit and an open-necked white shirt. His sparse grey hair was combed carefully across his skull, and his hands looked as if they had been soaked in vinegar. He looked like any one of the old men who passed their days in Washington Square with their singing canaries.

Henry Wing clapped his hands for *yum cha* and invited Sammy Chen to sit. They enquired politely after each other's health and families, their voices echoing around the great, empty room. They spoke at length of the political situation in China.

Finally Henry Wing said: 'I hear rumours that you are to come and live here in San Francisco.'

'There is much uncertainty in Hong Kong. In less than twenty years it will revert to Peking. I have to think of the future.'

Henry Wing watched him with tired, grey eyes. 'Your Hung Men brothers will join you here?'

Sammy Chen shook his head. 'I do not invite conflict, Grandfather,' Sammy said, using the honorific to show his respect, although Henry Wing was only a few years older than himself. 'I am sure there is a way that all our interests can be served.'

Henry nodded sympathetically. 'There are whispers that some of your people want to put blood on the street.'

Sammy shook his head sorrowfully. 'Hot heads. I am the voice of the Fei Lung, Grandfather, not the *fa'an gud rai* on the street.'

Henry Wing nodded his understanding. 'You know, things are different from when I was a young man. We had respect for our elders then. The Hung Mun was a democratic instrument. There was proper respect for ritual, and for our history.'

'I have found this also.'

Satisfied that he had a sympathetic audience, Henry Wing went on. 'But now the young men want everything, straight away. They are Chinese, but they have been infected with America. You know, for myself, say a sailor comes to me, he has just left his ship in the bay, he has a little white powder to sell. He says to me: "*Tai lo*, will you take it and sell it for me?" I say, "Of course." I sell it to the triad, and I give some of the money to him, and the rest to the society. That way everyone is happy. The *tong* should benefit everyone. But now the young men, they are so greedy. I think many of them have forgotten their ancestors and their oath to the Hung Mun.'

'I agree with you, Grandfather. I too have young men who do not respect the old traditions and want to be a *tai lo* in America, before their time. Everything is quick-time, hurry, hurry, like everything in America, like McDonalds. This is why it is important that we do not come into conflict. Perhaps an alliance would be beneficial to us both.'

'What do you propose, Chen Giai Han?'

'I have a son, well educated, intelligent, honourable. He holds the rank of Red Pole in the Fei Lung. One day he will be chairman, after me. You have a daughter who is also well educated, I hear she had just returned from the Roedean school in England. Would it not be very fortunate if they were to find each other interesting? A marriage would be beneficial to us both.'

'I can see how it is beneficial to you, Chen Giai Han. But how is it beneficial to me?'

'The world turns, Grandfather. You wish to avoid conflict. So do I. I would like to know that the future of my children is secure, that they will be free to tend my bones when I am gone. You will gain the alliance of a powerful triad, and the business connections which I can provide. Our interests no longer conflict. They coincide.'

Henry Wing was silent a long time. 'Is it not ironic how the West brought us opium and made us slaves to them for so long?'

'The world is a circle, Grandfather. Now we bring the opium to them, and it is our turn to be rich.'

Henry Wing nodded slowly. 'I think we can do business, you and I,' he said. 'We will arrange for your son and my daughter to talk to one another. I am sure they will find each other's company fascinating.'

'I am convinced also,' Sammy said. But then he chuckled and lowered his voice: 'And if they do not, he has another brother.'

125

Bangkok

If a man did not have a nose this place might appear romantic, thought Baptiste, as the air-conditioned black Mercedes
turned off Rama IV Road, and purred over a bridge and
into Chinatown. The klong was as thick and brown as some
pungent soup. The rowshops along its bank looked drab and
forlorn, paintwork faded by years of monsoon and pitiless heat.
Shacks jutted over its canals, stilts perched in the mud, piles
of garbage rotting in the oily water.

Yaowarat Road was choked with the coughing chaos of
trucks and tuk-tuks and buses. His driver found the address
on a corner between a *bac si* and a money changer. In the street
outside a scrawny Thai, wearing a T-shirt emblazoned with the
logo of the 1976 Montreal Olympics, crushed sugar cane and
hawked the juice from a rickety street stall.

The Hong Kong Gold Shop was one of the largest jewellers
in Bangkok, its vaults reputed to hold more precious metals
than many of the western world's largest banks. A guard
armed with a shot gun stood sentry outside a sliding iron
gate. Baptiste knew this was a dumb show, because no one
had ever attempted a heist here; even the most hardened
Bangkok criminal would not contemplate such an act because
it was owned by the Fei Lung triad.

He left his driver in the car. He had not brought protection,
had not considered it necessary. Besides, he wanted to demonstrate that he was not afraid. He wanted to show his contempt.

The shop's façade, brown marble and smoked glass, con-
trasted with the impoverished look and smell of the herbalist

next door. The inside of the shop was painted in lucky red and gold, the pilasters adorned with a riot of gilt dragons. Gold chains, charms and pendants gleamed in their cabinets of glass under the neon. This was more than a jeweller's, he knew. It was a bank. The Chinese had never put much faith in bank accounts, and invested their savings instead in gold chains of varying weight. This afternoon there were several wealthy Chinese at the counters making purchases.

Baptiste did not approach the counter. He stood in the middle of the shop and glared at one of the shop assistants, a thin young man with pockmarked cheeks.

'Baptiste Crocé,' he growled. 'I'm here to see Sharkfin.' Not Mr Ho; he spat the triad nickname with disdain. The man turned away and barked a few words in chiu chao.

Douglas Ho appeared around the corner from a back room. He gave a short nod of his head and disappeared again. *Espèce de con*, thought Baptiste savagely, and walked past the hostile stares of the other salesmen and into the back room.

'Kwo-chao,' said Douglas.

Baptiste had thought about walking straight in and breaking his neck. But there were two *sze kau* lounging behind Douglas' chair; one of them was trimming his fingernails with a razor, the other had a bulge in the left side of the jacket, hinting at a formidable weapon, a meat cleaver or a Magnum .357 perhaps.

Douglas was seated behind a metal desk. There was no other chair in the little office. The only furnishings were the desk, which had been shoved against the wall, a computer, a small calculator, and some cash books stacked on top.

Baptiste had never been here before. He made his deals with Sammy, had met Douglas only occasionally to discuss mundane matters of delivery and means of payment.

When the courier had brought him the message from Douglas, asking for a meeting, he knew who had taken Lucien.

'I want you to know Lucien is safe and well,' Douglas said.

'Where is he, you piece of shit?'

579

Douglas flinched, as if he had been struck. He's a vicious little bastard, Baptiste realised. Not much keeping him in check at the moment.

'You should be careful,' said Douglas softly. 'You are in no position to insult me. I am trying to help you.'

'Do you have my son?'

'I know how you can get him back.'

'Did you take him?'

'I can help you. That's all you need to know.'

'What do you think Sammy Chen is going to do to you when he finds out about this?'

'He is never going to hear about it. Not if you want to see your son again.'

'What is it you want from me?'

'Very little, compared with what you have to lose.' Douglas relaxed, once more in control of the conversation. 'I believe Lucien lives with his mother. But a son is always a son, is he not? When they are gone, they cannot be replaced, unlike daughters.'

'Just tell me what you want.'

'Kee Lung is in America right now. In San Francisco. I want you to convey to him a message. Tell him you have learned that Henry Wing plans to have him chopped. Tell him you have learned of the plan from your association with the Trincas.'

'What's all this about?'

'You don't need to know that.'

'Then why me?'

'Because he will believe it if it comes from you.'

'And if I convince Sammy of this conspiracy?'

'Lucien will be returned. If you do not he will die. By inches.'

Baptiste took a step forward with his fists clenched, an involuntary spasm of rage. The two *sze kau* immediately put themselves between him and Douglas Ho, the razor glinted in the light, the gun half appeared from the jacket. Only Douglas stayed absolutely still.

Baptiste took a step back.

There is no way out of this, he thought. Rocco had taught him the rules of manipulation. Once I've done what he asks

580

he has to kill me. Even if he took the risk it would not save Lucien. And he was not going to forfeit his life so easily, even for his son. He had to stall, give himself time to manoeuvre.

'Let me think about this,' he said.

'There is nothing to think about. As soon as I hear that Chen Giai Han's conversations in San Francisco have been concluded to my satisfaction you will have your son returned to you.' Otherwise you will have the pleasure of viewing him next on a slab in the morgue. It will not be pretty. You can go.'

You can go. Baptiste had never been spoken to that way. But he was in the unaccustomed position of being utterly powerless and so he turned on his heel and walked out of the shop, slamming into one of the astonished salesmen on the way out and knocking him to the floor.

The courtyard was ringed with halogen lamps, and at night the swimming pool mirrored the surrounding rock garden and sugar palms. May dived in, leaving barely a ripple on the water. She swam the length of the pool and back without breaking the surface, knifing through the electric blue water like a dolphin.

When she emerged, she stood on the edge of the pool for a long time, smoothing back the short bob of jet hair, enjoying the feel of the water cooling on her skin. She was as lithe and muscular as a boy. She had nothing else to do with her time now but enjoy the luxuries that Douglas made possible: the facials, the manicures, the personal trainers and masseurs. She was his personal accessory, and he insisted that she be maintained to flawless perfection.

May did not bother to dry herself with her towel. She wandered around, her body still gleaming with water, leaving wet footprints on the marble floors. It is not a house, she thought, it's a palace, a mausoleum, a jumble of expensive styles and hideous taste; Aubusson-backed chairs that had never been used were arranged around a table topped with pink Italian marble; a Louis Quinze sofa upholstered with French brocade was propped against a wall under an oil by Géricault and a portrait of the King and Queen of Thailand; a crystal chandelier hung suspended above Persian silk carpets. Sounds echoed around the rooms like a vault.

May went to the long, mahogany bar, poured some Hennessy XO into a brandy balloon and went back outside, to stare at the glow of the city above the walls. Have I really left the bars and the brothels behind? she asked herself. I am still a whore, I am still not free. Otherwise, why do I walk around this great house every night, drinking my expensive liqueur, getting drunker and lonelier?

My life, thought May: I no longer worry about starving to death, as I did in Saigon and the Economic Zones; I don't have to sell myself to strangers, as I did at Ranchoi and Le Palais. I have expensive clothes, I live in a luxurious house with servants and have a beautiful car to drive in. It is a wonderful life, a life I could never have imagined.

So why am I so unhappy?

She thought about the endless hours spent on jet airliners, between Bangkok and Singapore and Hong Kong, swept along in the wake of a vicious and lonely man, whose business she could still only guess at. He did not love her, sometimes she wondered if he even liked her. Her life was spent negotiating the minefields of his temper, trying to fathom what it was he wanted from her and wondering when he would have had enough.

Sex was always unsatisfactory. For Douglas it was frequency that counted. He was on a marathon, with himself the only timekeeper. Sometimes she felt he forced himself to each act. He could have bought what he had from May, but then any man could buy a whore and Douglas did not like to share. He used her beauty to taunt other men; he insisted that she wore provocative clothes whenever they went out, sometimes even around the house in front of his own bodyguards. He did not love her, but he did enjoy having something everyone else wanted and only he could have.

She could not walk away now. He would kill her, she was convinced of that. One day he would grow tired of her and release her, find some other beauty to take her place. She could only hope he would do it in a fit of boredom, and not in the midst of one of his raging tempers when he might make good his oft-repeated threat to tear her face off.

It's what you wanted, she reminded herself. When it's all over you will still have the jewellery and the clothes, enough there to start a new life, or enough to impress a new man. This is what you wanted. This is how you planned to survive.

If only she didn't feel Mai Koo's eyes on her all the time, his face twisted with loathing and disgust.

Mai Koo. If she had not seen him again perhaps her conscience might not trouble her like this. As long as she thought he had abandoned her, life made sense. It was the way things were. No one could be really trusted, not even friends like Noi, but you did your best to survive despite everything. But he said he had searched for her. He said he had not meant for her to be left behind.

Like Bich. A piece of the jigsaw that did not fit.

On an impulse she went to find Chang. She told him to fetch the car and then went up to the bedroom to dress. She had to get out of this house. She had to see for herself. She had to remember.

She had to be sure she was doing the right thing.

She told Chang to drive around Patpong, two narrow, sordid lanes of strip bars, massage parlours and brothels between the Suriwongse and Silom Roads. Disco music throbbed into the street, touts grabbed at the tourists, neon pulsed overhead: *Superstar Bar ... Spanish Harem ... Roxy Bar, spirits and hard waters served ... Girls! girls! girls! You want 'em, we got 'em ...*

Through an open doorway May saw girls in G-strings gyrating under smoky spotlights. Others clustered around the doorway, staring down the Westerners who passed in the street.

'Stop the car!' May shouted.

She knew one of those girls. It was Noi.

Chang braked to a halt and she jumped out, darting through the traffic to the other side of the street. Noi was outside the Nevada Bar, in the parody of a hooker's pose; one arm across the chest, the other extended, holding a cigarette. She had on too much make-up, wore a short leather skirt and a top that exposed small breasts pushed up by a half-cup brassiere.

As May got closer she saw the scabs on her arms. 'Noi,' she said.

The woman looked at her. May reached out to touch her and she jerked away.

'What do you want?'

'Noi?'

She stared at her in confusion and fear. 'I don't know anyone called Noi.'

No, not Noi. May realised she wasn't even like her. She was just one more prostitute in a city of thousands. My imagination did the rest.

'I thought you were someone else,' May said.

The woman flicked away her cigarette in disgust and went back into the bar.

Chang was standing behind her, watching. 'Who was that?' he said.

'I thought I knew her.'

Chang's face betrayed disbelief and scorn. May ran back to the Mercedes. It doesn't matter that it wasn't her, she thought. In the end they're all like Noi. We're all just good little Buddhist girls without a choice. But you're safe now. You escaped all that. That's the way the world is, if Noi was in your pretty little shoes right now she wouldn't look back. Why do you?

Because that wasn't the point. She had never been like Noi. She could never have smuggled drugs inside dead babies, no matter how desperate things had been.

And besides, there was Mai Koo.

When she got back to the villa, Douglas was there. 'Where have you been?' he asked her.

'I went for a drive.'

'Get your clothes packed. Tomorrow night we're leaving for Hong Kong.'

That night he made love to her three times. After the first time he fell quickly asleep, but woke her twice more during the night to repeat the act.

She imagined something good had happened for him that day.

126

A string quartet performs each afternoon in the lobby of the River Wing of the Oriental Hotel. The central court is tall, with graceful bamboos reaching for the skylights, which are hung with classical brass bells. Guests sit in elegant white cane armchairs and take afternoon tea or cocktails while they watch the rice barges and long-tailed boats sweep up and down the Chao Phrya river.

When Baptiste arrived Noelle was already there, waiting. She wore a black suit and no make-up, and looked pale and gaunt. As if she had just returned from a funeral.

She did not stand up to greet him.

He gave her his best smile. 'The black is a little premature,' he said.

'What have you found out?' she said, her expression withering.

'These things take time.'

'I said, what have you found out?'

He signalled to a white-jacketed waiter and ordered two Planter's Punches. He had pondered all morning on what to tell her. If he told her the truth, she would insist that he complied with Douglas Ho's demands, and that was out of the question. So he had decided that it was best that he remain vague at this point.

'I am still looking into this, Noelle.'

'You know something. I can see it in your face.'

'I know nothing for certain.'

'Tell me!'

'All right!' He took a deep breath. Noelle's eyes were liquid, her knuckles white on the arms of her chair. Careful, she could get hysterical. 'I think it's a rogue element in one of the triads,' he said, which was partly true. 'But they've gone to ground. That's all I know.'

'What do they want?'

'As soon as I know what they want, I can set about meeting their demands. But so far I have heard nothing.'

'So I was right. This has to do with you and your business.'

'I think so.'

'You bastard!'

'It's not my fault, Noelle.'

'He's innocent. All my life I have tried to keep him at a distance from you and your intrigues, and now this!'

'I could not know this would happen. If he was under my protection, if you had never taken him away, I could have ensured his safety.'

Noelle's hands were shaking. 'Do you have a cigarette?' she asked him.

He reached into his pocket, took out his Russian cheroots. He handed her one. 'They're strong.'

'I don't care.'

He lit it for her, but she barely inhaled.

'I promise you, I will do everything in my power to get him back. I love him as much as you do.'

'I wish I had never met you.'

'A little late for recriminations. We are what we are. History cannot be changed. For myself I love you today as much as I always loved you. Nothing will ever alter that.'

Noelle was not listening. 'What do you think is happening to him right now?'

'They will not harm him,' he said, with more confidence than he felt. 'They will lock him up somewhere while they decide what to do next. Trust me. I will get him back.'

'I should have gone back to France. I knew I should not have stayed here in Asia.'

'It's not your fault,' he said, and laid a hand on hers.

'No, it's yours, Baptiste. Yours.'

The Punches arrived. The waiter left them on the table and they sat in silence for a long time, staring at them.

'You know more than you're telling me,' she said, finally.

'I swear to you, I don't. They must contact one of us in the next twenty-four hours. Then we will know what to do.'

'He's such a nice boy,' Noelle said. 'He's not like Papa. Or like you. He's just a nice boy. Uncomplicated. Kind. Gentle. God knows where he gets it from.'

'Thank you for the compliment.'

Two huge tears ran down her cheeks. 'I'm going to go crazy. I just imagine him...' She stood up. 'I can't stay here, not in public.'

Baptiste took her arm. 'I'll drive you home.'

'No. I don't want anything from you. I'll get a taxi. Just get me my son back, and perhaps I won't cut your throat in the night.'

She walked away, her heels clicking on the marble. Her head was high, her shoulders back. Inside she was breaking, but she had her pride.

He sat down, and picked up her cigarette from the ashtray. Hard habit to break. His doctor said they were bad for his health. But when a man was in this position, there was nothing for it but to reach for the nearest addiction. Mother of God. He had had so many plans for Lucien, had always assumed that one day he could win him over, Noelle too. There still might be a way out of this. But he had to stall, at least until his own plans were in place.

Poor Noelle. She was right. She had lived a blighted life.

After Douglas had left the next morning May made a call to the US Embassy in Wireless Road. 'I want to speak to Mai Koo Dale,' she whispered. No need to whisper, she knew. Chang was downstairs in the foyer, and Douglas had gone into Chinatown. But her own fear betrayed itself in her voice.

'I'm afraid we don't have anyone of that name here, ma'am,' the male clerk told her.

'Someone there must know. Please. Is very urgent.' Perhaps he had gone back to the United States?

'Just a moment ma'am.'

She was put on hold. She waited for what seemed like an eternity, the phone trembling in her hands. What if Douglas walked through the door right now? What if Chang happened to listen in on another extension? But she was never allowed to leave the house alone, this was the only way.

'Paderewski,' a voice said.

'Mai Koo Dale,' she said.

'Who's calling?'

'Is he there?' May almost screamed into the phone.

A silence. 'Ma'am can you tell me what this is about?'

She wanted to weep with frustration. 'My name is May. You tell Mai Koo. Tell him May must talk with him.'

'May? Is that May Wong?'

'Please tell him,' she said and hung up.

127

San Francisco

It was like the headquarters of any bank or commodities
house, Dale thought. Through the glass windows of his office
he watched the throng of neatly dressed young men and
women hunched over computer screens, staring at printouts,
talking into phones; the hum of everyday commerce. One
of the young men was a moon-faced Chinese, laughing into
the phone that he held between the crook of his shoulder
and his chin. He sipped coffee from a polystyrene cup and
hammered figures into a calculator. Dale was perhaps the
only one in the office who knew he was Chiang Kai Shek's
grandson.

Dale's visitor sat in the chair across his desk, admiring the
panorama of the Bay and the Golden Gate bridge through the
smoked glass window behind Dale's head.

Dale returned his attention to the folder open on the blotter
in front of him. It consisted of twenty-three typewritten pages
on legal size white paper, single-spaced. It was the complete
order of battle for the North Vietnamese Army currently
deployed on the border with the People's Republic of China,
together with military and political intelligence, updates and
forecasts, the kind of thing any military strategist might dream
about holding in his hand before entering into a war. Pacific
Investments International relayed these sorts of documents to
Langley in Virginia about twice a week.

'This is very thorough, Sammy,' Dale said.

'Is one hundred per cent reliable.'

'I'll pass it through the normal channels, of course.'

Sammy nodded and smiled. He had dressed for the occasion, a Brooks Brothers suit, a sombre tie.

'If I remember correctly, the last time we met I passed on to you Gerry Gates' request for some verification of your source.'

'Cannot,' Sammy said.

'But intelligence like this has to be verifiable.'

'Is one hundred per cent reliable,' Sammy repeated.

'But where does it come from?'

'In Saigon still have many friend. After 'seventy-five, many die, but some now very high up in Army, in police. We still do good business.'

'Can we please have a closer identification than this?'

Sammy Chen shook his head. 'Cannot.'

In truth, Dale had not expected Sammy to be more forthcoming. After all, this was triad business.

'I make big contract with you soon,' Sammy said. 'For big contract is big discount, okay?'

'I'll talk to Gerry. I'm sure we can arrange something.'

The relationship had worked well for Sammy, Dale thought. He had already laundered twenty million dollars through Pacific International. The money had financed the acquisition of an entire new town near Sacramento, with its own industrial park and police and fire departments. Finally it was official: Sammy owned the police.

Gerry Gates was delighted with his new client. Sammy was providing top level intelligence without cost to the Company, and the percentages charged by the banks disappeared into accounts in Washington where they helped finance projects like the Border Patrol Police in Thailand, or Solidarity, or the Contras in Nicaragua.

The origins of these tributaries of money had begun to disturb Dale as much as their destination. Clients like Henry Wing had been introduced to the bank by one of Sammy Chen's sons. Henry Wing stayed loyal to Pacific International even when he regularly lost millions through his accounts every month. The reason was simple.

In March, for example, a company owned by the Chen family had purchased two contracts on gold in Hong Kong. On the same day another company – of whom Henry Wing was a major stockholder – purchased identical contracts in San Francisco. Gold had stayed high and in Hong Kong Sammy's low contract was torn up; in San Francisco Dale had himself shredded Henry Wing's high contract. Henry lost two million dollars, which was then deposited in Sammy's account, to pay out his high contract, less Pacific International's commission.

Dale knew, but could not prove, that the entire transaction had been payment for a heroin shipment. It seemed to him that somewhere along the line the dreams of the cold war warriors had turned into a nightmare.

'You know, I think one day we go back to Saigon,' Sammy was saying.

'Not me,' Dale said.

'Yes, we go back. Not with gun, not with soldier, but with money. Can fight wars all you want, make soldier die, yours, theirs. But in the end, is money that win.'

Waves slapped against the rocks. The light was fading. A tanker edged past the point, lights on the top spar and bridge. It was chill and a mist clung to Mount Tamalpais. Lights were blinking on in the clapboard houses nestled among the laurels and oaks and huckleberries.

Dale could not stop thinking about Sammy Chen, what he had said: 'Money wins.' He had never believed that when he was a young man. He had thought that a country had a moral life, the same as an individual. But it was not true. Countries were governed by fear, not morality.

He had believed, but what he had believed in was wrong. He had put his faith in one perfect governing principle; that democracy was right, and everything else was wrong. But you could not engrave truth and justice in stone. That was why lawyers like himself grew rich while the country fell into decay. A country was only as great as the sum of its individuals.

He did not recognise the America of his middle age. He felt like an astronaut who, coming back from a week's journey to the moon, discovered that two hundred years had elapsed on earth. He had tried to make his home in the land he called home, but instead he felt alien and alone. His home had been Magsaysay's Philippines and Sukarno's Indonesia and the Indochina of the sixties. There had been castles then.

Now he had to face the fact that he had given half his life to an illusion.

And what was he doing now? Fighting a war he no longer believed in, helping gangsters and drug barons get rich. In the name of foreign policy. In the name of democracy.

It was growing chill. He shivered and made his way back across the rocks, racing the veil of rain that swept across the bay from the Golden Gate.

When he got back home, he found a battered brown Toyota parked in the driveway. Jennifer's. She was sitting on the porch steps, her elbows on her knees, waiting for him. He wondered what she wanted now. Money perhaps.

She stood up. He could not see her face, it was in shadow. 'Hi Dad,' she said.

It had started to rain. 'You'd better come inside,' he said.

She was straight. Her eyes were clear, her hair had been brushed, although she still looked undernourished. She had on an old jumper and jeans. She reminded him for a moment of the way she had looked as a teenager. 'I came to apologise,' she said, while Dale stood at the bench in the kitchen making coffee.

'Apologise?'

'For last week. In the restaurant.'

He was not ready for this. There had been too many other times. 'What brought on this change of heart?'

'You were right. What you said to me.'

He handed her a steaming mug of coffee. 'I can't help you any more, Jennifer. It's up to you what happens from here.'

She held the mug close to her face and blew the steam. 'One day, it's just enough, you know. Nothing's changed. I've just had enough.'

'I wish I thought you meant that.'

'I do mean it, Dad.'

He could not meet her eyes. He was still too angry with her. 'You know, we've never seen eye to eye on anything very much, but in the end it doesn't matter. Because nothing can change what's done. You're either going to get on with

592

your life, or you're not. I know I've caused you pain, but I can't take it away from you, no matter how much I want to.'

Jennifer looked at the floor. The coffee dribbled out of her cup and splashed on the tiles. 'Oh, Dad, I'm sick of this life,' she said. She started to cry.

It took him by surprise. Suddenly it was as if there was a stone in his throat. The room got misty. He reached out and took her in his arms. Let this be over now, he thought. Let this be the price, fully paid. It was too high, much too high, but let it just finally be over.

'I love you, Dad,' she whispered.

128

In contrast to the tourist shlock and gaudy chinoiserie of Grant Avenue, the back streets of Chinatown are grey, sombre with the realities of human suffering in old and overcrowded tenements. Just a few streets from the stylised lion statues copied from the Forbidden City, the red and gilt wooden dragons coiling up lamp posts and the glazed green-tiled roofs no longer seen in the real China, there is another Chinatown; a place where rubbish rots in narrow alleys; where sewing machines hum in sweat shops in which Asian immigrants toil for the minimum wage; and washing poles sprout from tenements where whole families of Chinese live in one small room.

It was here that Jonathan Dale arranged to meet Robert Jordan for lunch, in a *dim sum* restaurant called, predictably, the Golden Dragon. It was not yet twelve o'clock and the only customers were two old Cantonese in trilbies. It was not the sort of establishment that Robert Jordan was accustomed to patronising for lunch, Dale realised, but it was one place they were certain not to be recognised.

Washington had been good to Robert Jordan. He was power-dressed in a three-piece tailored suit with a two-toned shirt and maroon silk tie. There was more of him than there had been in the days when Dale knew him in the Embassy in Saigon, mostly around the middle. He had been fresh out of Yale then, a young man with a quick mind and a bright future. Dale realised he was now looking at the bright future. It had wingtips of grey at the temples, and the vague frown of a man with too much on his plate.

'You're looking well, Bob,' Dale said. He felt it was what the younger man was expecting to hear from him.

Jordan seemed satisfied with the compliment. 'I jog. I work out.' He patted his middle. 'Not that it does me much good. You know Washington. Twenty per cent bullshit, twenty per cent lunch, twenty per cent tips.'

'What's the other forty per cent?'

'Lies.'

Dale wondered if this was a joke. What seventeen years of success, promotion and influence can do to a man, he thought. Makes him cynical and fat.

'Thanks for coming up to meet me,' Dale said.

'Well, I had business in LA, like I told you, Jack. And you made it sound as if it was pretty important.'

Dale nodded. 'I think so.'

Jordan did not seem disposed to move on to business just yet. 'So I hear you're trying your hand back in private enterprise.'

'Fills in a few hours,' Dale said carefully. 'Retirement didn't really suit me.'

'Never thought it would.'

They chose prawn dumplings and spare ribs from the *dim sum* cart. Jordan spread his napkin carefully on the waistcoat of his suit. Mustn't get any juice on that silk tie, thought Dale.

'Been a long time,' he said.

'Last time I saw you ... must have been ... fifteen years ago. Just before you left Saigon.'

'I think I left a few bits behind in the café that day. I never bothered going back for them. I figured they must have gone.'

It was meant as a joke, but Jordan took it seriously. 'Those sons of bitches,' he said.

'It's a long time ago.'

'So, how are things with you?'

'You heard about me and Susan?'

Jordan seemed discomfited that Dale had brought this up. He flushed, as if Dale had just wiped his mouth with the tablecloth. 'Yeah. I was sorry to hear about that,' he murmured. 'Must have been hard.' When Dale did not respond, he said, 'I got three kids now. All boys.'

'Boys are easier,' Dale said. 'I had one of each. Believe me, boys are easier.'

There was an awkward silence. Jordan found something of particular interest in his prawn dumpling. 'These sure are good,' he said.

'I didn't bring you all the way up here to talk families,' Dale said. He put down his chopsticks and reached for the crocodile skin briefcase on the floor beside him. He snapped open the locks, reached inside, and put a plain manila envelope on the table. The contents were one inch thick.

'What's in there, Jack?'

'Evidence.'

'Of what?'

'Of a massive money laundering operation involving hundreds of millions of dollars of drug money every year. Taking place right here in San Francisco.'

Jordan looked at Dale, then at the envelope, as if it was a rattlesnake. He swallowed his dumpling. 'This is a joke, right?'

Dale shook his head.

'Does this have anything to do with this company you're with? What is it ... Pacific Investments?'

'It has everything to do with it.'

It seemed the room was suddenly too small and airless for Jordan. He pulled at his tie. 'You know, Jack, there are some rumours in Washington. I thought you knew.'

'That the Company owns this company?'

'They're just rumours. Hey, not even that. Nobody's saying anything. Just the name gets mentioned now and then, and it has a certain cachet, if you know what I'm saying here. People say the name, then they kind of raise their eyebrows a little.'

'That's why I came to you.'

'Why?'

'I could have handed this to the FBI. They kiss my ring, interview me a dozen times in a dozen different rooms, tell me this case is going to bust America apart. A couple of months later, I ring them back, ask them when they want me in the witness stand, they tell me they never heard of me before, how do you spell your name again? You know what happens when this sort of thing goes upstairs. It can get lost in an in tray somewhere. I need maps, Bob. I need to know exactly how to find my way through the maze with this little bag of goodies.'

Jordan nodded his understanding. He threw his napkin on the table. Suddenly he seemed to have lost his appetite. 'This is a poisoned chalice, Jack. You know that?'

Dale leaned forward. 'I want you to remember, these are photocopies. The originals are safe. So, have a look at them tonight, then eat them, burn them, whatever it is a good State Department lawyer does with evidence that is too hot for him to handle. Then make some enquiries for me. Find out how far the protection goes for Pacific International. Because if it's all the way to the top, then fuck America.'

'Why me, Jack? You know the Company better than I do. You were with them for twenty-five years.'

'I've been away a long time.'

Jordan touched the envelope with his fingertips, as if testing the temperature. His eyes lingered on it for a long time. 'Who are you laundering for?'

'Pacific International has offices in San Francisco, Hong Kong, and Vancouver, among other places. What does that tell you?'

'Holy Christ.'

'Exactly. It also helps to talk a little Italian. Are you getting the Big Picture?'

'I don't understand, Jack. You've been a Company man since before I was born. Why are you doing this?'

'I haven't changed. America has. They switched sides, I didn't.'

Jordan picked up the envelope. He turned it over a few times, a prospector examining a rock. He grimaced, replaced the envelope on the table. 'I'll do what I can. But don't expect miracles.'

'I never expected miracles, Bob. Just justice.'

129

Chinatown, Bangkok

The two men leaned against their motorcycle, smoking cigarettes, their eyes fixed on the smoked glass doors of the Hong Kong Gold Shop. They were Thais, dressed in T-shirts and dirty trousers; one of them affected a drooping moustache to disguise the fact that he was barely out of his teens.

Anyone watching them closely would have noticed that they became instantly alert when a black Mercedes limousine pulled up at the front doors of the shop. The man with the moustache jumped on the motorcycle and kick-started the motor. Across the road a tall Chinese strode out of the shop, and one of the salesmen ran ahead of him to open the car's door. Another ran behind, carrying the man's attaché case. He got into the car, and, with an exaggerated bow, the man passed the case to him.

Yaowarat Road was a valley of carbon monoxide, choked with traffic even this late in the evening. As the limousine moved off into the traffic, the two men on their motorcycle had to weave their way through the press of buses and trucks to position themselves directly behind.

They did not make their move until they reached Rama IV Road. Night had fallen, the long tail of lights snaked towards the floodlit white tower of the Dusit Thani. The limousine was stalled at a stop light in front of a dilapidated Victorian bungalow, its verandahs and fretwork concealed by a three-storey movie poster, lurid with scenes of violence and sex.

The pillion passenger reached behind him, and thrust a hand into the rattan basket of rambutan that was strapped to the back of the motorcycle. He pulled out a 7.62 millimetre Makarov

598

automatic pistol and a .357 Magnum revolver. He handed the revolver to the man with the moustache. Almost casually, he took it and got off the motorcycle, stood the Yamaha on its stand and walked with the other man to the limousine in front.

The man with the Makarov fired his entire clip through the windscreen of the Mercedes, and then reloaded. The man with the moustache stood beside the rear passenger window and fired through the glass. The other man joined him and emptied a second clip into the slumped and gory figure of the man in the back seat.

They ran back to their motorcycle, pushed it to the other side of the road, and weaved back through the traffic towards Chinatown.

The windscreen of the Mercedes hung in crumpled shards, smeared with gouts of dark blood. Its two passengers were sprawled at grotesque angles in the interior, almost unrecognisable as human beings. The leather appointments of the luxury car were sodden and ruined.

Pak Sha Wan, Hong Kong

Douglas Ho's home at Pak Sha Wan had been built into the hillside, raw white concrete hidden away from the road by high walls. Men with pump-action shotguns, with trained Kamoy dogs on metal leashes, patrolled the grounds and the private water frontage where Douglas' thirty-five-metre motor yacht, the *Hammerhead*, was moored.

On their second night back in Hong Kong, Douglas took a phone call from Bangkok. After he replaced the receiver he fetched a bottle of Hennessy XO cognac and went out on to the balcony alone.

So, Baptiste had given his answer. He had tried to kill him. Now there was only one choice left. Perhaps it was best this way, he thought. The risks are greater, but the stakes made the gamble worthwhile. If he succeeded, he would wrest control of an enormous business empire, and astronomical profits from the triad heroin business.

Sammy is too old. He has lost his hunger, and grown soft. He does not have my vision. We could build a vast empire, but instead he wants to make deals with Henry Wing and the Italians.

It was time for a new generation. It was time for Douglas Ho.

130

Berkeley, San Francisco

Dale knocked on the door of Jennifer's apartment but there was no answer. Her car had broken down and he had agreed to pick her up early and take her across town for an interview with a law firm. He hammered on the door again, louder this time, feeling his heart race. Perhaps she had just slept in. A fat man came out on the landing in his dressing gown and told him to keep the noise down. Dale ignored him.

'Jennifer!'

There was something else now, a faint smell, something he recognised from another life, when a body bag started to leak in the back of a Huey.

He threw himself at the door.

'Call the police,' he heard the man in the dressing gown say to his wife. 'Guy out here's gone fuckin' crazy.' The voice seemed to come from a long way away, and it was as if Dale was seeing everything through a long tunnel.

He launched himself against the door again and the wood splintered. He kicked at the lock with his boot and the door broke open.

She had been dead no more than a day, and the smell was not so bad that you would really notice, despite the heat. She was lying on her back on the sofa, her eyes staring sightless at the ceiling, her skin mottled a greasy blue colour. She was wearing a greyish T-shirt with a slogan printed on the front: MAKE LOVE NOT WAR, the letters almost faded away with age. Underneath she wore a pair of cotton underpants. There was a syringe lying on the carpet, next to a pizza box. The tourniquet was still loose around her arm.

Dale knelt beside her, took her head in his arms, and began to rock her. 'Oh, baby,' he murmured, 'oh, baby.'

You were right, darling, I never loved you when you were a kid. I had other things to do. I only learned to love you when it was too late. I tried to make it up to you, but you can't undo history.

'Oh, baby.'

So cold, so grey. Just a shell left. Wherever Jenny was, he imagined she must finally be satisfied. She had lied to him for the last time, had set him up for this, had had her final revenge. She had got what she wanted. She had broken his heart, as he had broken hers.

131

Jennifer Dale was buried next to her grandparents in the local churchyard. The funeral service was held inside. The musty interior, the wooden pews and the white-painted walls reminded Michael of those Sundays when he and Jennifer had crammed in here with Susan and their grandparents, he in his grey shorts and black knotted tie, Jennifer in her straw hat and printed frock, both fidgeting and bored, united by their discomfort. He remembered how she deliberately feigned hay fever attacks or fainting spells during the sermon, exacting measure for measure from those who had forced her to come against her wishes. He felt a tightening in his throat when he remembered. Strange how a child's games become the adult's destiny.

His father had met him at the airport the night before. On the drive home Dale had given him the gritty details of Jennifer's death. Dale had found her himself, in the living room of her apartment in Berkeley. An overdose, he had said, probably accidental; as if that made any difference. Dad had been eerily composed, as if he was giving a lecture. 'Most of the dope these kids use is adulterated with milk sugar,' he had said, 'it's very weak. But the stuff she was using, it was too pure, over seventy per cent. Perhaps one of her friends smuggled it back themselves from Asia. Jenny put it straight into her bloodstream undiluted and she just died.'

There were a lot of faces in the congregation Michael did not recognise. Jennifer's friends, her companions in desperation, were clustered near the back of the church. He knew only one of them, Scott, or the eighties version of him, dissipated and thin and sallow in a borrowed suit. There were a few of his father's friends from the golf club, some old family friends from Tiburon. He wondered if there was anyone from Pacific International.

His father, in a breaking voice, read a eulogy. The priest said something about the pressures of today's society on its young people. His grandmother and his aunts wept, his father sat like stone, Susan beside him in a black veil, not touching. Michael could not concentrate on any of it. Afterwards he helped carry the bier to the churchyard and dropped a handful of earth on the polished walnut coffin, but he could not imagine that his sister was really inside. It all seemed unreal, an elaborate charade.

He grieved for a sister he had never had. He knew that even if she were standing beside him, right now, they would still have nothing to say to each other, and that knowledge depressed him. They were a family of misfits, opposites thrown together into the same house to spit and fight. Regret sat on his shoulders like a wet, grey shroud. It should have been raining. Instead it was a clear blue day, warm and pleasant.

He drove back to Tiburon, with his father and an uncle, none of them speaking. At the wake people stood around in small groups, the conversation subdued and stilted by embarrassment; they left early.

Finally only Michael and his father were left. They stood on the deck, the ice melting in their whiskies, and tried to avoid each other's eyes. As the sun set, the bay shimmered gold, reflected from thousands of windows in Berkeley.

'Can you stay on for a few days?' Dale asked.

Michael shook his head. 'I have to catch a flight to Hong Kong tomorrow morning.'

'She was your sister. Surely it can wait? No one's indispensable.'

'It's a big case. I've got a connection to it no one else has. Sorry.' He drained his glass. 'I'd stay if I could.' He turned to go back inside.

'You blame me for this.'

'No, I don't blame you.'

'Then what is it? Why this silence?'

'Is it that hard to figure?'

Dale looked hard at him, then turned away. 'You don't understand.'

'That's it, tell me I don't understand the Big Picture. That's the classic response from you people, isn't it?'

'What do you mean, "you people"?'

'You know who runs Pacific Investments. It's your old pals in Virginia. It's not a brokerage, it's a Chinese laundry.'

'I can't talk about it.'

'Sure you can't. It's classified. Like your whole life. I just don't understand how you can work for a drugs bank after what happened to Jennifer.'

'I have my reasons.'

'You always had your reasons. When you run Old Glory up the pole, you're liable to do anything.'

'You think what you're doing is making any damned difference? Taking the high moral ground may make you feel a lot better, son, but it isn't actually solving what's happening to Jennifer and kids like her.'

'She wasn't a kid, Dad, she was thirty-four years old. She had her own agenda. She died because she didn't want to face up to her life. Maybe it was even deliberate, you ever considered that?' He could see by Dale's face that he had. But when his father still did not comment, he added: 'That still doesn't mean I want people making their first million out of it.'

'Neither do I.'

'Then what the hell are you doing at Pacific International?'

Dale did not answer.

'I never thought I'd say this, Dad, but you make me sick.'

'Michael!'

'Flight leaves at six-thirty. I think I'll have an early night. Goodnight.'

132

Hong Kong

Douglas Ho had a private box high above the stands at Happy Valley. On the table in front of him were the remains of his luncheon, mud crab and lobster and prawn shells scattered in a bed of green lettuce. A bottle of VSOP Remy Martin was at his elbow. He cupped a brandy balloon in one hand and a race card in the other. His eyes flickered between the track and the closed circuit television mounted in one corner of the room.

Baptiste was only allowed admittance after submitting himself to the indignity of a body search; even then two of Douglas' bodyguards flanked him on either side as they ushered him in.

Douglas was resplendent in charcoal pin-striped trousers, dark blue knitted tie and a tailored beige silk blazer. A diamond and ruby ring glittered on his little finger, there were more diamonds in the face of his gold Rolex and his belt buckle.

He did not look up when Baptiste entered. 'You've come a long way to watch a horse race, Kwo-chao.'

'We have some unfinished business to discuss.'

'Lucien,' said Douglas, smiling, as if at some pleasant reminiscence.

I'm going to kill you, Baptiste promised himself. Not now, not yet, but I will kill you. Even if I get Lucien back, your life is still forfeit for this humiliation, this suffering. I promise.

'You left Bangkok very suddenly.'

'Double lucky for me, Kwo-chao. The very night I left my car was in a very serious accident.'

'I know nothing about that.'

Douglas looked up from his race card for the first time. 'Of course you do. It is why you raced here, to Hong Kong. You know you have had your chance and wasted it.'

Baptiste felt the first thrill of real fear. He had been sure he could beat this vicious little bastard. He had underestimated his ruthlessness. 'Where's my son?'

'I thought we made an agreement, Kwo-chao. What have you done about your part of it?'

'I've done as you asked.'

'Then why is Sammy Chen still in San Francisco? No, I think what has happened, you thought you could wash me, and that would solve your problem. This did not work, and you are desperate. So now you have to make your decision. You will either keep our contract or lose your son. It is your choice, Kwo-chao.' He looked back to the race track. 'The race is about to start. Are you a gambling man, Kwo-chao?'

'I never lose.'

'Neither do I. It should be interesting.' He turned away and fixed his binoculars on the field. Baptiste knew there was nothing more to discuss. He turned around and pushed his way past the two bodyguards, shaking with helpless rage.

133

Hong Kong

The Hopewell Centre soars sixty-four storeys into the Hong Kong skyline, above the shops, restaurants and Suzie Wong bars of Wanchai. On the directory beside the elevators are listed the offices of banks, trading companies, and real estate firms; but the name of the tenants on the fifty-seventh floor is not included.

Ray Schultz sat behind a wide oak desk with a view over the Hong Kong harbour. There was a bright green metal filing cabinet against one wall and a sixteen button red phone on his desk.

Schultz stood up as Michael entered and thrust out a huge paw. He was a beefy, red-faced man in his early fifties with little hair, an expensive taste in suits and a ready smile.

'Mike,' he said. 'Pleased to meet you. Ray Schultz.' His accent was mid-west.

'Hello, Ray.'

'Want some coffee? Sit here and enjoy the view and when I come back we'll talk about Douglas Ho.'

Ray Schultz put his feet on his desk and leaned back. In contrast to his tailored suit, his shoes were scuffed and unpolished. 'So this girlfriend of Ho's has had a change of heart,' he said.

'It would seem that way.'

'This is a big break, Mike. I don't want you to underestimate the importance of this case for us. Douglas Ho is a big name on our wish list. We believe he's a lieutenant to a guy called

608

Chen Giai Han, also known as Sammy Chen, the 489 of the Fei Lung triad. If we got a CI this close to the top, it could bust the whole syndicate wide open.'

'I'll do my best.'

'This May Wong's taking a big risk. Does she realise this?'

'I don't know. I guess so.'

Schultz chewed on his bottom lip. He picked up a manila folder. 'I read the file on your association with this girl. Can we trust her?'

'I'll be honest with you, Ray. I don't have a clue right now.'

Schultz considered. 'Well, I guess we've got nothing to lose.' He opened the file. 'Our first problem is how to make the initial contact. She never leaves his little palace at Pak Sha Wan without him.'

'I managed to get to her in Chiang Mai and Bangkok.'

'He's tightened up on his security since then. Could be he's suspicious, could be a hundred other reasons. Bottom line is we can't arrange a meeting outside, so we got to find a way to get you inside.'

Michael grinned. 'I could pretend to be a Mormon?'

'Budget don't stretch to bicycles, Mike,' Schultz answered, deadpan.

'Then what?'

'Well, we keep Pak Sha Wan under surveillance whenever our friend Ho is in town and we got a list of the regular visitors.' He took a sheet of white paper out of the file and handed it to Michael. 'Kind of service people you'd expect for a place this size. Pool maintenance man once a week, two gardeners, they come in every day, an army of domestics. None of these people is any use for our purposes. But there's one guy that does have access three times a week, as well as social contact with the lady in question.'

'A personal masseur,' Michael said, shaking his head.

'Yeah, right. Okay, we got a beautician down here too, plus a hairdresser, but I don't think you could quite cut it in that department. But maybe we could lick you into shape for a few back rubs. What do you think?'

'I think you're crazy.'

609

'No, I figure this has possibilities. One, the guy she hired is a Chinese-American. So if you came on the scene as an emergency replacement, it's not going to look too suspicious. And two, the guy has gambling debts. According to the local cops he likes to play fan tan and he's got himself in too deep with the loan sharks. 14K of all people. We can offer to bail him out with some cash.'

'You really want me to masquerade as her personal masseur?'

'It's called going undercover, Mike. You've done it before, according to your file.'

'I normally impersonate drug dealers.'

'Well, you don't want to get typecast. Got to extend yourself, Mike, test your range.'

'Thanks, Ray.'

'Hey, it's what I'm here for.' The smile fell away and he leaned forward, elbows on the desk. 'I mean it, Mike, this is important. She wants to talk to you, we want to talk to her. She could be the most important CI we ever had.'

'Well, I'd better not rub her up the wrong way then.' It was a weak joke, but Schultz laughed, dutifully. Michael laughed along with him, but inside he was cold with fear. He thought about the little Hmong girl with the huge, staring eyes, sitting on the bar of the hootch at Long Tieng. He didn't want to do this to her.

Yet finally, he reminded himself, it had been her choice. And above everything, over the fear, for himself and for her, there was another emotion that now slowly began to override all else.

Desire.

'I want him washed,' Douglas said. 'Kee Lung and both his sons.'

At the bar young Chinese in white T-shirts flexed their muscles for China dolls in heavy make-up and sheath-tight dresses. The nightclub was a triad favourite, ultra-modern, with exposed air conditioning ducts writhing across the ceiling, speakers and video screens mounted on exposed chrome scaffolding. A strobe pulsed in time to the thudding bass of the disco music. The Swatow Disco was the place where the young *sze kau* came to spend money and get face.

Douglas Ho and his guest were separated from the crowds by a circle of empty tables; no one approached, out of fear and respect. Douglas lounged on a banquette, his feet on a glass-topped cocktail table.

'How much?'

'Half a million dollars. A hundred now. The rest when the job is done.'

Tran van Li's face barely registered any interest at all. 'That's a lot of money,' he said. These days the former Butcher of Saigon looked like a retired Asian businessman. His pearl grey suit appeared a size too large and hung loose on his sparse frame, and he had affected a goatee beard which was rapidly greying, together with his hair. To a casual observer he would have appeared almost innocuous.

But the Butcher of Saigon was still very much in business. He now organised teams of Vietnamese refugees into for-hire soldiers for the Chinatown triads of San Francisco, including Henry Wing.

'We are talking US dollars?'

Douglas gave a harsh laugh. 'Of course. Who do you think you are talking to? Some gangster?'

Tran van Li sipped his orange juice – he had become an exemplary Buddhist in middle age, and would not corrupt his body with strong drink – and considered. 'You are taking a great risk, Sharkfin.'

'With Sammy Chen and his two sons dead, there will be no one to challenge me. I will be the next 489 of the Fei Lung. I also have control of Sammy's drug business.'

'You invite war with the Chuen Chung Wa.'

'A war is what I want. It will make me master of Chinatown.'

'You will have to make peace with the Six Companies.'

'Those old fools! You know as well as I, if you hold a man by the balls, he will shout to the world that you are the greatest friend he ever had.'

'If you are going to fight Henry Wing, you will need soldiers.'

'Whatever he is paying you, I will pay double.'

Tran van Li shrugged his shoulders. 'I have known Chen Giai Han a long time. We have done business for many years.'

611

'Loyalty is not something you keep, it's something you bid for on a regular basis. It's up to you. Half a million dollars. For one life. No one ever paid so much. They shot Kennedy for less.'

'It's tempting.'

'It's too good to refuse.'

'You're right.' Tran van Li nodded and smiled. 'Half a million dollars. I would have killed the Pope in Rome for that.'

'If he ever gets in my way, I'll call you.'

The next morning Tran van Li boarded China Airlines Flight 004 from Hong Kong to San Francisco. Before he left he deposited the sum of one hundred thousand dollars with Pacific Investments International.

134

There was not one moment in the day that May did not think of the phone call she had made before they left Bangkok. She wondered if the message had got through or if it had been lost somewhere in a clerk's in-tray; if someone at the embassy might intercept it and betray her to Douglas Ho; or if the man she had spoken to had hung up, shrugged his shoulders and dismissed the whole conversation.

There was no way to know because it now seemed almost impossible that Michael would be able to contact her, even if her message had found its way to him. She was virtually a prisoner at Pak Sha Wan, and the only people allowed inside were gardeners and domestics. When she did go out, Chang was under strict instructions not to allow her out of his sight for a moment. Douglas' car had been ambushed in Bangkok and his driver and a decoy murdered. Ever since he had become obsessed with security.

But she had witnessed Michael's ingenuity before. If her message had got through, she sensed there might yet be a chance.

Every morning she worked out in the gymnasium from nine to ten o'clock, and then swam fifty lengths of the pool. At ten-thirty precisely, on Mondays, Wednesdays and Fridays, Howard Tan, her personal masseur and trainer, arrived. Tan had been Douglas' idea. I am like the garden, or the swimming pool, or the Rolls-Royce Phantom in the driveway, May thought. Douglas wants all his possessions to be maintained in immaculate condition.

Tan usually stayed for half an hour, discussing her fitness regimen while he worked and pummelled her muscles and joints. The session often contained as much pain as pleasure. She submitted to the routine on one of the benches in the gymnasium, under the watchful eyes of Chang and the security cameras.

That Wednesday, Howard rang at eight-thirty to say that he was unwell, but was sending a replacement, a Californian, highly qualified, with excellent recommendations from an exclusive Malibu gymnasium.

At ten-thirty precisely, while May was still in the pool, Chang ushered in the new masseur. He was wearing a freshly pressed white linen T-shirt and black shorts that barely covered his groin. His skin was tanned the colour of honey and his hair was platinum blond.

Chang was smirking.

'Some new strain of California fruit,' he whispered to May out of the corner of his mouth, and resumed his post by the pool.

The new instructor put down his Adidas sports bag and waited for instructions. 'My name's Michael,' he said.

May bit her lip, assailed by both fear and a sense of the bizarre. She wanted both to shriek with laughter and scream with terror. She was aware of Chang watching her from the pool. She pretended to dry her hair with a towel, to hide her face and give herself time to think. Mai Koo. *Mai Koo!*

'This way,' she said, and lay face down on the sun chair on the terrace.

Mai Koo!

May unfastened the string of her bikini, put her arms above her head, and tried to relax. She heard him unzip the Adidas bag, take out bottles and towels. He began to rub some oil into her back, working it into the muscles along her spine with his fingers. May turned her head towards Chang. He was now deeply engrossed in a Kung Fu comic.

She turned again so that her face was towards Michael. I have crossed the river, she thought. I can't go back now.

'Mai Koo,' she whispered.

'Like the hair?' he whispered.

'Chang thinks you are bum boy.'

614

'Perhaps I should offer him a quick massage and make him worry.'

'You have many nice clothes, Mai Koo. The pineapple shirt, now this short short. If you wear together you will stop traffic.'

'Next time.'

'Also have nice hands.'

'I bet you say that to all the boys.'

May looked back at Chang. If she spoke too much, she would attract his attention. She would have to keep her voice dull and even. 'I have a lot of fright,' she murmured in a monotone. She might have been commenting on the weather.

'I'm scared too, if that helps.'

He worked for a while longer. His massage was not at all like Howard's she noticed. The fingers did not knead as deeply, and he was too slow and sensuous in his movements. But she did not imagine Chang would notice. Or the cameras.

'Must make it hurt,' she whispered.

'Why?'

'Don't know. But this is what Howard does. If Chang thinks I like too much, he will be suspicious.'

'Do you like it too much?' he said, and grinned, but before she could answer he had worked his knuckles into the soft muscle along her spine and she cried out and gripped the sun chair with her fists. 'Like that?'

It took her a few moments to get her breath back. 'How do you arrange this?' she asked him.

'We came to an understanding with Howard. He is being suitably compensated for his loss of income.' She relaxed again as his hands moved up to her shoulders. He became gentle again. He massaged oil into the tight muscles of her neck, gentle as a lover. She felt the buds of her nipples spring up. This was not how Howard worked at all. 'Do you normally talk to Howard?' he asked her. 'Is Chang going to get suspicious?'

'Howard talk to me. Like hairdresser. All gossip.'

'Well, I won't mince, I told them that. I'll wear shorts halfway up my butt, I'll bleach my hair, but I won't mince.'

May suppressed a giggle. 'Must not make me laugh, Mai Koo. I have too much fright already. Douglas kill me dead if he find out.'

'You don't have to do this.'

I don't have to do this. Yes, but you were the one who sowed the seed. You were the one who came to me.

'Okay,' she said. 'Not help you then. Much more easy this way.' She turned her head away again. Chang was dozing in the sun.

'No, you don't have to do it. You can live off other people's misery and pain. It pays for the swimming pool. It pays for the bracelet on your wrist. It pays for the massage.' He pinched the skin of her shoulders hard and she stifled a cry of pain. 'If you can live with that, then you don't have to do anything.'

She turned back to him, looked up into his face. 'Too much scared.'

'We all have to do things we're frightened of some time. I remember you in the hospital in Long Tieng. You must have been real scared then, but you got through it. I don't know how, but you did. And you can do this, May. If you want to. It's real important that you do.'

She had already made up her mind. They both knew that. She nodded her assent.

He leaned closer. 'Does he have an office here? A private area? Somewhere locked?'

'Next to the bedroom.'

'Can you get inside?'

'Can try.'

'Look in my bag,' he said. She looked down. The Adidas bag was open and there was a Zippo lighter beside it on the marble tiles. 'See the lighter? I'll leave it there when I go. That way you can return it to me next session, and it won't look suspicious.'

'Want me to set fire to the house?'

'It's a camera. Look at the lighter carefully, and you'll find a small view-finder. You just point the thing and press the shutter release at the top. Get into his office and photograph as many of his papers as you can. Do you think you can do it?'

'Can try.'

'Next appointment's Friday. It gives you two days.'

616

I can't do it! she thought. I can't! 'Douglas kill me dead for this,' she whispered, almost too choked to speak.

'He won't know.' He gave her further instructions on how to use the camera, and the best way to photograph many papers at once. As he spoke his hands pummelled her back, her buttocks, her thighs. He was hurting again, as if he could pound a new resolve into her. 'We'll get you out if it gets messy. We'll protect you. You have my word.'

'Cannot protect from Douglas. Never can. Even you, Mai Koo.'

When the massage was over, she jumped off the bench and dived into the pool. Michael packed up his oils and towels and Chang showed him out.

May forced herself through twenty-five more laps, working the fear and adrenaline out of her muscles through sheer physical exhaustion. Crazy. Why do you want to do this? You have survived so much and now you are going to throw it all away!

Perhaps because of Bich, she thought. Perhaps because he sacrificed so much for you. You owe something back. Perhaps because of Noi.

But most of all she would do it for Mai Koo.

135

San Francisco

The black stretch picked him up on Montgomery, its smoked glass windows ensuring anonymity. The only clue to the identity of the occupants were the government licence plates. As it pulled alongside the kerb Dale heard the electric locks on the doors click open and he climbed in.

Robert Jordan sat in the corner, one arm along the back of the seat. He was in full uniform, dark blue tailored three-piece, gold collar pin, a knitted claret tie, a matching silk handkerchief in his breast pocket. He pressed a button and a smoked glass perspex screen slid up between themselves and the uniformed chauffeur, ensuring complete privacy.

'How you doing, Jack?'

'Hi, Bob. I wondered if you'd forgotten about me. I was about to give you a call.'

Jordan tried to smile but it came off as a grimace. 'I've been working hard on this one, Jack.'

'I never doubted it.'

Jordan dropped all pretence at easygoing good humour. 'This is a real mountain of shit, Jack. You have to drop this.'

'Drop it?'

'Remember Nugan Hand? Remember that? The government can't have another piece of crap like that landing in the rotors. This is not a wildcat operation. This is sanctioned. At the highest levels.'

'So drug running and money laundering in our own country are okay now. Is that what you're telling me?'

'Don't be naïve, Jack.'

'I'm not naïve, as you call it. I understood we did this in Asia. I understood the rationale then. It was: Everybody does it, so we do it too. Okay, so we run drugs around Indochina. Okay, we go to bed with the local bandits, it's for a cause. But I don't see this, Bob. We're fucking our own economy and our own people. And you tell me this is sanctioned?'

'It's a question of the devil you know. There's no easy choices between black and white any more. This deal has to do with national security, for Christ's sake. The Third World War started thirty years ago, you know that. We've been at war with Russia and China ever since. That's our priority.'

The limousine was snarled in traffic on Kearney. Dale saw a bumper sticker on the Plymouth in front:

STRIKE A BLOW FOR JUSTICE. PUNCH AN ATTORNEY.

Yo for that, Dale thought. Let's start with Robert Jordan.

He no longer felt angry, just bone weary. 'I used to think that Russia and China were our number one priority too. Now I think our biggest enemy is ourselves.'

'Bullshit, Jack.'

'Bullshit? We're making drug runners our silent partners and you tell me worrying about our national identity is bullshit?'

'The British Empire was the biggest fucking drug runner in the world's history, Jack, and they're our allies. Hell, your pals in the Company got into bed with the fucking Mafia when it suited them, for Christ's sake. Look at the Sicily Invasion. Look at the Bay of Pigs. Don't fucking lecture me about national identity. I'm telling you what's possible and what isn't. And it is not fucking possible to prosecute International Pacific because it would be like bending right over and shooting ourselves up our own ass. All right?' Robert Jordan was shaking with rage. At Dale, at his job, at his country's predicament.

'And what if the Russians and Chinese went away?' Dale said quietly. 'Is anything going to change?'

'Hypothetical question.'

'Hypothetical answer. The gorillas are in charge of the monkey house.' Dale shook his head and looked out of the window. Rain spattered down, grey thunderheads rolled over the

Golden Gate. They turned left on to Union. 'You're looking at a dying breed, Bob. One of the believers. I believed in Reagan's Evil Empire. I thought that was what I was fighting. I didn't know I was helping to make another one. Let me out, will you?'

'It's raining, Jack.'

'So I'll get wet. I've gotten wet before. It beats getting pissed on every time.'

'Promise me you'll drop this?'

'What choice have I got?'

'If you take my advice you'll destroy those copies you took.' Jordan leaned forward and tapped softly on the glass. The driver slowed and pulled over to the side of the road. Dale got out.

'Take it easy, Jack. Sorry I couldn't have been more help.'

'Shove it up your ass,' Dale said and let Jordan shut his own goddamned door. He walked blindly away across Washington Square, letting the rain plaster his hair across his skull, not caring where he was going.

Sanctioned at the highest levels.

It was a bad time to be a believer, a bad time to be a father, a bad time to be anything but a man of expedience.

A bad time to be a patriot.

The evening rush hour traffic crawled across the Golden Gate towards Marin. Dale drummed his fingers on the steering wheel of his Mercedes. He flicked through the radio channels, caught the six o'clock news. Government soldiers in El Salvador had been accused of murdering five American nuns. So much for our allies, Dale thought, our champions of democracy in Latin America. Good to know that Sammy Chen's money is going to a good cause.

'Do you have to do this, Dad?' Jennifer said.

He turned to look at her. She was just eight years old, a tomboy with grazed knees and a torn skirt. She was wearing the blazer from the Convent des Oiseaux in Manila. They had all still been together then.

'What happened to you has to matter. It has to make some sense,' he said.

'I don't want you to get hurt.'

'I know how to look after myself.'

'Don't do it for me. I'm a silly girl sometimes.'

I'm not just doing it for you, he thought. I'm doing it for me. 'I don't know when it changed,' he told her. 'I don't know if there was ever one particular moment when we stopped being right. But I've lived my whole life thinking I was on the side of the angels. I can't stand it if I was a fool my whole life. I can do at least one thing right.'

When he turned again she was a young girl in a fringed suede jacket, a red bandana keeping the lank, sandy hair from her face. There were dark bruises under her eyes.

'I'm sorry,' he whispered. He heard the hammering of car horns and realised he had stalled in the traffic. He re-started the engine and drove on.

When he looked back at her, her eyes were glassy and dilated, there were purple blotches on her cheeks. He understood that she was dead. He pulled across two lanes, ignoring the curses and the clamour of the horns, and skewed to a halt on the hard shoulder. When a motorcycle patrolman stepped up to the car he found Dale slumped over the wheel, fat globs of tears rolling down his cheeks.

Jonathan Dale spent the evening alone with a bottle of Bushmills. Fifty-five wasn't old, he reminded himself, but tonight he felt it. His life was in hiatus, stalled on regret. When he picked up the newspapers in the morning, or watched the television news at night, he saw urban crime and drugs and decay, and still Viet Nam, Laos and Cambodia in communist hands. He wondered what it was all for. His crusade had been futile, and brought him nothing but misery. Those he had treasured he had lost.

The night outside the windows was raging. Small branches, torn from the trees by the wind, littered the deck. The house was in darkness, except for a single yellow light that burned in the study, where Dale entertained the cast of his life.

The ghost that had come to haunt him this evening was not represented among the gallery of photographs above the log fire. She was a raven-haired woman in her middle-twenties, wearing a dress of white muslin, and when she spoke her voice was mellifluous, softly accented with French.

'Dale,' she whispered. 'Why do you look so sad?'

'Everything is wrong,' he answered her. 'Even if we win now, we've lost. Stalin and Mao and Ho and Kruschev were all straw men. The real enemy was ourselves. We made a pact with the devil and now his legions are running through our house. And I was one of the gatekeepers, Noelle. I am one of the damned.'

'You knew it would come to this. When I warned you about Baptiste that day in the park, you knew.'

'I'm a fool, Noelle. My whole life has been a folly.'

A sudden slash of rain slapped against the windows, like a barrage of small stones. An oil tanker sounded its horn as it passed under the Golden Gate.

He stood up and went to the window. A black night. No stars, no light. His own reflection stared back at him from the glass, an ageing warrior fighting for a cause he no longer believed in. 'I did everything I thought was right. But if you make one small compromise, you find yourself making another, and then another. You can't fight the devil with his own weapons.'

He turned around. The chair was empty. A lonely old man shouting at phantoms, he thought. How damned sad.

Well, he could rail against the night or he could stand up and be counted. An old warrior he might be, but there were still a few weapons in his arsenal. He might yet snatch a victory from an improbable cause.

136

Hong Kong

From his apartment Baptiste Crocé looked down on the carbon monoxide corridor of Queens Road, the neon banners of Japanese cameras and French perfumes and Swiss watches shimmering in the wet night. The white lights were the ferries and junks and freighters scurrying for shelter in the face of a coming storm. The penthouse occupied an entire floor of the building, his inner sanctum furnished with long sofas upholstered in dark blue silk, watercolour panels of Chinese landscapes by Hong Kong artist David Wong occupying one entire wall. A white Ming Dynasty Nephrite bowl appeared to float in the phosphorescence of a spotlight.

Noelle was ushered into the room. She wore a black gaberdine raincoat over a navy blue silk suit, her hair tied back from her forehead. She looked at once unutterably sad and breath-takingly beautiful.

She looked around her, one eyebrow raised in surprise. 'Is this an apartment, or a harem?'

'It can be both.'

'I imagine.'

'Can I take your coat?' It was damp with rain. 'A drink perhaps?'

'No, thank you, Baptiste.'

'You don't mind if I do?'

'I don't mind what you do any more.'

He went to the bar and poured three fingers of Remy Martin VSOP into a brandy balloon. 'We have come a long way.'

'You take up a lot of space on the lobby wall. Do all those companies belong to you? You should have your own phone book.'

'Precious stones, textiles, air freight, import and export. And this is just a branch office. It's a long way from those three Cessnas we owned in Vientiane.'

'That my father owned,' she said.

He brought his drink and sat beside her on the sofa.

'Where's Lucien?' she said.

He shook his head.

'You know more than you're telling me.'

'You did not have to follow me here, Noelle. I would have called as soon as I knew.'

'You left Bangkok and you did not tell me where you were going. I have to assume it has something to do with Lucien.' Her bottom lip trembled for a moment, and she almost choked on his name.

A flurry of rain spattered on the window.

'Are you going to tell me?'

His shoulders slumped. 'I would trade all this if I could...'

'Let us just keep to the subject, Baptiste.'

He took a deep breath. 'There is a man called Douglas Ho. He is a business acquaintance.'

'Precious stones? Air freight? Or heroin?'

'He wants me to do something for him.'

'What?'

'Manipulate. Lie.'

'That should not be too difficult.'

'Thank you.'

'Are you going to tell me all of it?'

'He wants me to influence certain negotiations.'

'Well?'

'If I do as he asks, he will have to kill me. It would not be in his interests to let me live.'

'But if you don't...'

'I realise that. I am trying to stall him.'

'Have you thought of anything else?'

'I have tried once to kill him.'

'Brilliant.'

624

'You understand, there are not many options.'

She bit her lip, her eyes liquid. She was quiet for a long time. When she spoke again, she had regained some measure of control. 'You have to save Lucien.'

'What do you suggest?'

'That you do as he asks.'

'It's a death warrant.'

'For him. Or for you?'

Baptiste was silent.

'You continue to astonish me, Baptiste. I thought you had plumbed the depths of craven depravity, but it seems you have an endless talent for it.'

He lit a cigarette. His hands were shaking. She had never seen him like this. 'I have to stall him,' he said. 'While the negotiations are still going on, Lucien still has a chance.'

'For God's sake, Baptiste. He's our son.'

'What can I do?'

'Get him back.'

'I can't! There's nothing I can do!'

She hit him as hard as she could, again and again. Baptiste just sat there. When her rage had spent itself, there were red welts on his face from her hands, and a trickle of blood spilt from his lip. He dabbed at it with his handkerchief. 'I'm sorry Noelle. This is my fault.'

'Of course it is! Do you think I ever doubted that?'

'I promise you, I will do all I can.'

'Except risk your own life!' She stood up, snatched her coat and walked out. Baptiste stared at the night. The storm was coming on. He made up his mind.

He placed a call to San Francisco, traced Sammy Chen to his son's home in Pacific Heights. The conversation was brief, and when he replaced the receiver he could not be sure that Sammy Chen had believed a word of what he had said.

137

The problem with Sammy Chen, Douglas decided, was that he was an old man getting ready to meet his ancestors. He could not see the future, because he was still trapped in the past, in a time when opium meant a few poor coolies smoking in a divan in Ladder Street. He couldn't envision a future where heroin was the drug of choice for an entire generation of Americans, when the triads must assume an unassailable place among the American crime élite.

The Mafia had been softened by years of living in America, their codes of discipline eroded. Sammy Chen was still paying them obeisance as if they had reason to fear them. And then there were the American hongs, like those of Henry Wing, whose ancestors slaved on the American railroads. More old men, the grandchildren of coolies, shackled by tradition.

The time was ripe to expand. Triads had never done business outside their own ghettoes, there had never been the need nor the opportunity. So western authorities knew nothing about them, had no infiltration at all. They were at the same point of opportunity as the Italians during Prohibition.

Instead of bootleg liquor, their bedrock would be number four heroin. Triad lieutenants would purchase it, triad cooks manufacture it, triad couriers transport it, and now they were in America the triad itself would wholesale it. Once they controlled every facet of the operation, the potential profits were vast, beyond comprehension. It just required vision and courage. It was time for a new generation. It was time for the sons of China to be emperors again.

The North Beach area of San Francisco had long been

known as Little Italy, though by the early-eighties it had more in common with Hamburg's Reeperbahn and London's Soho. On both sides of Broadway there were strip joints, jazz clubs, peep shows and hot dog palaces, the street patrolled by freaks and punks and crazies. But behind the sleaze, the Italian community still thrived, living in crowded, riotous streets as they had done since the early days of the century.

Sonny and Aldo Trinca arranged a lunchtime meeting in Coluzzi's, an anonymous Italian restaurant just a block away from Broadway. Sammy Chen and Henry Wing arrived together, the smiles they exchanged with the Trincas in heavy contrast to the hostile glares of the protection, who stared each other down from opposing sides of the restaurant.

Giorgio, the proprietor and a distant relative of Sonny Trinca, put up a sign on the front door: CLOSED. The four men settled down to swap business gossip, as if they were lawyers or stockbrokers or corporate executives; who had married; whose wives had had children; who had divorced; who had been forced into retirement by the government; who had died. The only difference was that the nature of their business was never mentioned.

After the meal Giorgio brought a tray of espressos and the real business was done; previous tentative agreements were ratified.

Finally, Sonny Trinca leaned back in his chair. 'We agree on no overlapping of markets then,' he drawled. 'You get everything west of Grant, plus you also wholesale to us for our market.'

Sammy looked at Henry, who nodded his assent.

'Agreed,' Sammy said.

Sonny and Aldo exchanged the amiable smiles of men who think they have got their own way. Sonny raised his glass to Sammy Chen and Henry Wing.

'Here's to business then,' Sonny said.

Sammy Chen grinned back. He had his foothold in America. And not a drop of blood had been spilt.

Yet.

Douglas was in high spirits. In fact, his mood bordered on elation. His cheeks were flushed, like polished bronze, and his dark eyes glowed with some private victory. He led her upstairs and made love to her with characteristic violence; there was never any tenderness in his lovemaking. He forced her through the usual catalogue of positions that he carried around in his brain, watching himself in the full-length mirror at the end of their bed. It went on for almost two hours, without climax. An endurance test, a marathon.

Finally he reached his moment with the gods, the muscles of his neck and arms taut as whipcord, his face mottled and contorted into a grimace. He shuddered and his weight settled on top of her. After a few minutes she wriggled from under him, and pushed him away. She felt as if she had been split apart.

'I need a drink,' she whispered.

The sweat was running into his eyes. He rolled over on his back and grinned at her. 'Hurry back. Maybe I haven't finished with you yet.'

There was a mahogany bar in the corner of the room. She poured some brandy from a bottle of Hennessy. The bottle's seal had been broken that afternoon, when she had crushed a bottle of Mogadon into it. One glass of this should keep him out for the rest of the night.

She poured in five fingers and dropped in some ice, took a Coke out of the refrigerator for herself. Then she lay down on the bed beside him. He was propped on the pillows, his hands behind his back, inviting her to admire him.

He must know how much I fear and loathe him, she thought. But he probably enjoys that. When she was with him, she experienced the same awe and terror she had once felt watching a shark circle an aquarium. He was so cold, so efficient. She remembered in the convent in Saigon the canonesse had told her that every child had a redeeming soul; but she no longer believed it. There was nothing of value left in this man. Any kernel of humanity had been cauterised from his spirit, perhaps by poverty, or by cruelty, or by hunger. All that had been left was the predator.

And here she was, in the water with the shark.

He gulped down the brandy, kept one of the ice cubes clenched between his teeth. He grinned at her and pushed her on to her back. He ran the ice over her nipples, her stomach, down to her vagina. She was still wet from his seed. He didn't seem to care, he was drunk with himself.

She whimpered. The ice was unpleasant, and she tried to push him away. He spat it on to the sheet and entered her again, suddenly.

And it started all over again, on and on. She pushed him away. 'I can't,' she whispered.

He came out of her, laughing, still erect. He got up and went to the bar, poured himself another large Hennessy, drank half of it in one swallow, as if it was beer. For the love of Buddha! There was enough there to kill a horse!

Douglas sat on the edge of the bed, his glass leaving a ring of condensation on the black silk sheet. 'You'll have to do something about this,' he said.

'Please, Douglas.'

'*Tai lo*. Call me *tai lo*.'

'Please, *tai lo*.'

He grabbed her by the hair and forced her head down between his legs. 'Do it! No, over here, so I can watch in the mirror.' He drained the rest of the glass while she worked on him. May prayed to Buddha, to Jesus, to the *phi* that watched her from the carved Ganesha. It had never been as bad as this. Let this torture be over soon!

Douglas lay on his back, spreadeagled, snoring. May got up, painfully, and went to the shower, letting the hot needles of water ease the pain from her body. She slipped on a black silk kimono and came back to the bed, leaned over him and slapped his face as hard as she could.

He did not stir, but the imprint of her palm and fingers showed livid against his cheek. Perhaps the Mogadon would kill him. She didn't give a damn.

Douglas' jacket lay on the floor by the door. She picked it up, found his keys, went back to her bedside drawer, and took out the Zippo lighter Michael had smuggled in for her. There was a dressing room off the bedroom, as large as an ordinary room. On the other side of the room was the door to Douglas' office. She hesitated, her heart banging against her ribs. She took a deep breath. Too late to go back now.

There were perhaps three dozen keys. She went through them one by one, until she found the one that fitted the lock. The door swung open.

The blinds were open. The moon hung over the water, lights bobbed in the darkness. May closed the blinds, in case Chang or one of the guards patrolling the gardens should see her. Then she turned on the light.

The office was not large; unlike the rest of the house, it was compact, functional. There was a tubular steel chair, a large office desk with two racks of three-tiered filing trays, and a three drawered steel filing cabinet.

She wondered if she should photograph the papers on the desk, or find something in the filing cabinet.

The ones on the desk.

She reached into the first tray, laid out all the papers like playing cards, as Michael had instructed her. There were no letters, or typewritten documents, as she would have expected to find in an ordinary office; instead there were just lists of figures and numbers and names that meant nothing to her. Code names, perhaps.

She removed the base of the Zippo lighter, armed the tiny camera inside and peered through the miniature eyepiece. Hopeless. What had Michael said? The lens was fish-eye. Spread the fingers of both hands to estimate the range. She stood back until she guessed that the whole desk was in focus.

Shoot.

She repeated the process until she had photographed everything in the trays, then carefully replaced them. She turned to the filing cabinet, found the right key, threw open the drawers.

She flicked through quickly, taking two files at random; Deutschbank, and Fragrant Investments. The file on Fragrant Investments contained a number of letters and accounts. She laid these out on the desk also and photographed them. The film was finished.

She opened the Deutschbank file anyway, and stared at the contents. It contained just three pages of statements, from the Deutschbank in Geneva, and a piece of paper in Douglas' handwriting with two five-digit codes. Triad money, she thought.

She was so tense it was difficult to breathe. Any moment Chang might walk through the door, discover her; or Douglas himself might be standing there, with that malicious golden smile, somehow recovered from the drugs in his brandy. She forced herself to stay calm, keep her nerve. She ripped a clean sheet of paper from the writing pad on the desk, sat down, and carefully copied the code numbers, and noted the account number and dates and amounts of all the transactions on the third page of the statement.

When she had finished, she stood up, and slipped the piece of paper into the pocket of her dressing gown. She returned the two files to the cabinet, and locked it. She checked the room, to satisfy herself that everything was as she had left it. She carefully removed two of her hairs from the polished surface of the desk, then turned off the light, remembered to open up the blinds. Then she locked the door, the Zippo still clutched in her right fist, and went back to the bedroom.

Douglas was still snoring. Even asleep he frightened her. No innocence on that face in repose. His body was knotted with muscle, a fighting machine, the livid scars on his thigh and his arms, pale and grotesque. What twisted road brought me here? May thought as she watched him. And where will that road lead me now that I have this terrible man's secrets pressed in the palm of my hand?

631

138

Michael arrived on time in a white vest and red silk running shorts. He wore a gold identity bracelet on his wrist and two gold chains around his neck. May felt her terror evaporate. It was all she could do not to laugh out loud. Michael was playing his role to the hilt.

She watched him from the pool. He was smiling at Chang, who stared back at him with cold derision. As a concession to the heat Chang was dressed today in Bermuda shorts and a blue polo neck shirt, but he still did not look anything other than what he was: a street thug.

'Hello, Miss Wong,' he said.

'Hello, Mai Koo,' she answered. She was aware of Michael and Chang watching her as she pulled herself out of the pool, and she was not displeased with the sudden air of tension. She casually picked up her towel and wrapped it around her middle. 'Too much hot out here,' she said, and walked straight past them.

French doors led off the terrace into a gymnasium. May threw herself face down on one of the benches. The two men followed her inside. Chang took up his post against one of the mirrors in a corner of the room. She could feel his eyes on her.

'Get me a Coke,' she said to him.

Chang scowled but wandered off to do as she asked.

'He keeps staring at me,' Michael said.

'Perhaps he love you too much,' May said. 'Where do you get such brown skin so sudden?'

'Out of a bottle.'

She reached behind her, loosened the towel, and untied the drawstrings of her bikini top. Michael began to smooth some oil into her back. 'Where is it?' he whispered.

'Left hand,' she said, and opened her fist.

'You had it with you in the pool?'

'You think I'm stupid? It was in the towel. I pick it up while I am taking off the wetness.'

Michael, conscious of the security cameras behind him, took the lighter from her, transferred it deftly to his Adidas bag while towelling the excess oil from his hands. 'You're a natural,' he whispered.

They heard Chang's footsteps. Michael worked her back muscles with sudden vigour that made her gasp. Chang gave Michael a hostile stare, and handed the Coke to May.

'Put it there,' she told him, pointing to the end of the padded bench.

He did as she asked and resumed his post against the mirror, still staring. May jerked her head around. 'Aiy-aaa! Chang! Why you stare like that, okay?'

'I'm not ... it is the *tai lo*'s instructions,' Chang said sulkily.

'Can do *tai lo*'s orders outside. What if I tell him you make sweet eyes at me, Chang? He cut your little thing off and hang it round your neck.'

'I wasn't ...' Chang protested, confused.

'Out!' May snapped.

Chang flushed with anger, stood up slowly, and went out.

Michael began the massage, feeling Chang's eyes on the back of his neck from the terrace. Had he done something to make him suspicious? It was hard to concentrate on what he was doing, to forget the erotic possibilities, even with Chang so close. Ly May's skin was like satin. He remembered that she was just nine years old when he had first met her, and felt a guilty flush. But there was no doubt that she was a woman now. Sweat inched between his shoulder blades, oozed from his forehead into his eyes. Christ. She was clenching her bottom, first one cheek, then the other, to draw attention to it. The scrap of her swimsuit barely covered anything.

Her face was shielded in the crook of her arm. She was smiling up at him. When their eyes met she winked.

A big game.

He squeezed the muscles in her neck as hard as he could.

'Chang!'

He leaped to his feet and ran in from the garden. 'Yes, Miss Wong?'

She pushed herself up on her elbows, holding the slip of the bikini top across her breasts. She held out the Coke can. 'Too warm.'

Chang knew she was taunting him. He took the Coke from her and sulked away.

'Do you enjoy making his life a misery?' Michael whispered.

'He is just a piece of dog business. Douglas say do it, he pull out all my toenail.'

She allowed the bikini top to slip away but stayed in the same position, resting her weight on her elbows. Her breasts were perfect tear drops, the nipples erect. He saw her watching him in the mirror.

She gave him an elfin smile. 'You like me then, Mai Koo, just a little?'

'Oh, May.'

'Maybe you think I'm cheap stuff. Because I live in so much badness. A lot you do not know about me, Mai Koo. I do much badness too. You will not like me so much if I tell you.'

'I don't care what you've done.'

'There is bad *phi* in me. Follow me everywhere and makes me too much trouble.'

'I'm going to get you out of here,' he said.

'One day I think you can massage front of me, not just back. You like that, Mai Koo?'

'For God's sake, just lie down and behave.' He stole a quick glance at the security camera in the corner of the room. Did someone watch? Did they record?

'Lie down!' he hissed.

She obeyed. 'You come back for me, Mai Koo?'

'I'll burn down the gates of hell for you.'

'You do not get killed this time?'

Chang returned with another can of Coke. Michael went on with his charade, working his knuckles into her back muscles so that she yelped and complained. At least it stopped her dangerous games. When he had finished she rolled the ice cold Coke can against her forehead, watching him in the mirror, but he dared not meet her eyes again. He knew he would give himself away to Chang.

He wanted to drag her away from the house now, not leave her here with these gorillas.

This time you mustn't let anything happen to her.

The film was in his bag. She had put her neck on the line for him, he would not let her down again.

139

They arranged to meet in Gaddi's, in the Peninsula Hotel. Dale had already decided that this might be his last trip to Asia, might even be his last really good meal. He ordered fillet of sole and a bottle of Chassagne Montrachet. Life was short, and getting shorter all the time.

He had not recognised Michael when they met in the lobby. He had bleached his hair, and the effect was unsettling, for his eyelashes and eyebrows were still dark. Michael mumbled something about his work, but did not elaborate.

As they ate Dale noticed too the fine lines that had been etched into the corners of his eyes, that spoke of long hours and too much emotional strain. Well, join the club, son.

Michael toyed with his food, his eyes wandering around the restaurant as if his mind was somewhere else. 'So what are you doing in Hong Kong, son? Are you allowed to tell me?'

'I've been seconded by Centac.'

'Centac?'

'It's a division of the DEA. They've picked up a file they think I might be able to help with. I've been transferred to the case for the duration. What about you? Is this business or pleasure?'

Michael seemed cool. Dale remembered that he had not sounded thrilled when he had tracked him down through his contacts at the embassy. The memory of their last encounter at Jennifer's funeral was still fresh in his mind. 'It's not business or pleasure,' he said.

'What then?'

'I came to see you.'

Michael looked uncomfortable. 'Let's just leave all that for now.'

'It's about Pacific International.'

Michael leaned closer. 'It's a drugs bank. I know it, everyone in the DEA knows it. Just because you can't see the shit on your shoes doesn't mean you can't smell it.'

'I didn't know just what they were doing when I joined them, Michael.'

'It doesn't matter any more. Can we talk about something else.'

'I want you to understand. It's important to me.'

'Understand what?'

'That I thought what I was doing was right. That I never did any of this out of greed or cynicism or anything else. I really thought it was right.'

'Yeah, well, you know what they say. About the road to hell, and all that.'

'Michael, I know I've disappointed you. But for my own part I'm very proud of you. I think you know that.'

He shrugged off this intimacy. All his childhood and early adolescence Jonathan Dale had been his hero, a god-like figure who returned from fighting great battles to regale him with stories and exotic souvenirs. He had assumed a mythical importance, a crusader king enshrined in his memory.

He did not know exactly when all that had changed. But some time in his early high school years, as the world became smaller and less mysterious, he discarded the need for an icon, wanted instead someone to throw a ball to, to take him to see the Giants at Candlestick Park like all the other dads.

And that was when his idol became a flawed father. There were times, later on, when he had hated him. When Dale returned on his occasional leaves, he had distanced himself even further and now any sort of intimacy between them left him feeling irritable and suffocated.

But despite his secession, he still carried his father's banners into life every day. He had not yet surrendered the colours to the enemy, as Jennifer had done. If he was an idealist, if he too was a warrior monk, then it was because of his father.

'I love you too, Dad,' he mumbled. 'I just wish we were fighting on the same side.'

'Perhaps we are.'

'It doesn't seem like it to me.'

'Michael, you see the briefcase under the table?'

He nodded.

'When we've finished lunch, I'm going to get up and walk out of here without it. Take it with you. Your friends in Centac may be interested.'

Michael pushed his plate to one side. 'What? What are you talking about?'

'One of my clients is a man named Sammy Chen. I think you've heard the name.'

'Sure I know him. The guy exports more dangerous drugs than ICI.'

'With what I have under the table, you may not be able to nail him on narcotics offences, but I think you have some very clear-cut indictments on currency violations. It's the Al Capone solution, Mike. It doesn't matter what you get them for, just get them, right?'

'Jesus.' Michael had turned pale. 'You mean this? Why?'

'Why what?'

'Why the sudden change of heart?'

'It's not sudden. I've been thinking about this for a long time.'

Michael shook his head. 'Well, son of a bitch.'

Dale leaned forward, gripped Michael's wrist. 'You'll have to be careful. I've tried this stuff with Justice. They bounced it right back. Don't forget, these are Company files.'

'We'll make it stick.'

'Just be careful, all right?'

'I'm sorry, Dad. About what I said ... at the funeral. I never ... I never thought.'

'That I'd turn cannibal?'

Michael's smile fell away, as other consequences played themselves out in his mind. 'What's going to happen to you?'

'No pension from the bank, I guess.' He raised his glass. 'A toast.'

Michael touched his father's glass with his own. 'Hearts and minds,' he said.

Dale smiled. 'And to America. May she rest in peace.'

*　　*　　*

Dale left first. As he was walking through the lobby he saw Baptiste Crocé.

Both men stopped and stared. Baptiste had two other men with him, trying hard to look like business associates, though it was painfully obvious what they were. When they saw Dale staring at their patron, one of them reached inside his jacket, an instinctive reaction that left the concierge wide-eyed with fright. Baptiste stopped the man with a piercing glance, then walked over, leaving his protection at the desk.

If he needs muscle, he must still be in the drugs business, Dale decided. By the look of his clothes and the diamonds on his fingers he was doing well at it, too. Who wasn't? He wondered if Noelle was with him, and the thought of seeing her just once more made him feel sick with desire. Had she changed? Was she the blowsy woman waiting by the reception desk, too much lipstick, too many pearls, holding the poodle with the diamond collar?

'Monsieur Dale,' said Baptiste, and held out his hand, smiling, as if they were former business partners who had lost touch.

Dale did not take the proffered hand. 'They'll let anyone in here these days.'

Baptiste's smile did not falter. 'Apparently. Even Americans. What are you doing in Hong Kong, *mon vieux*?'

'A little duty free shopping. Same as you, right?'

'Of course. Why else would anyone come to Hong Kong?'

'Is Noelle with you?'

'Why, would you like to see her?'

More than anything else in the world, right now. He watched the other man's reaction. He was still smiling. 'She might not want to see me,' he said.

'She's dead,' said Baptiste.

Dale felt sick. He's lying, he thought. I could always check, I can always find out. But is there a point? 'I'm sorry to hear that. But I'm sure she prefers the company.' He looked at his watch. 'I have to go.'

'*Au revoir, mon vieux*.'

'See you around.'

He walked out into the barrier of heat, past the white-gloved

639

doormen and the waiting taxis, turned blindly on to the crowded Nathan Road. She couldn't be dead, couldn't be. But did it matter any more? He had already signed his own death warrant, and if there had ever been a time for them, that time had long since passed.

140

The Royal Hong Kong Police Headquarters was in Arsenal Street, Wanchai, close to the waterfront, two monolithic high rises hidden away behind concrete gun emplacements and forbidding spike-topped walls. The headquarters of the Narcotics Bureau occupies one of the upper floors.

That May afternoon there were three men in the room. Raymond Schultz and Michael Dale were there representing the DEA; the other man was Chief Inspector Lau Chi-fen, or Teddy Lau as he was better known.

It was not yet seven o'clock in the morning, and as they spoke the horns of ocean-going ships woke the commercial heart of the city for another day.

Teddy Lau was studying the copies of the documents May Wong had photographed in Douglas Ho's office just three days before. After a while he sat back and put his hands behind his head, studying the two men on the other side of his desk. 'How did you get these?' he said.

'We have an agent in place,' Schultz said carefully.

Teddy Lau shook his head. Most of the documents were useless. Almost all were in code, a jumble of indecipherable names and numbers in Chinese characters. Like hieroglyphics, he thought ruefully. From their origin they might well contain records of the Fei Lung's entire heroin shipments in and out of Hong Kong, but without a Rosetta stone to decipher them they were useless.

And yet ...

It was the final documents that were intriguing. They demonstrated a clear link between a company called Fragrant Investments and China Sea Trading, whose major shareholding was held by Douglas Ho. Fragrant Investments owned a factory at Clearwater Bay, making a perfume with the intriguing name of Addiction. The documents also showed records of payments made from China Sea Trading to a Buddhist monastery on an island just half a mile from the factory.

'What conclusions have you drawn?' Teddy Lau asked aloud.

Schultz shook his head. 'The perfume factory would give Douglas the cover to legally obtain the chemicals he needs for large scale heroin production. That much I figured. But the monastery?'

'This has been done once before in the seventies,' Teddy said. 'A man called Limpy Ho used the idea to smuggle in morphine.' Schultz and Michael stared at him. 'A tunnel,' he explained. 'The monasteries were traditionally breeding grounds for rebellion, ever since the Manchus took power in China. They were raided so often by government soldiers they all had secret escape tunnels. I would guess that this place has a similar tunnel leading across to the mainland. It would mean triad junks could land the raw morphine at the island at night, and take away the finished number four. This way they would never have the problem of having to move narcotics across Hong Kong.'

Michael leaned forward. 'So can we raise a search warrant?'

Teddy Lau sat forward, collected the scattered documents from the desk, and replaced them in the file. He handed them back to the Americans. 'My theory is just that. A theory. And Mr Ho employs some very expensive lawyers. I would like to be certain we're going to find more than a few joss sticks.'

'What other reason would a man like this have to fund a run down monastery?'

'Philanthropy?' Teddy Lau said, but he did not smile. He sat for a moment, staring at the harbour, then seemed to make up his mind. 'I suppose the scenario does have a certain logic to it. All right, gentlemen. I'll see if I can organise some action on this.'

'And the girl?'

'If we find opiates on Mr Ho's property, we can write a warrant for his arrest. We can then protect your informant.

If we find nothing, Mr Ho may be left to wonder where we got our information.' He paused. 'It's a risk.'

Michael looked at Schultz but he shook his head. 'There's nothing else we can do, Mike. We have to go with what we've got.'

Michael slumped in his seat. He experienced a cold and greasy dread. He hoped that they had not made a terrible mistake.

141

San Francisco

On the other side of the Pacific Sammy Chen was sitting down to dinner.

Waiters burst in and out of the kitchens like tag wrestlers. The noise was deafening, the air rich with the aromas of garlic and anise and ginger. The restaurant sprawled over two levels, bronze dragons coiled up the red-lacquered plaster columns, the walls a riot of mirrors and gold leaf paper.

There were five people at the circular table at the top of the stairs. Sammy Chen wore a bow tie and tuxedo for the occasion, his sons either side of him looking like lawyers in their striped shirts, pagers and YSL double-breasted suits. Henry Wing sat opposite, with his daughter beside him. She was an unremarkable-looking girl, with a broad, flat face, and was overdressed in crimson taffeta and gold.

A grey Toyota pulled up outside the restaurant. Four Vietnamese youths climbed out, wearing black zippered jackets, joggers and jeans. One carried a shotgun, another a .357 Magnum; the third youth had a black assault rifle with a banana clip; the last boy carried a 9-millimetre Smith & Wesson automatic pistol, loaded with Super-Vel hollow points. Strollers on the sidewalk screamed and ducked away.

The four youths ran inside the restaurant.

Conversation stopped as the four walked in, their weapons held in front of them in the classic firing position. They started screaming instructions in Vietnamese, their eyes glassy with adrenalin. Everywhere diners scrambled for cover, dived under tables, shrieking in desperation.

One of the youths ran over to a table of five Chinese, an immigrant family celebrating the engagement of their daughter to a Cantonese from New York. The gunman kicked away the table they were sheltering behind and emptied his pistol into the huddled mass of humanity on the floor. By the time he had realised his mistake his jeans were wet with the blood of his victims. The pistol emptied and he jammed another clip in the magazine.

Meanwhile two of his colleagues had run upstairs. One of them carried a Double O Buck 12-gauge shotgun powerful enough to lift a refrigerator into the air. A waiter was trapped on the landing, frozen with horror and unable to retreat. He was blown out of the way. The shotgun blast toppled him over the stairs, and sent him crashing on to the marble floor below, a tray of empty plates shattering around him.

Henry Wing and Sammy Chen had positioned two pairs of bodyguards at separate tables between them and the stairs. These four men were already on their feet, aiming their pistols. As the first Vietnamese reached the top of the stairs they fired their handguns, more than half a dozen bullets hitting his body in the space of a few seconds. The youth would have fallen but the boy behind him held him upright, using him as a shield. He brought up the assault rifle, and emptied the entire clip of heavy bullets in panic. The effect in the confined space of the restaurant was devastating. Plates and glasses and mirrors exploded into shards, as the violently kicking rifle sprayed bullets everywhere. Two of the bodyguards took bullet wounds to the head, and fell. A third, despite being hit five times, continued to fire his pistol. As the Vietnamese gunman fumbled to reload, a bullet took him in the chest. He slid down the stairs, his dead companion slumped over his body.

The third youth took careful aim with his .357 and the last of Sammy's bodyguards reeled back, hitting the mirror behind him with a sickening crack, leaving a smear of dark blood down the shattered glass.

Sammy Chen had thrown his sons under the table and sheltered beside them, confident that his protection would deal with the intruders. When he heard the bark of the assault rifle, he lost control of his bowels.

He saw one of his bodyguards lying among the rain of broken plates and spilled food, pawing desperately at his shotgun wounds, geysers of blood exploding between his fingers as a lacerated femoral artery pumped his lifeblood onto the floor. Someone put a pistol against his head and his face disappeared.

His Beretta had spun across the marble floor just inches from Sammy's hand. He had never had to use a handgun before, but he knew this might now be his only chance to save himself and his sons.

Henry Wing had pushed his daughter towards the toilets at the back of the room. The gunmen were high on their own adrenalin now, and one of them, holding the heavy .357 Magnum in both hands, blazed away at the running figure. The gun was loaded with 265-grain hollow points, and the gun kicked back so hard the slightly built Vietnamese could not keep his aim. The first two bullets slammed into the mirrors at the back of the room, one smashed into an upturned table and wounded an Australian tourist sheltering behind it. The final two bullets hit Henry Wing just as he reached the door, one entering just below the left shoulder blade and blasting a hole in his chest the size of a soup plate as it exited his body; the other all but severed his left arm just above the elbow. His daughter screamed and tried to grab him. He shouted at her to run. But she froze, and just stood there and screamed hysterically until another of the Vietnamese calmly walked over to her, placed his Smith & Wesson pistol against her head and blew off the top of her head.

Henry Wing cried out in rage and pain. The man stood over him, aimed the gun straight at Henry Wing's face and pulled the trigger.

At that moment Sammy Chen kicked over the table and fired the Beretta blindly in terror and panic. His sons rushed for the unguarded stairs, a pistol coughed twice and then there was nothing.

One of Sammy Chen's bullets took the gunman with the Magnum in the belly and he lay doubled over on the floor, kicking and writhing. His comrade, shocked at the carnage around him, panicked at being the last of his group still standing, grabbed the wounded youth and dragged him on the stairs. He fired twice more, screaming for everyone to stay out of his way.

He bundled his wounded colleague into the back of the waiting Toyota and they sped away through the back streets of Chinatown.

The devastation inside was terrible. The tiles were slippery with bright blood. There was a long and shocked silence, and then men as well as women began to weep openly, and their weeping mingled with the cries of those maimed and wounded by the stray and ricocheting bullets. It smelled like a charnel house.

Sammy Chen made bubbling sounds as he lay on his back at the top of the stairs. There were four holes in his suit, and his shirt and trousers were soaked with blood. But he was alive.

When the police and first emergency crews arrived he was still conscious, his face a white mask of grief and shock and pain. He kept repeating one word over and over.

'Douglas.'

142

Hong Kong

At three o'clock in the afternoon, armed police and Narcotics
Bureau detectives blocked off the entrance to the perfume
factory at Clearwater Bay and conducted a thorough search
of the buildings. In a simultaneous raid, a Royal Hong Kong
Marine Police patrol boat landed a search party at a Taoist
monastery half a mile offshore. Although no narcotics were
found inside the factory, searchers at the monastery discovered
vats and filtration equipment similar to those used in the
preparation of number four heroin.

A stairway at the rear of the main shrine led to an under-
ground passage. It was clearly more than a historical curiosity.
Modern electric cables provided power for lighting, and the
ceiling had been reinforced with steel struts.

They followed the tunnel for over half a mile. At the far
end they found what they were looking for; fifteen hundred
kilograms of raw opium, packed in burlap sacks; two hundred
and ten kilograms of morphine bricks; and eighty kilograms
of number four heroin, bearing a Tiger brand stamped in red
on the face of the plastic wrapping, a brand often found on
Customs seizures in air terminals and ports across the western
seaboard of the United States. A barred iron door led to a fake
distilling vat in the factory above.

In the DEA office in the Hopewell Centre Michael Dale and
Ray Schultz received the news by telephone and exchanged
high fives. They knew they had finally broken Douglas Ho.

Douglas stood in front of the mirror in the gymnasium, his eyes closed, his body still, hardly breathing. He wore only a pair of red nylon training shorts. His body was a pale yellow ivory and gleamed with sweat. The muscles on his compact frame could have been sculpted by an artist. It was not the body of a forty-year-old man, thought May, as she watched him. Every muscle was perfectly defined, an anatomy lesson of sinew and ligament and bone. His physical perfection made the scars on his left thigh and across his forearms more shocking. It was as if he had been beautifully carved from a piece of wax then held for a moment too long near a flame.

He opened his eyes and attacked the man in the mirror. It was part of his training. Although he now had soldiers to do his killing, Douglas Ho remained a predator by instinct and inclination. Every day he performed this ritual, shadow fighting in the mirrored gymnasium, anticipating and blocking his own attacks, trying to defeat his own guard, pitting his reflexes and speed against a mirror, defying reality as he had done all his life.

His movements were a blur, dozens of separate blocking movements and blows all in the space of a few seconds. Then he returned again to his meditation, eyes shut.

'Someone tried to assassinate Sammy Chen,' he said, knowing she was there, though she had entered the room as silently as she could.

'You, Douglas?'

'A gang of Vietnamese went crazy with guns in a restaurant. Henry Wing is dead, and one of Sammy's sons. But one of them lived. And so did he.' He attacked the mirror again, shadow fighting with sudden, vicious anger. When he had finished his chest heaved with the expended effort.

'What does this mean for us?'

'It means we are renegades, May.' His eyes blinked open and he fixed her with a glacial smile in the mirror. 'They will try and kill me. You too, May.'

She could think of very few things she might wish to die for. Douglas Ho did not number among them.

'You must not leave this house until this is over. Even with Chang.'

'Will you win?' she asked him, hardly caring.

649

'I always win.'

Chang entered from the terrace. 'A phone call for you, *tai lo.*'

Douglas picked up the extension in the corner of the room. He listened for a long time, barking out his questions in chiu chao. She saw the muscles on his back stiffen. He replaced the receiver and turned around, fixing her with his black eyes.

'Is anything wrong?' she said, as calmly as she could.

'We have to leave Hong Kong.'

'We are going back to Bangkok?'

'Taiwan. We sail as soon as possible.'

'Sail?'

'I can't use the airport.' Without warning he tore the phone from the wall and flung it at the mirror. 'Come here, May.'

He's going to kill me. He's going to break me with his bare hands. She forced herself to stay calm, not to run blindly away. Where was there to run to? 'What's wrong, Douglas?'

'I said, come here!'

She took three faltering steps towards him, trying to control the trembling in her limbs. As soon as she was within reach his arm snaked out and he grabbed a fistful of hair, twisted, forcing her to her knees. 'It was you,' he said.

'Stop it!'

'It was you!'

'What is it? What have I done?'

He leaned closer to her, his breath strangely sweet with the spices he had eaten with his lunch. He wrapped a coil of hair around his wrist like rope and jerked her head back. He moved behind her. His thumb and index finger found the nerves in the muscles of her neck and shoulders and squeezed. The world exploded into a red shock of pain. 'The police have raided my factory at Clearwater Bay. You gave them the information, didn't you? Or do you want me to give you to Chang? He'd enjoy getting all the details.'

'Stop it!'

'Just tell me!'

'Please, it hurts ...'

'Was it you?'

'Yes, yes, yes!'

He released her and she fell on to the floor. 'I knew it was you,' he said. 'That was one of my people in Arsenal Street. They said your name.' When she looked up, Douglas had resumed his position in front of the mirror, eyes closed, as if she did not exist.

She knew he was going to kill her. The only questions were when and how. She thought about Michael. Will he know what has happened, will he try to get me out of here?

'Kuan Yin is angry with me,' Douglas said. 'So much bad luck in one day. Sammy Chen still alive, now the police have found the heroin at Clearwater Bay. I will have to give her a sacrifice to win back my joss.'

I am not going to beg for my life, thought May. It would be pointless, and I still have my pride. She got to her feet, watched his face in the reflection of the mirror. 'What now?'

'You are a ghost, May. You are not living, but you are not yet dead.' She searched the gymnasium for a weapon. She saw the piles of weights by the bench press, imagined crushing his skull.

She started to move, but suddenly he was watching her in the mirror. 'Do you want me to break your arms?' he said softly.

'What are you going to do with me, you vicious chicken-humping piece of monkey shit!'

He laughed. 'So much spirit! I like that, May, I always liked that. Why did you do it? Why did you risk your life to betray me? Not for money. I gave you all the money you wanted.'

Stay calm, May. Think. There must be some way out. There always has been before. When the pirates attacked your boat, you thought that was the end. You were patient. You clung to life. The *phi* of the water protected you.

'Why did you do it?' he repeated.

'For fun,' she said.

He knew she was mocking him. He called for Chang, and told him to tie her hands and feet and lock her in the bedroom until they were ready.

651

143

Baptiste Crocé was holding a glass of brandy and studying the view across the harbour from Noelle's suite in the Peninsula Hotel. 'I've heard they're planning to build a planetarium over there,' he was saying. 'Have you ever heard of anything so barbaric? They're Philistines, the Cantonese. Everything is money to them. They're going to ruin the view from here entirely.'

'You didn't come here to discuss the view,' said Noelle.

Baptiste turned around. His face was grey. 'Bad news,' he said.

Noelle had guessed as much. It was as if something inside her broke, a part of her heart that was at once luminous and fragile, shattered into a thousand pieces, too delicate ever to be mended, too precious to be replaced.

'How did you find out?' she asked him, and was surprised at how calm she sounded.

'Perhaps I can get you a drink. To fortify you?'

'Just tell me.'

Baptiste turned back to the window, as if he could not bear to watch her face as he told her. 'A few hours ago in San Francisco there was a shooting. An assassination, if you like. It could not have happened if Lucien was alive. It means all deals are off.'

'Is there some chance?'

'He is no longer a pawn in the game. Will the man who took him now just hand him back, with his apologies? I would not have you lose sleep over such a remote possibility.'

'But there is a chance.'

'There is no chance.'

'You don't know he's dead.'

'I know the man who took him.'

The room was spinning. Noelle gripped the arm of the sofa, until the moment had passed. Baptiste was standing over her.

'Are you all right?' he asked her.

She nodded, and got to her feet. She smoothed down her dress, her head held high. Life might break her heart, she would not let it humiliate her in public.

He took her shoulders. 'Please, Noelle. This is my sorrow too.'

She shook herself free. 'Please don't touch me, Baptiste.'

'He's a dead man, Noelle. I swear I'll avenge him.'

'What difference does that make?'

'Please, Noelle. I still love you. Now we have lost Lucien, you're all I have left.'

'You have your money, don't you?'

'Come back to me. Please.'

She took a step towards him, brushed the comma of hair from his forehead, touched his cheek. 'It is my one and lasting fervent hope, that you fry in hell,' she said.

Later, he thought about what she had said. She did not mean it. She could not. One day he knew he would get her back. After all, everything he had done, he had done for her.

Michael paced Schultz's office in the Hopewell Centre, waiting for confirmation of their victory. When the call came through Schultz snatched up the phone on the first ring. The conversation was short. When it was over he dropped the receiver on its cradle and slammed the desk top with the flat of his hand.

'Have they issued the arrest warrant?' Michael asked him.

Schultz shook his head.

'What the hell are they waiting for? They have the stuff, it was right there in the factory.'

'I don't know what the problem is. Teddy Lau won't say.'

'If they don't take him today, he'll run. He must have been warned by now.'

'There's nothing we can do, Michael. You know that.' He rubbed the corners of his eyes with his thumb and forefinger. 'It's out of our hands. You did a good job. Go home and have a couple of days' rest.'

'My source is still in there. I have to get her out.'

'I told you, there's nothing we can do.'

Michael wanted to punch the walls. Punch Ray. Punch Teddy Lau. Punch someone, make them understand. 'My CI! She's still inside the house! We can't just walk away!'

The phone rang again. The conversation was brief, Schultz's replies monosyllabic. The last one was a crude oath.

The receiver was returned to its cradle with so much force the handset cracked.

'What's happened?'

'Douglas Ho is getting ready to go on vacation,' Schultz said. 'Jesus Christ.'

'He's loading supplies on board the *Hammerhead*. Getting ready to sail off into the sunset.'

Michael felt hollow. 'They're going to let him go?'

Schultz shrugged. 'It's not Teddy's fault. You know how these things work. They have a big bust, they have some heads to parade in court. But someone up the chain has decided Douglas is too much of an embarrassment. He can name too many names. It's just like the Ma brothers back in the seventies. They're giving Douglas a few hours to get the fuck out.'

'So that's it?'

'That's it.'

Michael was on his feet. 'But what about Ly May?'

Schultz spread his hands. 'There's nothing we can do, Michael.'

'She put her life on the line for us! If someone inside Teddy Lau's department has ratted this deal to Douglas Ho, he'll tear her to bits with his teeth! Ray, we have to do something!'

Schultz was on his feet too. 'Like what? Tell me what I can do, for Christ's sake!'

Michael walked out. He did not know where he was going, or what he was going to do. He only knew he could not sit cursing in Ray Schultz's office while Ly May was left to suffer alone.

For the second time.

144

He was kept waiting outside Teddy Lau's office for almost half an hour. When the door finally opened, the man he had spoken to just twelve hours before seemed to have aged ten years. The weight of the world's problems were on his shoulders. The pouches under his eyes had sagged, and his face was pale and taut with stress. Michael's fury evaporated in the face of Teddy Lau's obvious exhaustion.

'Come in, Mr Dale,' he said. 'Drink?'

He opened a grey metal cabinet. There was a small bar refrigerator inside. He reached in, took out two cans of San Miguel and two glasses, set them on his desk.

He poured one of the cans into a glass and took a long swallow.

Michael did not touch his. 'What's going on?' he said.

Teddy Lau sighed. 'I don't have to do this, you know, Mr Dale. There's no need for anyone to give you explanations. No need at all.'

'We gave you Douglas Ho on a platter.'

'Don't hector me. I want Douglas Ho as badly as you. Perhaps more, because I have been chasing him for a lot longer. We have both just come face to face with an unpleasant reality.'

'Which is?'

'That if you pursue international criminals successfully, you finally reach a certain rarefied level where the trail turns icy cold. Suddenly you are no longer talking about criminals. You are talking about politics and diplomacy. That is hallowed ground, Mr Dale. A place where policemen like ourselves are not allowed to tread. That is when our masters turn on us, when they tell us to go back to the streets and arrest the people who look like criminals, and not the rich businessmen in smart suits who sit next to them at charity dinners, who attend their cocktail parties and are numbered among their personal friends.'

'You've been told to let him go?'

'Indeed.'

'Who gave you those orders?'

'I cannot tell you.' He poured more beer into his glass. 'You can see why it is hard for a policeman to be honest, Mr Dale. When his own masters compromise their morals so thoroughly, a man starts to wonder what benefits there are in being decent. I will tell you now, I have never taken a bribe in my whole career. But then I think I am a fool, and so does my family.'

'If we don't get Douglas Ho, this whole thing is just a fucking pantomime. Why did I let my informant risk her life for this?'

'A good question, and one for which I have no answer. But I am sure the police commissioner will be satisfied. You have led us, after all, to a great deal of heroin which we can parade before the press to show them we are doing our job. We have some very evil-looking men whose photographs will appear in the newspapers. Officially, I am very grateful for your department's co-operation.'

'The number two man in this whole conspiracy is still dangling his toes in the water at Pak Sha Wan. I want his ass.'

'It is not possible. I am told his arrest will compromise the interests of Hong Kong and her allies.'

'The United States?'

'Precisely.'

'For Christ's sake, Teddy, how many crimes are we willing to overlook in the name of national security? And who makes that decision?'

Teddy Lau finished his beer, crushed the can in his fist and threw it in the metal waste bin next to his desk. 'Not you, Mr Dale, and not me.'

'And what about the girl?'

'Your informant?'

'She just has to take her chances, right?'

'I wish I could help you,' he said. He turned around in his chair and stared out of the window at the harbour. Michael got up and walked out without another word.

*   *   *

The two Corsicans cut the Zodiac's outboard and paddled around the heads into the bay at Pak Sha Wan. The *Hammerhead* was moored at a private jetty below the villa, the superstructure illuminated with halogen lamps. Steps had been cut into the side of the rocks and three Chinese in white ducks came down carrying cardboard cartons.

It was clear they were loading the yacht for a long sea voyage. Baptiste had told them the loading would continue all night.

They anchored the Zodiac in the bay. The moon had not yet risen, and the water was black. A strong onshore wind stirred the surface, creating a chop that would camouflage their air bubbles. They watched the *Hammerhead* for several minutes through field glasses, noting the guards positioned fore and aft. Then they donned scuba tanks and vests over their wet suits, and unpacked the limpet mines from the canvas bag that lay on the deck of the rubber boat. The fuses were set for six hours.

They slipped into the water and dived straight to the bottom, using compasses to navigate. Forty-five minutes later they were back in the Zodiac, cold and shivering but each fifty thousand dollars richer. They again used the oars to get out of the bay, so they would not attract attention, then started the outboard and skimmed across the surface of the water, beaching below Hiram's Highway. They were at the airport at seven that morning for the Air France flight direct to Paris.

While the two Corsicans were checking in their bags, Jonathan Dale was on the other side of the terminal staring through the crowds at Noelle Crocé. She was waiting at the Thai International first-class counter, booked on that morning's flight to Bangkok. She looked pale, exhausted, and was dressed in black. She was alone.

Dale stopped and stared, making sure. He felt the same way he had when he first saw her; a hollow feeling in his stomach, his chest tight, his mouth dry. He almost shouted her name across the terminal.

But he didn't.

What could he say to her? Was there really anything left to say? There was something forbidding about her appearance, she looked like a mourner at a funeral. She was as beautiful as he remembered, but now her beauty seemed pale and fragile, like a porcelain doll's.

He watched her take her boarding pass and ticket, slip them into her wallet and walk slowly towards the boarding gates. He followed her for a few steps, and then stopped. It was best left alone. After all, he was a fugitive now. He checked in his own luggage for the Pan Am flight to San Francisco and let his ghosts be.

145

Michael watched the *Hammerhead* from the bridge of the *Police 78*, almost half a mile distant. Her white hull glistened like bone in the early-morning light. Above Pak Sha Wan, the misty peaks of the New Territories were dotted with early lights, street lamps hung like strings of pearls. There were still stars in the western sky.

Michael heard the *Hammerhead*'s twin eight-cylinder Gardiners throb to life, the sound carrying to them clearly. The commander of the *Police 78*, Inspector Ian Thorn – Thorny to his men – picked up his field glasses. 'There she goes,' he said.

A thread of blue vapour rose from the exhausts at the stern. Two men in white ducks jumped on to the jetty to free the guide ropes. The screws churned the water and with engines at slow the *Hammerhead* moved away from the jetty, manoeuvring towards the middle of the channel.

Douglas Ho appeared on deck for the first time, and climbed up the companionway to join the skipper on the fly bridge. Still no sign of May.

Thorn ordered the *Police 78* half speed ahead and followed the yacht out to sea.

'She's going to get away,' Michael said. He had been praying for some last-minute reprieve. Schultz had been making phone calls to Washington all through the night. Now all hope had gone.

'My orders are to observe but not intercept,' said Thorn. 'Short of him committing an act of piracy inside Hong Kong waters, I doubt that there's anything I can do.'

I've lost her. Michael was desolate.

They tailed her out of the bay. Her engines rose to a higher pitch as she accelerated south across Port Shelter. Ngau Mei Chau loomed from the morning mist. The *Hammerhead* turned south and headed towards the Poi Toi islands and the open sea, a moustache of white foam around her bows. She sliced through the chop, the Red Ensign whipping from her masthead and stern. She sped past a fleet of junks on Tathong Channel, her smooth lines silhouetted against the brown ghosts of China and the torn grey clouds of dawn.

May felt the throb of the motors through the hull and the rolling movement of the sea and knew they had left Hong Kong. She had been left tied and gagged inside the house since the previous afternoon. During the night Chang and another man had carried her down to the yacht and threw her in the forward locker. No one had spoken a word to her since.

They were going to kill her and dump her at sea.

She tried to prepare herself. As a little girl she had been told that when a person died the spirits of the body returned to the place where their father had buried the birthing cord. Hers had been buried, by tradition, under the hut where she was born. A part of her now longed to return to the mountains, but she wondered how her souls would ever find their way back from here. It was such a long way and souls were notoriously wayward and stupid. She had made so many long journeys without a *basi*, a ceremony that would have tied her spirits to her body in preparation. She knew of no spirit that had ever had to cross the ocean. Perhaps hers would become scattered over the world and wander for ever.

Has it all been worth it? she wondered. I took such a big risk, and in the end it did not make any difference. It did not hurt Douglas, only me, and now Mai Koo has abandoned me again. I was stupid. I should have been more like Noi.

If only I knew what Douglas has devised for me.

She closed her eyes and willed herself to be strong.

Douglas Ho sat in a deckchair on the aft sundeck. He wore a cable-knit white roll-neck jumper, canvas ducks and Sperry topsiders; he was sipping Hennessy VO and smoking a Havana cigar. The elegant Chinese gentleman out for a cruise.

A crewman stood directly behind him. Douglas gave him whispered instructions and the man began hauling buckets of mashed fish and offal from below and emptying them off the stern. Finally a fin broke the water and dived through the slick.

Douglas removed his sunglasses and returned his attention to his prisoner. Chang ripped the plaster off her mouth.

'My darling,' said Douglas.

May stared back at him.

'I imagine you're wondering how I'm going to do this?'

'I'm sure you've thought of something.'

He laughed. 'It's nothing all that novel, I'm afraid. I'm a traditionalist sometimes.' He drew on the cigar. 'These are terrible things. Addictive. One must try to avoid addiction.' He studied her with acute interest. 'Haven't you anything you'd like to say to me?'

May shook her head. He had already made up his mind to kill her, there was nothing she could say that would make any difference. The best she could hope for was that he would do it quickly.

'I'm curious to know. Was it money or principle?'

'Principle,' she said.

Douglas looked disappointed. 'If it was money, I could have understood that. It would just have been a bad bargain. But for principle? I always thought you were smart.'

She shivered in the cool of the morning, took deep lungfuls of salt air. The last few breaths, precious to her now.

'Strip her,' he said.

Chang put his fingers in the neck of her shirt and tore down, ripping out the buttons. He wrenched the thin silk down around her shackled wrists. Then he threw her face down on to the deck and cut away her shorts and underwear with a knife.

He yanked her back to her feet.

Douglas was standing in front of her, holding a knife. He tested the blade with his thumb. He held it to the light and she saw the blood well from the thin cut.

'Death is a symbol, May. Killing alone is easy. It serves a purpose – it eliminates someone who is dangerous to your future plans or punishes an enemy. But there is another

661

dimension; it also serves as a warning to others, to those who oppose you, and elicits respect from your followers. That is why a good manager endeavours to make each end as symbolic as possible. One needs a sense of theatre, of ritual. One needs to introduce an element of the supernatural. The triad taught me that, at my initiation.'

He held the knife in front of her face. 'Also, like you, I believe in the spirit world. Our luck, our good joss, comes from the spirits, *neh*? Kuan Yin saved my life once, she has been my good luck all my life. Now my joss is not so good. So I will give her a sacrifice. I will give her you.'

He touched the blade of the knife between her breasts. 'I am not a sadist, May, I take no pleasure in this. But it has to be done.' He turned to Chang. 'Throw her on the deck.'

Chang kicked out, striking her behind the knees so that she buckled and fell. He put his knee between her shoulder blades to keep her down. Douglas leaned forward and with great precision tracked half a dozen incisions across her buttocks, her thighs and her back.

May writhed desperately on the deck, thrashing against the pain. Not this way! Just kill me and get it over with! She tried to grit her teeth against the agony of each burning slash but finally she filled her lungs with air and screamed.

Ian Thorn put down his field glasses, his face dark with rage. Michael snatched them from him and focused on the deck of the *Hammerhead*. The sound in his throat was barely human.

'You have to stop this!'

'We're in international waters. I'd have to fire on her to stop her, and I'd need permission from God knows who to do that. They'd want it in fucking triplicate, it would take all week, and then they'd say no!'

'Stop him!'

Thorn's face was twisted with impotent fury. 'I can't! We have to turn back.'

Michael closed his eyes. Like Vietnam, like Laos, like the Triangle; all manner of barbarity taking place in front of him and still they were telling him there was nothing that could be done.

'I'll kill him,' Michael said, and his voice was a rasp. 'I'll find him in Taiwan and I'll kill him. Fuck the job, fuck everything. I'm going to kill him.'

Thorn looked shaken, for Michael and for himself. 'I have to turn back,' he repeated.

May could not get her breath. The pain twisted her body in spasms, she was helpless with it. She only dimly realised they were forcing her to her feet. Chang was holding her upright, gripping her under the arms. Her blood was slippery under her feet.

Douglas was standing by the buckets that were lined up at the stern. The crewman delivered the contents of the last of them into the water. 'Offal,' Douglas said, turning back to her. 'From a pig. It attracts the sharks. They come for the offal, and then hang around, like greedy little children, waiting for more. There's three of them out there now. You can see their silhouettes in the water if you watch carefully.'

He nodded his head and Chang brought her to the stern.

'We tie you to this rope and then tow you behind us. The sharks will smell the blood and come racing in. Sometimes it takes a few minutes, because they're cowards and they can be cautious, even now. If you are sensible you will not try to fight the rope. Let yourself drown. It will be easier on you. As I said, this is not for your benefit. It is for mine. And for joss.'

May was only barely aware of what they were doing. She did not see them attaching the rope to the metal bracelets that held her wrists. Chang carried her to the stern and then she was dropping into the ocean.

Douglas wiped the blood from his hands with a towel. A few spots had stained his pullover. A pity. He sat down in the fishing chair, took out his binoculars and settled down to watch the show. The rest of the crew were gathered around him. He wanted them to witness this. He wanted them to repeat the story again and again when they reached Taiwan.

May tried to scream as she hit the water, the salt making each wound a tearing agony. Water rushed into her mouth. She jerked on the end of the rope and despite the advice

Douglas had given her she instinctively kicked for the surface, struggling for life.

The rope jerked taut and she was pulled along on her back. I must drown before the sharks find me, she reminded herself. But it is so hard to die. So hard...

The *Police 78* stopped dead in the water. Michael watched the *Hammerhead*, in despair and disbelief. It was over, and he had failed.

He no longer cared what happened to Douglas, all he could think of was Ly May.

He knew he would never forgive himself for this.

Douglas scanned the horizon, saw the *Police 78* stop her engines and prepare to turn back to Hong Kong, as he knew she would. He waved, hoping someone on deck would see him. Then he returned his attention to the figure bobbing in the water fifty metres from the stern. He tested the tow rope, waiting for the jerk and tug as the sharks came to take the first chunk of warm, living flesh.

146

On the *Police 78* they saw the flash seconds before the thunder of the explosion rolled across the ocean. A mushroom of black smoke rose into the morning sky.

The *Hammerhead* was gone.

Thorn stared at the sea in disbelief: debris all over the water, heads bobbing in the swell, the white bellies of fish killed or stunned by the explosions; and over everything, the smell of cordite.

'What the hell happened?' he said, to himself as much as any of the gaping officers on the bridge.

The *Police 78* cut through the water, racing the dark shapes that arrowed, fins erect, through the water. The crew worked frantically to pull the living from the sea.

Michael saw her floating face down, black hair fanning around her in the water, the knife slashes raw against her skin. She was twenty yards from the boat, a length of thick manila rope trailing from her wrists on the surface of the ocean. He launched himself over the side before Thorn could shout a warning to his crew to stop him.

A desperate fear sent him ploughing through the water. Please let her not be dead. Please ...

As soon as he reached her, he rolled her over on to her back, treading water as he tried to breathe air into her lungs. He heard the shouts from the crewmen of the *Police 78*, as Thorn tried to manoeuvre the patrol boat closer. He kicked desperately at the water.

At the periphery of his vision he saw a crewman from the *Hammerhead* swimming desperately, no more than a few yards away. Then his body rose out of the water as a shark piled into him. He saw the ugly blunt nose and the flash of a fin.

If he could save May, at least. He owed her that much.

They had thrown a net over the side of the launch. One of the crew scrambled down and hauled May out of the water. Michael felt something slam into him, a shark, a small one, confused and excited. It cannoned him into the hull, winding him. He flapped helplessly at the water.

He saw the gaff in front of his face, grabbed it, thinking he could not make it. They pulled him clear of the water, and other hands closed around his wrists, hauled him from the boiling and terrible sea.

May felt a racking spasm in her chest and when it was over she was lying on her side vomiting seawater on to the deck. Her wrists were still shackled and each retching spasm in her chest was a new agony. Someone was yelling at her to stay awake, stay awake, but the pain and the exhaustion were just too great and she let the blackness envelop her once more, followed the souls of her body to a wonderful darkness where pain recedes and everything is floating and warm.

Michael had May's head cradled in his arms. 'Stay awake!' he shouted. 'Stay awake!'

He looked around. There were five bodies on the deck. Two were dead, and two crewmen were working desperately to revive another. He was unconscious, face white, jaw slack. One of the constables bent over him to breathe air into his lungs.

Douglas Ho.

And Michael thought: No. No more Romeos. No more international borders. No more playing by gentlemen's rules. This time justice is going to be done.

He pushed the two Chinese crewmen out of the way, grabbed the body under the armpits and dragged it to the side.

'Dale!' he heard Thorn shouting. 'No!'

Douglas rolled in the swell. One of the constables ran to fetch the gaff they had used to hook the bodies from the water. Michael wrestled with him, pulling him off balance. They fell sideways on to the deck.

A dark shape came out of the water. A hammerhead. Douglas Ho disappeared, a cloud of blood welled up. The fish backed away, shaking its great head, its teeth pink with blood.

The crew were silent, watching the grim show, as other sharks raced in to finish the feast.

Justice, thought Michael. Arbitrary, natural and cruel. The only kind there was left.

147

The doctor asked to see him alone. He was a young man, Cantonese, with prematurely greying hair.

'You wanted to know the condition of Miss May Wong?' he said.

Michael nodded.

'You are a close friend?'

'I've known her since she was a little girl,' he said.

He waited, trying to decipher the doctor's expression. She has to be all right, she has to!

'The greatest danger in the case of near drowning is secondary infection from the seawater that enters the lungs. We will have to keep her on antibiotics for a few days, watch her very closely. As for her other injuries, she has one hundred and twenty-three stitches in her body. She will never be quite as beautiful again. But the incisions were clean and straight and the scars will fade in time. Perhaps only her husband will ever really notice.'

'So she's going to be all right?'

'We will have to wait and see.'

'Well, can I see her?'

'She is sedated. But you may see her for a short while. By the way, who did this to her?'

Michael hesitated. 'Everybody.'

May lay on her side, her face deathly pale. There were purple shadows under her eyes. An intravenous tube fed morphine into a vein on the back of her hand.

'May,' he whispered.

Her eyes fluttered open. 'Mai Koo.'

'How are you doing?'

She took a long time to answer, the sedatives slowing her responses. 'Okay.'

'I'm sorry, May.'

'I still be beautiful, Mai Koo? Boys still want to make sweet eyes at me?'

'The doctors said you're going to heal just fine.'

'Think I lose jewellery he give me. For my wrinkle time.'

'I'll take care of you.'

Her eyes watched him for a long time. 'Maybe. I don't know. More better we wait and see.'

She slipped into the sudden, dreamless sleep of morphine. Michael brushed a lock of hair from her face, kissed her gently on the forehead, and left the room.

148

San Francisco

Jonathan Dale was alone in the den. He took a bottle of Bushmills from the bar and sat down to drink it. Pockets of fog appeared in the bay as evening fell; a freighter passed under the Golden Gate, the foghorn echoing around the harbour. A lonely sound, haunting, whispering of other ports, other countries, other lives.

He wandered around the den, occasionally stopping to pick up the souvenirs of his life. A Chinese SK bolt action rifle taken from a dead Viet Cong near Pleiku; some photographs of Vietnamese regulars found in a bunker in Sam Neua; a bronze statue of Ganesha bought in a junk market in Vientiane; a bamboo opium pipe given to him by a Hmong chief in Northern Laos.

And absolutely nothing of his life with Noelle.

But you pays your money and you takes your choice, as someone had once said to him. He had married the wrong woman and committed himself to the wrong cause. On the way he had lost his children, lost his faith.

'Well,' he said aloud, 'you can't be right all the time.'

The bottle was half empty when he heard a noise behind him and realised there was someone else in the room.

'Hello, Gerry,' he said.

'Jack.' Gerry Gates sat down in the wing-backed chair next to him. 'Lost none of that old sixth sense.'

'Want a drink?'

Gates shook his head.

'Not even for old time's sake?'

'Especially not for old time's sake.'

Dale studied him. He realised he had never liked Gerry all that much. They had just happened to be on the same side.

Kind of.

'Come to give me a lecture?'

'We're both getting a little old for that.'

'Speak for yourself.' Dale swallowed some more of the Bushmills. It burned on the way down. Felt good.

Gerry looked awkward. As if he had to break the news of the death of a close friend. Which in a way was exactly what he was about to do, Dale thought.

'Jack, I've been hearing some things that have disappointed me a whole lot. Your appointment to Pacific International was an act of great personal faith. I hung my ass on the line for you there. I thought I could trust you.'

'Just goes to show.'

'Goes to show what?'

'That you never know.'

Gates' face was immobile, frozen in an expression of sullen ill humour. 'No, I guess not.'

'The way I look at it is this.' Dale paused and sipped a little more of the whisky. 'You're an ignorant asshole and I'm not.'

Gates flushed but his body remained motionless. 'You knew we'd find out.'

'Not until I spoke to Jordan the second time.'

'Jack, you've let the team down. I can't believe you could turn on us like this. We were your family. We were on the same side.'

'No, we may have been allies at the beginning, but I don't think we were fighting for the same thing. Not really.'

'I thought you understood.'

'Understood what? That we're condoning the destruction of our society in order to protect it?'

'Sammy Chen, the Trincas ... those guys aren't the problem,' Gates said, as if explaining something to a small child. 'They hate the communists more than we do. They're natural allies. Always have been, it's nothing new. Been happening since the Sicily landings in the war. It's just a fact of life. Guys like Sammy Chen have huge networks of agents in place for their business. We need to tap in.'

'Their business is drugs, Gerry.'

'Shit, a few boogaloos frying their brains in the ghettoes.'

'Like my daughter?'

'Hit by friendly fire, Jack. I told you that.' He shook his head, like a tutor trying to understand how his star pupil failed the examination. 'Was that why you did it?'

'Part of it. The real reason is, I think we're our own worst enemy. Every empire crumbles from the inside out, not the other way around.'

'And that's it?'

'What we're doing is wrong. Simple as that.'

'Morality is not a good basis for making choices, Jack. Shit! What did it achieve? The file you gave Michael. It's not going anywhere. We stopped it. Maybe fifty years, some wannabe from the *Post* will find it mouldering in a vault some place. We'll all be dead by then.'

'And some will be deader than others. Right?'

Gates sighed. 'Jack, I've got a couple of boys waiting outside in the car. They want you to come with us. We need to talk.'

Dale finished his whisky and put the bottle and glass on the carpet beside his chair. He stood up, a little unsteadily. 'Oh, Gerry, how the fuck do you manage to sleep at nights?'

'It's a cool evening. You'll need a coat.'

'The fuck I will. Not where I'm going.'

Queen Elizabeth Hospital, Hong Kong

It was vanity that had May back on her feet so quickly. Michael found her in the hospital corridor, trailing a mobile intravenous unit, breath-taking in the short white hospital gown. It seemed she had persuaded a nurse to buy her some cosmetics, and when Michael got closer he could smell perfume. Her hair was freshly washed and brushed out.

'Like my new dress, Mai Koo?' she said when she saw him, and tugged at the hem of the gown.

'You'll start a riot,' he said.

'Want to come to my room? See all of Kowloon through the window. Let you look if you promise me you don't try no dirty business.'

Michael held up his hands in mock surrender. He helped her wheel the IV unit back into her room.

'You save my life.'

'I was the one who put you in danger.'

She shook her head. 'My choice, Mai Koo. Can make danger all by my own self, not need help, okay?'

'I think you're a remarkable woman.'

She giggled at that. 'You just want to make dirty stuff with me.'

'Yeah, I do. But that's not why I'm here.'

'I think it is why you are here. For a man dirty stuff is everything. Believe me, I know. Do a lot of badness in my life.'

'I don't care what you did before.'

'Ly May do not care either. Why should you?' She was suddenly serious. 'You really want me, Mai Koo?'

'I can't think about anything else.'

She gave him a mischievous grin. 'Me too.'

He realised he did not know this girl at all. His nine-year-old orphan had turned into a seasoned and world-weary woman. He was awed by her courage, intrigued by a past that was inextricably linked with his own. He had never met any woman like her, and he wanted her more than he had ever wanted anything.

'What are you going to do, May?' he said.

'*Beaucoup* things a pretty girl can do. Lot of rich Mandarin men in Hong Kong.' She put her head on one side. 'How much money you got, Mai Koo?'

Her candour caught him off balance. 'I'll never have as much as guys like Douglas Ho.'

673

'Maybe you can.'

'I don't think so.'

She lowered her voice in a theatrical whisper. 'When I take picture of papers, I find other things too.'

'What other things, May?'

'Access code.'

'To what?'

'Maybe to Douglas Ho's money in Switzerland.'

'You mean drug money, May?'

'But who will take money if I do not take?'

'That's not up to me to decide. The Hong Kong government . . .'

'You crazy, Mai Koo?'

'May, that's not your money.'

The mischief went from her eyes. She gave him a cold stare. 'I don't know how you live so long when you are this good. Maybe too good for me, Mai Koo.' Her voice was suddenly very sad. He realised that his being too good for her was not a criticism of herself. It was her personal indictment of him.

'I don't think I can learn to be poor again,' May said in Vietnamese. 'Besides, I earned this money.'

'What was that?' Michael asked her.

'I say I am tire. I think I sleep now. Maybe more better you go now, okay?'

When he got back to his hotel later that afternoon there was a message waiting for him, to ring the United States urgently. The number was the homicide desk of the San Francisco Police. His father had been found dead in his car.

The Mercedes had been found beside a lonely track in the Tiburon National Park by bushwalkers. Dale was slumped over the wheel, the fingers of his right hand still coiled around the trigger and guard of a .38 Smith & Wesson revolver. There were powder burn marks around the entry wound and a lot of blood on the driver's door and the floor well.

He was buried beside his daughter four days later. It was the second time in as many months Michael had been forced to return to the United States to bury one of his family. He thought that life had done its worst, but when he returned to Hong Kong a week later there was one further body blow. Ly May had checked herself out of the hospital two days before. There was no message for him and no one had any idea where she had gone.

EPILOGUE

149

In the first-class compartment of the Thai Airways 727, Baptiste Crocé drank champagne and watched the angry green hills of Hong Kong dip from sight below the wings. His business was concluded; Douglas Ho was dead. But the knowledge of his revenge was like dirt in his mouth. Without Lucien and without Noelle, there seemed little point to any of it.

Noelle...

My trouble, he decided, is that I am a hopeless romantic. I loved her too much. Everything I did, I did for her, and she was too vain to appreciate it. Noelle and her precious conscience! See how much good it had done her.

It had cost her their son. *His* son.

They should all have anticipated this. Sammy Chen should have removed Douglas Ho a long time ago. A man has to keep his own house in order. Rocco had taught him that much, God rest his rotten soul. Sammy had paid the price. He was still breathing through a tube in some American hospital, one son dead, and his empire a shambles. There was just one consolation. Baptiste had heard that his old friend Colonel Tran van Li had finally miscalculated. His body had been found in the San Francisco harbour yesterday. Parts of it, anyway. Information was that he might still have been alive when certain vital organs went missing.

A great tragedy.

But that would not bring back his son. So what did he have left to strive for?

His mind returned to the problem of Noelle. Why did it still gnaw at him this way? She was no longer young, of course, although she had aged with the grace of an angel, damn her. Through chastity hopefully, or more possibly out of sheer spite.

Why could he not remain indifferent to her, as she did to him? He had his own stable of mistresses now, God knows he could afford as many as he wanted, so it was not a physical need.

So why?

If he was honest with himself he would have to say it was because he was lonely. She was his one link with his own past, and his glorious youth. She knew him, understood him. They had history. In his life there had never been any woman quite like Noelle.

But it wasn't over. Nothing was over until he said it was over, and one day she would come back to him.

There had to be some way...

The black Toyota turned off Sukhumwit Road and raced down the Tanon Sapphankwai. It screeched to a halt in the alley, and Lucien Crocé was kicked out of the back door. The Toyota quickly reversed and was gone.

Lucien groaned and rolled on to his side. He rubbed his wrists, which were torn and swollen from the shackles he had worn ever since they had kidnapped him. He climbed painfully to his feet, but his left leg would not support his weight. His knee had twisted when they threw him from the car.

But he was alive. Mother of God, *he was alive*.

There were lights on in the villa. He imagined Noelle sitting inside, alone. By now she must imagine him dead. He himself had never expected to survive, the last weeks an endless night caged in a stinking warehouse waiting for them to kill him. When they finally came for him and threw him in the car, he had supposed it was to take him to his place of execution. Now, suddenly and unexpectedly, the nightmare was over.

He breathed in the steamy, gasoline air; a Bangkok night had never smelt so good.

From the transit lounge at Kai Tak, Michael stared at the teeming slum of the Walled City, a swarming nest where the triads spawned their armies of workers and soldiers.

The procession of 747s swept in to the city over its roofs, passengers lured by the shimmering duty free bazaar. One day they would pull the Walled City down. But it would be too late. The infection had already spread.

Michael felt his shoulders stoop under the burdens of despair and loss. Hong Kong had beaten him, and it had beaten his father, as it had beaten so many others. He knew how Dale had died, of course. The pain of it was still raw, and he winced whenever he thought of it. It was not suicide, he was sure of that.

'Jesus, I'm sorry,' he heard himself say aloud, when he thought of the things he had said to the old man over the last few years. He had misjudged him. Dale had always backed his commitments with courage, even when those commitments changed direction. It took a special kind of man to do that.

There was so much Michael had not said to him, and there was both comfort and pain in the knowledge that even if the old man was standing next to him now, he would maintain his silence. It had always been their way with each other.

And still he had not cried for his father.

He wondered if the old man's sacrifice was worth it. The file had been lost somewhere in Washington. Sammy Chen would never face trial. The last Michael had heard, there were doubts that he would survive; he was still on a ventilator in the intensive care unit at San Francisco General.

Michael had been offered compassionate leave, but it had not been necessary. He had written out his resignation while he was still in San Francisco. There no longer seemed any point to his job. The big bosses always got the last train out of town, and the department was left with the fall guys, the soldiers who were too stupid or too scared or too confused to run.

And the game went on.

Travellers trooped past him, the mass of humanity that travelled the skies every day; Chinese in T-shirts and baggy trousers, flying back to Canton, their bags stuffed with clothes and liquor and duty free cigarettes; British businessmen in powder blue shirts and sharp suits; tourists overburdened with the detritus of their luggage; Sikhs, Arabs, Thais. Any one of

681

them could be a courier, he thought. How could you ever sift this great tide?

There was only one way the trade could be stopped, and as his father had found, that way conflicted with the politics of the western world.

He found himself thinking once again about Ly May. He had no doubt she had caught a flight to Zürich, that she had used the access codes she had found. He wondered why he should feel so bitter. He had painted a romantic picture of her in his imagination; that kind of girl could not have survived as Ly May had done.

He heard his name announced on the public address system, asking him to report to the service desk. He wondered what had gone wrong. Perhaps a ticketing problem. He rose wearily to his feet and made his way down the corridor.

As he approached the desk she saw him and flashed a smile. She was wearing a full-length leather coat and there were Porsche sunglasses nestled in her glossy black hair. Gold gleamed at her throat. She had never looked so beautiful.

Or so rich.

The coat swung gracefully about her legs as she ran towards him. She rose on tip toe to kiss him. 'Think I miss you,' she said. 'Think I must go to Bangkok to find you.'

'May,' he said.

'*Aiii-ya*, don't look like cheap stuff no more, okay?'

He shook his head. 'I thought I'd lost you too.'

She frowned, confused. 'What is wrong? You look so sad.'

Dale shook his head. How could he tell her about his father? How could he tell her what they had done to him?

'What is wrong, Mai Koo?'

He put his head on her shoulder, and suddenly the grief wanted to spill out of him. But not here, not in public. She encircled him with her arms and held him. The airport crowds brushed past them, some staring then quickly turning away again, seeing just another airport farewell.

She did not understand why he looked so sad. They had survived. The good-luck Buddha she had given him had saved his life, and hers too.

For herself, she had never been so happy. She had Mai Koo, she had her life, and for the first time she had her freedom. And best of all, she had three and a half million dollars of Douglas Ho's money.

Patriotism is the last refuge of the scoundrel.
                                      - Samuel Johnson

COLIN FALCONER

FURY

'If I forget thee, O Jerusalem . . .'

For two thousand years the Jews recited these words in prayer.
By 1933, it was impossible to forget.

Germany:
Netanel cannot forget the girl he loves is Catholic; the Nazis will not let him forget he is a Jew.

Palestine:
Rishou cannot forget his forbidden affair with a beautiful Jewish kibbutznik; a girl whose fellow Jews have come to destroy him and his homeland.

From the horrors of the Holocaust, to the bloody birth of modern Israel and the climactic siege of Jerusalem, *Fury* is a superb, unflinching epic of survival, tragedy and triumph, of ordinary people trapped in a modern apocalypse, and of events that still reverberate through the Middle East today . . .

HODDER AND STOUGHTON PAPERBACKS

COLIN FALCONER

HAREM

It began with a man and a woman.

Süleyman the Magnificent: Lord of the Lords of this World, Possessor of Men's Necks, Allah's Deputy on Earth, absolute ruler of the mighty Ottoman Empire.

At his pleasure, his vast harem, scented, pampered, hushed, waiting only to be summoned to his bed. And among them, Hürrem, daughter of a Tatar, sold into slavery, lovely, ruthless in her desire to captivate and use him.

So began a story of obsession and agony that was to cost him his closest friend, his sons, his sanity and finally his dynasty.

Harem brings to breathtaking life a world of intrigue, sensuality and violence, where an empire can be controlled through one man's desire.

HODDER AND STOUGHTON PAPERBACKS

COLIN FALCONER

VENOM

'I will survive', he promised the black silence. 'I will survive and I will come back to haunt you. All of you . . .'

It began like a page from the Kama Sutra. A beautiful French girl and her Indian lover locked in the white heat of illicit passion.

The result was Michel. Thrown out on to the dangerous streets, he grew to ferocious manhood in the alleys of Saigon. He survived to wreak the most extreme vengeance for every beating and all the betrayals. Possessed of a raw sexuality and the flair of a master criminal, driven by a pitiless hidden violence, he left a trail of blood that stretched from the backstreets of Bombay to the boulevards of Paris.

When the judge's gavel cracks across a Delhi courtroom and the world waits for justice, his destiny will hang on one last ironic twist of fate . . .

'Exotic, exciting, darkly suspenseful – a splendid novel'
Campbell Armstrong

HODDER AND STOUGHTON PAPERBACKS